DERMATOLOGY - LABORATORY AND CLINICAL RESEARCH

ADVANCES IN DERMATOLOGY RESEARCH

Dermatology - Laboratory and Clinical Research

Additional books in this series can be found on Nova's website
under the Series tab.

Additional e-books in this series can be found on Nova's website
under the e-book tab.

DERMATOLOGY - LABORATORY AND CLINICAL RESEARCH

ADVANCES IN DERMATOLOGY RESEARCH

JAMES P. VEGA
EDITOR

NOVA BIOMEDICAL
New York

Library of Congress Cataloging-in-Publication Data

ISBN: 978-1-63482-226-8
Library of Congress Control Number: 2015932293

Published by Nova Science Publishers, Inc. † New York

Contents

Preface

Advances in Dermatology Research presents original research results on the leading edge of dermatology. Each chapter has been carefully selected in an attempt to present substantial advances across a broad spectrum. Some topics discusses in this book include pemphigoid; cyanosis, and acne.

Chapter 1 – Bullous Pemphigoid (BP) is an autoimmune blistering disease, preferentially affecting elderly subjects and rare in childhood. BP is characterized by widespread tense blister formation and rarely involves mucosa. In the skin biopsy, BP shows subepidermal clefting as a result of injury caused by autoantibodies against structural components of the hemidesmosome. The diagnosis is confirmed by immunofluorescence studies. Corticosteroids (CS) are the mainstay of treatment. Mycophenolate mofetil, azathioprine, methotrexate, cyclophosphamide are some of the steroid-sparing agents that can also be used. Despite multiple treatment options, there are few studies supporting their use.

Chapter 2 – Bullous pemphigoid (BP) is a rare skin condition with tense, fluid-filled blisters, and urticarial or other lesions on areas of the lower abdomen, upper thighs or armpits (flexoral areas). BP has highest incidence in people older than 60. In BP, the immune system attacks the basement membrane zone (BMZ) of the skin at the junction of the epidermis and dermis; however, current data indicates that the BP autoimmune pathology may also attack dermal blood vessels, some stromal dermal areas, nerves, sweat glands and the BMZs of skin adnexal structures. The BP pathologic immune response that initially was thought to be predominately focused on IgG and Complement/C3 deposition at the cutaneous BMZ; however, recent data indicates that B and T lymphocytes, other immune system cells and inflammatory markers may be involved. In some cases, clinical lesions resembling classic BP can be triggered by taking medications; however, the immunopathogenesis of this disorder seems to be quite different. In BP, direct and indirect immunofluorescence of the skin usually shows reactivity in a linear pattern along the BMZ with IgG, Complement/C3 and sometimes IgE; other immunoglobulins and complement may also be present. Multiple markers have been also described in the BP blisters; however, the data is not always consistent. A number of immunoblotting (IB) analyses have indicated that two major antigenic proteins of epidermal extracts are targets in BP; specifically, the 230 kilodalton (kDa) BP antigen I (BP230 or BPAG1), and the 180-kDa BP antigen II (BP180, BPAG2 or Type XVII collagen). These antigenic proteins are detected by sera from patients with BP in various IB patterns; however, other putative antigens have also been documented. Including an 84 kDa protein and others. Enzyme-linked immunosorbent assays (ELISAs) have confirmed the immunoblotting assays. Some studies have shown that BPAGII has an extracellular domain; polyclonal rabbit antibodies raised against an extracellular, non-collagenous domain of the murine BP180 antigen were documented as pathogenic in a passive transfer model. Several investigators have suggested a relationship between clinical findings and laboratory data in BP. The clinical and pathologic BP differential diagnosis includes lichen planus pemphigoides, and pemphigus vegetans.

The treatment of BP usually includes corticosteroids such as prednisone, and other drugs that suppress the immune system. BP can be life-threatening, especially for older people who are already in poor health. The disease may have significant impact on the patient and their family, and have important economic consequences due to their disability and via complications in the immunosuppressive therapy. The diagnosis of BP is challenging for primary physicians, nurses and other health care providers, especially when they lack of the proper laboratory techniques for the diagnosis of BP. In vitro and *in vivo* animal models for BP are available, but many of them do not seem reproduce the *in vivo* clinical disease. The current medical literature offers an arsenal of biological medications, but none have therapeutically surpassed corticosteroids. The long term treatment of BP patients' needs to have a multidisciplinary and comprehensive approach, including therapists and nutritionists.

Chapter 3 – Bullous pemphigoid (BP) is a bullous disease of autoimmune origin. These disorders are the result of an inflammatory process that causes skin lesions, with local increases of pro-inflammatory mediators. Alterations of the vessels, nerves or/or neurovascular structures have been previously described in BP. Here the authors aim to confirm reactivity to vessels and nerves in a case of BP.

Case report: A 68 year old Caucasian male presented with a sudden appearance of erythematous papules, plaques and few blisters on the abdomen, back, arms, and thighs; focal excoriations were present, with some itching and burning sensations.

Materials and Methods: Skin biopsies were taken for hematoxylin and eosin (H&E) staining and immunohistochemistry (IHC), and for direct and indirect immunofluorescence (DIF, IIF) with 1 M NaCl split skin studies.

Results: The H&E staining demonstrated a subepidermal blister with luminal cells including eosinophils, lymphocytes, some monocytes and rare neutrophils. Partial re-epithelialization of the blister base was appreciated. A mild, superficial, perivascular dermal infiltrate was present, with similar cells as those present within the blister lumen. Some dermal blood vessels seemed be damaged and/or dilated. DIF and IIF showed positivity for anti-human IgG, IgA, IgE, Complement/C1q, fibrinogen and albumin. These same antibodies were positive against the dermal blood vessels and some neurovascular structures as well as at the BMZ of sebaceous and eccrine sweat glands. IgM and complement/C3 were negative. IHC demonstrated thrombomodulin, von Willembrand factor, vascular endothelial growth factor, Complement/C5b-9/MAC, HLA-DP, DQ, DR, antigen, HLA-ABC, BCL-2, cyclo-oxygenase 2, and CD8 to be positive around dermal blood vessels and on the basement membranes of some skin appendices.

Discussion: Although the reactivity to vessels and/or neurovascular structures and the BMZs of skin appendices has not been extensively studied in BP, the authors' case and other cases indicate that these BP positive autoantibodies colocalizing with neurovascular markers could explain the clinical skin burning, pain and/ or itching sensations described in BP patients with BP, as well as also some neurovascular structural alterations in patients with BP.

Case report: A 68 year old Caucasian male presented with a sudden appearance of erythematous papules, plaques and few blisters on the abdomen, back, arms, and thighs; focal excoriations were also noted. Some of the lesions were violaceous and itchy. The patient was taking only vitamin supplements.

Chapter 4 – *Background:* The clinical presentation of bullous pemphigoid (BP) is variable; blistering skin lesions may be present, but an urticarial or erythematous rash may also precede the appearance of the blisters. The patients themselves may also traumatize blister lesions, and spontaneous ulceration of the skin may occur.

Aim: The authors sought to compare the immune changes in intact bullous pemphigoid lesions, versus ulcerated lesions. Here they aim to describe these changes, utilizing a skin biopsy containing both intact and ulcerated bullous pemphigoid lesional areas via hematoxylin and eosin histology (H&E), as well as direct immunofluorescence (DIF) and immunohistochemistry (IHC).

Results: The findings in these areas demonstrated distinctly different patterns of the immune response. In the intact blister areas, markers such as HLA-DP, DQ, DR antigen, cyclooxygenase-2 (COX-2), B-cell lymphoma 2(BCL2), CD3, CD68, alpha-1 antitrypsin, mast cell tryptase, von Willembrand factor and Factor XIIIa demonstrated positive staining in some areas of the blister and around adjacent dermal blood vessels. However, in ulcerated areas, most of these markers primarily compartmentalized in a linear manner at the base of the ulcer. The authors interpreted the ulcerated area pattern as evidence of the immune system attempting to phagocytose or extrude the ulcerated tissue. P53 demonstrated positive staining in nascent blister areas, but negative staining within the ulcer. CD4, CD20 and GFAP demonstrated negative staining in intact blister areas and in ulcerated areas.

Conclusion: The authors suggest that the immune response that is present around the ulcerated areas is acting as a secondary immune response, for the purpose of removing damaged tissue. Thus, the authors suggest the primary bullous pemphigoid immune response creates the blisters, and the secondary immune response forms as a result of ulceration of the tissue. Further studies are warranted to confirm these immunologic possibilities.

Chapter 5 – *Background:* Bullous pemphigoid (BP) is an acquired autoimmune disease characterized by subepidermal vesicles, with clinical macules and bullae. In contradistinction, drug induced bullous pemphigoid (DBP) may be triggered by medications and other agents. Presently, minimal pathologic differences have been documented to differentiate between these two entities. The authors present a case of a drug-induced bullous pemphigoid-like reaction, and review critical aspects that seem to differentiate these entities.

Case report: A 68 year old male was consulted for the presence of erythematosus plaques, papules and tense blisters on the abdomen and thighs, after the intake of multiple medications.

Materials and Methods: Skin biopsies were taken for hematoxylin and eosin review and immunohistochemistry, and for direct immunofluorescence studies.

Results: The H&E histology showed small subepidermal blisters with minimal fibrin and some eosinophils within the blister lumens; no epidermal vacuolar degeneration or acantholysis were noted. Not significant edema was noted in the epidermis or dermis. Direct immunofluorescence revealed dotted Complement/C3c and linear, discontinuous IgG deposits along the basement membrane zone (BMZ). In addition, cells strongly positive for CD20 and BCL-2 were noted within the lesional inflammation.

Conclusion: Some histologic clues favoring a bullous pemphigoid-like allergic drug reaction may include absence of epidermal vacuolar degeneration, edema, fibrin deposits, blister festoons and a significant luminal eosinophilic infiltrate. In addition to these findings, CD20 cells are normally not found in most cases of classic BP; in classical BP, HLA-DPDQDR is often strongly expressed in the lesions, which was not the case here. In addition, in contrast to classic BP, the authors noted discontinuous staining at the BMZ with immunoglobulins and complement.

Chapter 6 – Anti-tumor necrosis factor-α (TNFα) agents are increasingly being used for rapidly expanding number of autoimmune diseases, principally cutaneous, rheumatic and gastroenterological. With this use and longer follow-up periods of treatment, there are a growing number of reports of the development of autoimmune processes related to the use of anti-TNFα (cutaneous vasculitis, lupus-like syndrome, systemic lupus erythematosus and interstitial lung disease). Despite anti-TNFα can be used to treat severe forms of autoimmune bullous skin diseases, few cases of pemphigus vulgaris and bullous pemphigoid occurring under anti-TNFα therapy have been described. The triggering role of anti-TNFα blockers remains unclear but it can not be excluded that they could be an immunologic trigger for autoimmune conditions in predisposed individuals. These drugs may act as triggers by either modifying the immune response or altering the antigenic properties of the cutaneous antigens. Based on authors' experience it seems that different type of anti-TNFα blockers influences the immune response in different way.

The authors propose their personal experience and a review of the cases of autoimmune bullous skin diseases induced by anti-TNFα agents reported in literature.

Chapter 7 – Mucous membrane pemphigoid (MMP) is one of a group of autoimmune, subepithelial blistering diseases that predominantly affect mucous membranes. Desquamative gingivitis (DG) is a common manifestation of MMP. Both histopathological examination and direct immunofluorescence testing are essential to establish a final diagnosis. Early recognition and treatment of MMP can improve the prognosis, but diagnostic delays are common in DG because obtaining a diagnostic biopsy is technically challenging. The stab-and-roll biopsy technique is designed to prevent the epithelium from being removed from the biopsy specimen. The complications caused by scarring and associated loss of function often require surgical intervention in MMP patients. Early diagnosis of MMP is critical, and immunosuppressive treatment may prevent serious complications in mucous membranes.

Chapter 8 – The correlation between bullous pemphigoid (BP) and internal malignancies has been argued over for more than half a century, and remains controversial. In this chapter, the authors review the literature in three categories. First, they examine the historical perspective of the association between BP and malignancies; the first case report was probably mentioned by Forman in 1960, and the first case series (seven cases) was described by Parsons and Savin in 1968. Second, the authors look at the incidence of malignancy in BP patients; among 17 previous studies, six concluded that BP carries an increased risk of internal malignancy, while nine denied such an association. The most recent cohort study found no correlation. Third, they examine the incidence of BP among cancer patients; one cohort study reported no evidence of overall correlation, but a sub-analysis in the study suggested that kidney cancer alone was linked to an elevated risk of BP. Considering the results of these studies, an overall association between BP and malignancies is not shown, while restricted associations depending on the type of cancer or ethnic background of the BP patient might be possible.

Chapter 9 – Perinatal cyanosis is the expression of pathological low arterial blood oxygen saturation in children surrounding the time of birth. The birth process is very complicated and through many different mechanisms can lead to low oxygen levels in the fetus or newborn. The passage through the birth canal and potential placental or umbilical cord issues can interrupt CNS blood supply. Moreover, after birth the newborn must oxygenate its own blood for the first time and many newborns have lungs which are not sufficiently mature for this process. Thus, any respiratory immaturity or cardiac anomalies may quickly diminish efficient oxygenation. While acute medical issues can often be corrected with the newborn appearing fully intact, a brief period of insufficient oxygen to the brain can result in issues which are not readily apparent. Research suggests that instability of circulation or oxygenation is the leading cause of perinatal brain damage (1 – 6 out of every 1000 newborns) and can result in long-term neurological consequences, significant cognitive dysfunction, and subsequent academic challenges. Although medical practitioners often investigate the cause of a cyanotic event, parents and educators are frequently ill-informed as to the future developmental and long-term learning and social implications. This chapter will investigate perinatal cyanotic populations (i.e., cardiac, respiratory, prematurity, and hypoxic-ischemic) and their distinct neurocognitive and behavioral profiles. Specific focus will be placed on empirical literature which identifies cognitive, academic, and emotional deficits. The impact of perinatal cyanosis on all domains of cognitive functioning (i.e., intellect, language, motor, memory, attention and executive functioning) will be explored. Finally, general developmental and academic recommendations will be reviewed.

Chapter 10 – Laryngomalacia is the most common congenital laryngeal anomaly and the most frequent cause of stridor in pediatric age. The disorder involves 45–75% of all infants with congenital stridor. Signs and symptoms appear usually within the first 2 weeks of life and the spectrum of disease presentation, progression, and outcomes is variable. Most cases are mild and resolve spontaneously without surgical procedures. Such patients undergo only medical treatment for the gastroesophageal reflux that is generally associated with this disease. Only severe cases with intolerable symptoms such as dysphagia, failure to thrive, dyspnea, cyanosis, intermittent complete obstruction and/or cardiac failure must undergo surgery. Surgical therapy is in relation to the type and severity of laryngomalacia. The authors describe the different clinical pictures that every clinician can observe and summarize the different treatments available.

Chapter 11 – The use of pulse oximeters has minimized the need for the visual recognition of cyanosis. However, there are times when this is still valuable. Lighting is important for this visual task and it is also a difficult task for some people with color vision deficiencies. There were fluorescent tubes that permitted the accurate recognition of cyanosis but they used less efficient halophosphate technology. In the 1990s the change in fluorescent tube technology to give greater energy efficiency introduced tri-phosphor technology. This created some problems most notably for anesthetists. A standard for lighting to permit the accurate identification of cyanosis was written (Australian/New Zealand Standard 1680.2.5:1997) based on measurements of isolated blood that were later confirmed by measurements of lips, nail beds and palm creases. Using these data, the basis of the problem for people with color vision deficiencies was also illustrated. The standard introduced the concept of the Cyanosis Observation Index (COI), its calculation and compliance values. Since then, there have been many attempts to produce complying sources for hospital lighting using fluorescent tube technology. The solutions tended to be energy inefficient (using halophosphate technology) or expensive. As a consequence, there was no successful solution to the problem using fluorescent lamps (straight tube or compact fluorescent). The other, less demanding, visual tasks in clinical observation (like observation of rashes etc.) were satisfied using modified tri-phosphor technology. The future of lighting is now firmly with light emitting diode (LED) technology. LEDs are more efficient than fluorescent sources and have advantages of compactness and no warm-up time. There are a number of white LED products available that have a COI that easily complies with AS/NZS 1680.2.5. As a consequence, there has been a renewed interest in the COI as an appropriate and achievable measure in hospital lighting.

In this chapter the basis of the COI will be reviewed. The issues with color vision deficiencies will be discussed. The reasons why tri-phosphor technology fails to deliver a good solution will be outlined and the results of suitable LED sources will be provided.

Chapter 12 – Cyanosis refers to the bluish discoloration of the skin, nails or mucus membrane due to an increased amount of reduced hemoglobin [> 5 g %] in capillary blood. Cyanosis is broadly classified as being central, peripheral or differential but can also be caused by abnormal pigments circulating in the blood. Central causes of cyanosis are mainly cardiac or pulmonary while peripheral causes arise from local vasoconstriction or lack of peripheral blood supply. Differential cyanosis happens in specific cardiac conditions. Cyanosis is usually a sign of an underlying condition rather than being a disease in itself.

Patients with cyanosis may have other features like breathlessness, shortness of breath, bluish or purple discoloration of the oral mucous membranes, rapid and shallow breathing etc.

There is general tiredness or weakness in patients who suffer from long term cyanosis. There may be episodes of headaches as well.

Treatment of cyanosis focuses on the underlying disease rather than the symptom alone. Initial stabilization requires oxygenation. Treatment of central cyanosis due to congenital heart defects may often involve surgery. Peripheral cyanosis brought about by exposure to cold may be treated symptomatically using gentle warming of the fingers and toes.

Antibiotics are prescribed for treatment of pneumonia and other infections. The chapter analyses the various causes of cyanosis and the possible treatment options for patients when they are cyanosed.

Chapter 13 – The treatment of acne continues to be a challenge to practicing clinicians and dermatologists.

Among the available treatment oral isotretinoin remains the more effective acne medication and oral antibiotics the more prescribed treatments. Given the restrictions placed on the use of isotretinoin and the increase in antibiotic resistant strains of *P. acnes*, there is a high clinical need for new treatment.

Acne pathogenesis is a complex mechanism in which different factors play a role. In the recent years the increased knowledge of the acne pathogenesis lead to the development of new and targeted drugs such as drugs blocking the activation of Toll-like receptor, PPAR antagonist, inhibitors of IL-1α and leukocyte chemotaxis, the antagonist of pro-inflammatory cytokines, the inhibitors of the production of reactive oxygen species and so on. A number of molecules named with abbreviations are studied and registered in the official sites.

Another problem is the tolerability of the currently available topical. In order to increase tolerability of these topical and of consequence to improve the patients' compliance, new vehicles have been tested.

Finally, also a vaccination killed *P. acnes* may lead to an innovative approach of acne management.

This indicates that the research in the field of acne is very active and so it is probably that in the next years several new drugs will hit the market.

The authors propose a review of the emerging treatments in acne field.

Chapter 14 – *Background:* Acne is one of the major reasons that patients consult a dermatologist. Current recommendations for the treatment of juvenile facial acne suggest treating mild acne with topical treatments and moderate acne with a combination of topical treatments with systemic antibiotics. The aim of this investigational survey was to evaluate how European dermatologists in private practice currently manage acne.

Method: Dermatologists practicing in 12 European countries were asked how they manage patients with acne (except those undergoing isotretinoin treatment). Each dermatologist completed a written questionnaire, about patient characteristics, acne severity and the therapy they prescribed at baseline and after 2 months of treatment.

Results: In total, 5809 acneic patients were questioned. In 40% of cases (independent of severity), dermatologists prescribed up to 3 local treatments combined with up to 2 systemic therapies, and a cosmetic product. In 44% of cases, dermatologists prescribed only a dermocosmetic product for very mild acne; in 44% of cases of mild acne they prescribed one treatment, mostly topical one and in 48 and 58% of cases two treatments (mainly a combination of local and systemic therapy) to patients with moderate or severe acne respectively.

Conclusion: This observational study illustrates that dermatologists employ complex treatment regimens to manage acne. Seeing as complex regimens are harder for patients to comply with, this notably raises the question of adherence, which is a key factor in successful treatment.

Chapter 15 – Ocular rosacea forms part of the clinical spectrum of rosacea. It is characterized by a chronic and recurrent inflammation of the eyelids, conjunctiva and cornea. Approximately 50% of rosacea patients present ocular manifestations, and the condition is most frequently diagnosed when cutaneous signs and symptoms are present. However in 20% of patients, ocular manifestations may precede the cutaneous disease. Most frequent ocular symptoms are: red eyes, burning, foreign body sensation, photophobia and blurred vision.

Chronic blepharitis with meibomian gland dysfunction is the most frequent ocular manifestation of the disease, and produces evaporative dry eye with consequent ocular surface damage. Corneal inflammation and scarring may be a cause of severe visual loss. In addition to therapeutic strategies for the cutaneous disease, ocular rosacea treatment involves, lid hygiene, topical macrolides and tetracyclines as eyelid gels or ointments, lubricant eye drops, and short-term topical steroids, depending on the severity of blepharitis, conjunctivitis and keratitis. Prognosis and visual outcome depend on the severity of the disease, early diagnosis and appropriate treatment.

In: Advances in Dermatology Research
Editor: James P. Vega
ISBN: 978-1-63482-226-8

Chapter 1

Bullous Pemphigoid: An Overview

Alexandre Carlos Gripp, MD*[*,1], Aline Bressan, MD[2], Cândida Naira Lima e Lima-Santana, MD[3] and Daniele do Nascimento Pereira, MD[4]

[1]Assistant Professor of Dermatology and Chief of the Dermatology Ward at Pedro Ernesto University Hospital - State University of Rio de Janeiro, Brazil
Chief of the Dermatology Service at Pedro Ernesto University Hospital, Brazil
[2]Specialist in Dermatology by the Brazilian Society of Dermatology
Medical Assistant of the Imunobiologic Ambulatory and the Imunobiologic Ward at Pedro Ernesto University Hospital – State University of Rio de Janeiro, Brazil
[3,4]Dermatology at Pedro Ernesto University Hospital – State University of Rio de Janeiro, Brazil

Abstract

Bullous Pemphigoid (BP) is an autoimmune blistering disease, preferentially affecting elderly subjects and rare in childhood. BP is characterized by widespread tense blister formation and rarely involves mucosa. In the skin biopsy, BP shows subepidermal clefting as a result of injury caused by autoantibodies against structural components of the hemidesmosome. The diagnosis is confirmed by immunofluorescence studies. Corticosteroids (CS) are the mainstay of treatment. Mycophenolate mofetil, azathioprine, methotrexate, cyclophosphamide are some of the steroid-sparing agents that can also be used. Despite multiple treatment options, there are few studies supporting their use.

Introduction

Bullous pemphigoid (BP) is an autoimmune disease which affects mainly older individuals. It is more common in women and rarely occurs in childhood.

* E-mail: alexandregripp@yahoo.com.br.

Epidemiology

Data from the preliminary studies of BP estimated an annual incidence of 6 to 7 new cases per million people in Europe. [1,2] In a 2-year study involving the Swiss population, it was found an incidence of 12 cases per million people per year. [3] Another prospective study made in Germany found a similar result, with an incidence of 13.4. [4] Retrospective studies in England and France showed a trend of increased incidence of BP in the last decade. [5,6] It is a disease more common over 60 year with an increment of risk about 297 times higher over 90 years. [2]

Clinical Aspects

The most characteristic feature of BP is a tense bullae with widespread pruritus even in healthy or erythematous skin. [7-9] The bullae can persist for days, leaving eroded or crusted areas [8,10] and has negative Asboe Hansen and Nikolsky signs. [10] The lesions are generally symmetrical and can occur in any location. However, it occurs predominantly in the abdomen, extremities and trunk (Figure 1). [7,8,10]

Table 1. Clinical variants of bullous pemphigoid

Pretibial pemphigoid	Limited to pretibial area, reminding eczema, bullosis diabeticorum, contact dermatitis or drug rash
Dysidrosiform pemphigoid	Limited to palmoplantar region, reminding eczema, contact dermatitis, drug rash or dysidrosiform dermatitis
Pemphigoid nodularis	Excoriated nodules and papules in the limbs and trunk, which can develop scar, resembling nodular prurigo
Pemphigoid vegetans	Rare, with intertriginous purulent, erythematous, erosive, well circumscribed vegetating plaques
Erythrodermic bullous pemphigoid	Erythroderma with or without blistering
Vesicular pemphigoid	Small tense blisters with a symmetric distribution that mimicking dermatitis herpetiformis
Polymorphic pemphigoid	Vesicles and blisters, resembling dermatitis herpetiformis in association with bullous pemphigoid
Erosive bullous pemphigoid	Large eroded areas on the trunk, buttocks and flexures, without pruritus, blisters or urticarial inflammatory lesions, unwieldy
Lichen planus pemphigoid	Typical features of both lichen planus and bullous pemphigoid, it is speculated that the damage caused during the liquefaction of the basal layer in lichen planus induces the formation of antibodies against constituents of the basal membrane and has relatively benign course
Drug induced bullous pemphigoid	In general, the drug presents thiol group, acting as hapten in the lamina lucida
Bullous pemphigoid of childhood	It presents greater involvement of mucosae and palmoplantar region

Adapted from Khandpur S, 2011, Di Zenzo G, 2012; Walsh SR, 2005.

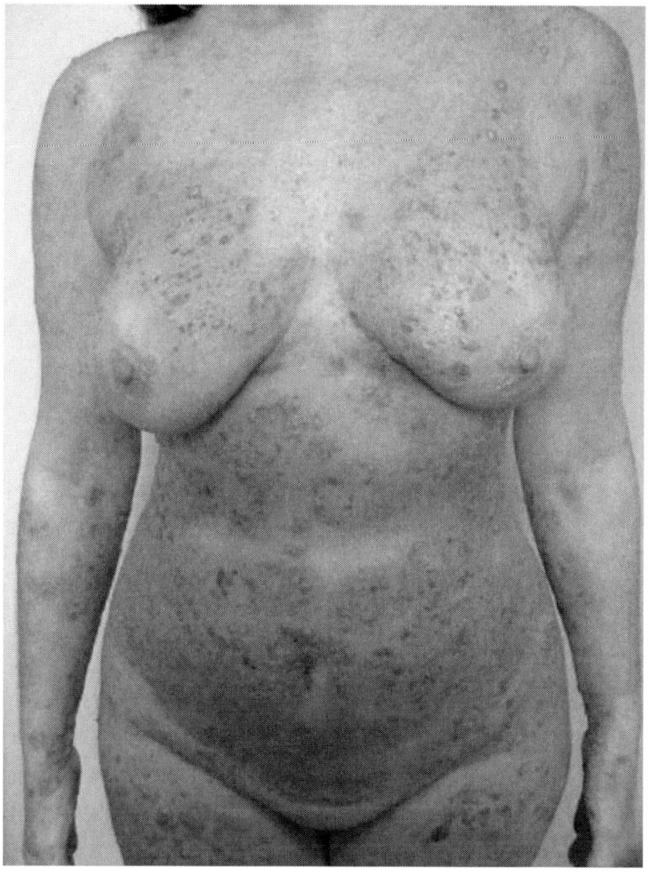

Figure 1. Bullous pemphigoid. Note the erythematous skin with tense bullae and eroded areas.

The blisters usually have clear content, but may be hemorrhagic. It is unusual scarring or milia and usually heals with post-inflammatory dyschromia. [7,8] The mucous involvement rarely occurs. [7]

The oral mucous membrane involvement occurs in 10 to 30% of patients, usually in newly diagnosed patients.

The ocular, nasal, pharyngeal, esophageal and anogenital mucosa may be more rarely affected [11] and has been reported a case of BP with the tracheobronchial mucosa involvement. [12]

In some patients, an initial assessment can occur on a stage without bullae, but with intense itching, and can express a variety of injuries like excoriated, eczematous, papular or urticarial lesions. [8,13] This observation implies the importance of considering the possibility of BP in patients with chronic itching without frankly blistering.

BP can remain localized, around stomas or in paralyzed limbs or irradiated areas, and may never reach the generalized form. [8,10] There are case reports associated with malignancy, such as renal cell carcinoma, gallbladder, colon, breast, and parotid malignancy and leukemia. [7] The clinical variants of BP can be evidenced in table 1.

Trigger Factors

Some factors have been associated to BP, as certain types of local aggression such as traumas, burns, radiation therapy and ultraviolet radiation, drugs, and certain autoimmune diseases, such as rheumatoid arthritis, Hashimoto thyroiditis, dermatomyositis, lupus erythematosus and thrombocytopenia. BP is also closely associated with neurological diseases such as dementia, Parkinson's disease, multiple sclerosis, psychiatric disorders and cerebrovascular injuries. This relationship can be explained by the fact that the Bullous Pemphigoid Antigen 180 (BP180) and Bullous Pemphigoid Antigen 230 (BP230), antigens related to BP, are expressed in central nervous system and, with the development of neurological diseases, there is the phenomenon of epitope spreading by the humoral immune system which affects the skin. [8]

Diagnosis

In the skin biopsy from a fresh blister, stained with haematoxylin and eosin, BP shows subepidermal clefting and inflammatory infiltrate mainly consisting of eosinophils. [14] These are results of injury caused by autoantibodies against structural components of the hemidesmosome. The known antigens in BP are BP180, also known as type 2 (BPAg2); BP230, also known as type 1 (BPAg1) and collagen type XVII. [10] The direct immunofluorescence of perilesional skin is essential for diagnosis and shows linear deposition of IgG, IgA and/or C3 along the basement membrane zone. In most cases of BP, the antigens are detected at the roof of the salt-split. [14]

The serum levels of autoantibodies to BP180 and BP230 can be detected by enzyme-linked immunosorbent assay (ELISA). The titles correlate with disease activity and can be used to monitor response to treatment in addition to the clinical status of the patient. [14]

Differencial Diagnosis

Includes bullous diseases such as linear IgA bullous dermatosis, bullous systemic lupus erythematosus, dermatitis herpetiformis, epidermolysis bullosa acquisita, gestational pemphigoid and cicatricial pemphigoid (also called pemphigoid mucous membrane). [7,8]

Management of Bullous Pemphigoid

The choice of treatment depends on age, severity of disease and presence of comorbidities, since there is increased risk of drug interactions and side effects. The major goal is controlling symptoms with minimum adverse effects. Multiple options are available, including immunosuppressive and immunomodulating drugs and agents that reduce pathogenic autoantibodies.

Corticosteroids (CS) are the mainstay of management; however, they are related to high incidence of side effects. Prednisone and prednisolone are the most used drugs. Daily dose higher than 0.75 mg/kg have no additional benefit and is related to larger frequency of side effects. [15] Patients with high levels of antibodies to BP180 and severe disease may require larger CS doses. [16] On the other hand, prednisone doses higher than 40 mg/kg at discharge are associated with increased risk of death in the first year after hospitalization. [17] Topical steroids are also safe and successful in treating BP and some studies have shown similar efficacy when compare to oral treatment. [18] Nevertheless, there are practical limitations and higher costs.

In refractory cases or in order to reduce CS doses due to associated side effects, other drugs can be added or used as monotherapy, such as azathiprine (1-3 mg/kg/day), mycophanolate mofetil (35-45 mg/kg/day) and methotrexate (7.5-25 mg/week). [14,19-22] Low doses of cyclophosphamide (50-100 mg/day) is also an option, as evidenced in a serie of twenty patients with beneficial results. [23]

Immunomodulatory antimicrobials are effective in controlling symptoms and preventing relapse. They are also safe and have more favorable side effect profile. Nicotinamide (500-2500 mg/day), tetracycline (500-2000 mg/day), doxycycline (200-300 mg/day) and dapsone (100 mg/day) can be used with or without CS. However, more controlled trials are necessary to improve knowledge about their use in the BP treatment. [14,15]

The intravenous immunoglobulin (2 g/kg/day during three consecutive days) should be considered in cases of treatment failure, significant adverse effects with conventional therapy, progressive disease and contraindications to the use of CS. The main mechanism of action is reduction of pathogenic antibodies. [14,21] In a case report about the use of immunoadsorption in the management of BP, that was evidenced an excellent clinical response, although more studies are necessary to prove effectiveness and to define treatment protocols. [24]

The use of monoclonal antibodies in the treatment of BP has also been demonstrated. Rituximab is a humanized antibody against CD20-expressing B lymphocytes which are involve in producing pathogenic autoantibodies. There is no specific protocol to patients with BP, but it has been used in refractory cases. [25] Case series of patients treated with omalizumab reported positive results. [26] The rational to the use is based on data that evidenced high levels of IgE in patients with BP. [27]

Despite multiple treatment options, there are few controlled trials supporting their use. The majority of related studies are uncontrolled trials and case reports with multiple definitions and outcome measures. In this context, an international BP definitions committee was organized to provide definitions for the stages of disease activity, define therapeutic end points and an objective disease extent measure. [28] Further studies are needed to compare the efficacy of BP treatment options and provide more consistent evidence.

References

[1] Bernard P, Vaillant L, Labeille B, Bedane C, Arbeille B, Denoeux JP, Lorette G, Bonnetblanc JM, Prost C. Incidence and distribution of subepidermal autoimmune

bullous skin diseases in three French regions. Bullous Diseases French Study Group. *Arch. Dermatol.* 1995 Jan;131(1):48-52.

[2] Jung M, Kippes W, Messer G, Zillikens D, Rzany B. Increased risk of bullous pemphigoid in male and very old patients: A population-based study on incidence. *J. Am. Acad. Dermatol.* 1999 Aug;41(2 Pt 1):266-8.

[3] Marazza G, Pham HC, Schärer L, Pedrazzetti PP, Hunziker T, Trüeb RM, Hohl D, Itin P, Lautenschlager S, Naldi L, Borradori L; Autoimmune bullous disease Swiss study group. Incidence of bullous pemphigoid and pemphigus in Switzerland: a 2-year prospective study. *Br. J. Dermatol.* 2009 Oct;161(4):861-8. doi: 10.1111/j.1365-2133.2009.09300.x.

[4] Bertram F, Bröcker EB, Zillikens D, Schmidt E. Prospective analysis of the incidence of autoimmune bullous disorders in Lower Franconia, Germany. *J. Dtsch. Dermatol. Ges.* 2009 May;7(5):434-40. doi: 10.1111/j.1610-0387.2008.06976.x.

[5] Langan SM, Smeeth L, Hubbard R, Fleming KM, Smith CJ, West J. Bullous pemphigoid and pemphigus vulgaris--incidence and mortality in the UK: population based cohort study. *BMJ.* 2008 Jul 9;337:a180. doi: 10.1136/bmj.a180.

[6] Joly P, Baricault S, Sparsa A, Bernard P, Bédane C, Duvert-Lehembre S, Courville P, Bravard P, Rémond B, Doffoel-Hantz V, Bénichou J. Incidence and mortality of bullous pemphigoid in France. *J. Invest. Dermatol.* 2012 Aug;132(8):1998-2004. doi: 10.1038/jid.2012.35.

[7] Khandpur S, Verma P. Bullous pemphigoid. *Indian J. Dermatol. Venereol. Leprol.* 2011 Jul-Aug;77(4):450-5. doi: 10.4103/0378-6323.82398.

[8] Di Zenzo G, Della Torre R, Zambruno G, Borradori L. Bullous pemphigoid: from the clinic to the bench. *Clin. Dermatol.* 2012 Jan-Feb;30(1):3-16. doi: 10.1016/j.clindermatol.2011.03.005.

[9] Ladizinski B, Lee KC. Bullous pemphigoid. *J. Gen. Intern. Med.* 2013 May;28(5):733. doi: 10.1007/s11606-012-2250-y.

[10] Walsh SR, Hogg D, Mydlarski PR. Bullous pemphigoid: from bench to bedside. *Drugs.* 2005;65(7):905-26.

[11] Di Zenzo G, Thoma-Uszynski S, Fontao L, Calabresi V, Hofmann SC, Hellmark T, Sebbag N, Pedicelli C, Sera F, Lacour JP, Wieslander J, Bruckner-Tuderman L, Borradori L, Zambruno G, Hertl M. Multicenter prospective study of the humoral autoimmune response in bullous pemphigoid. *Clin. Immunol.* 2008 Sep;128(3):415-26. doi: 10.1016/j.clim.2008.04.012.

[12] Bonifazi M, Zuccatosta L, Poidomani G, Ranaldi R, Gasparini S. Bullous pemphigoid with the unusual complication of tracheobronchial involvement. *Chest.* 2013 Jan;143(1):236-8. doi: 10.1378/chest.12-0226.

[13] della Torre R, Combescure C, Cortés B, Marazza G, Beltraminelli H, Naldi L, Borradori L. Clinical presentation and diagnostic delay in bullous pemphigoid: a prospective nationwide cohort. *Br. J. Dermatol.* 2012 Nov;167(5):1111-7. doi: 10.1111/j.1365-2133.2012.11108.x.

[14] Venning VA, Taghipour K, Mustapa MFM, Highet AS, Kirtschig G. British Association of Dermatologists' guidelines for the management of bullous pemphigoid 2012. *Br. J. Dermatol.* 2012;167:1200-14.

[15] García-Romero MT, Werth VP. Randomized controlled trials needed for bullous pemphigoid interventions.*Arch.Dermatol.* 2012 Feb;148(2):243-6.

[16] Miida H, Fujiwara H, Ito M. Association between effective dose of prednisolone, alone or in conjunction with other immunosuppressants, and titre of anti-bullous pemphigoid 180 antibody: a retrospective study of 42 cases. *Clin. Exp. Dermatol.* 2011 Jul;36(5):485-8.

[17] Rzany B, Partscht K, Jung M, Kippes W, Mecking D, Baima B, Prudlo C, Pawelczyk B, Messmer EM, Schuhmann M,Sinkgraven R, Büchner L, Büdinger L, Pfeiffer C, Sticherling M, Hertl M, Kaiser HW, Meurer M, Zillikens D, Messer G. Risk factors for lethal outcome in patients with bullous pemphigoid: low serum albumin level, high dosage of glucocorticosteroids, and old age. *Arch. Dermatol.* 2002 Jul;138(7):903-8.

[18] Joly P, Roujeau JC, Benichou J, Picard C, Dreno B, Delaporte E, Vaillant L, D'Incan M, Plantin P, Bedane C, Young P,Bernard P; Bullous Diseases French Study Group. A comparison of oral and topical corticosteroids in patients with bullous pemphigoid. *N. Engl. J. Med.* 2002 Jan 31;346(5):321-7.

[19] Daniel BS, Borradori L, Hall RP 3rd, Murrell DF. Evidence-based management of bullous pemphigoid. *Dermatol. Clin.* 2011 Oct;29(4):613-20.

[20] Bressan AL, Silva RS, Fontenelle E, Gripp AC. Immunosuppressive agents in Dermatology. An. Bras. Dermatol. 2010 Jan-Feb;85(1):9-22.

[21] Ruocco E, Wolf R, Caccavale S, Brancaccio G, Ruocco V, Lo Schiavo A. Bullous pemphigoid: associations and management guidelines: facts and controversies. *Clin. Dermatol.* 2013 Jul-Aug;31(4):400-12.

[22] Tirado-Sánchez A, Díaz-Molina V, Ponce-Olivera RM. Efficacy and safety of azathioprine and dapsone as an adjuvant in the treatment of bullous pemphigoid. *Allergol Immunopathol* (Madr). 2012 May-Jun;40(3):152-5.

[23] Gual A, Iranzo P, Mascaró JM Jr. Treatment of bullous pemphigoid with low-dose oral cyclophosphamide: a case series of 20 patients. *J. Eur. Acad. Dermatol. Venereo*l. 2014 Jun;28(6):814-8.

[24] Müller PA, Bröcker EB, Klinker E, Stoevesandt J, Benoit S. Adjuvant treatment of recalcitrant bullous pemphigoid with immunoadsorption. *Dermatology.* 2012;224(3):224-7.

[25] Shetty S, Ahmed AR. Treatment of bullous pemphigoid with rituximab: critical analysis of the current literature. *J. Drugs Dermatol.* 2013 Jun 1;12(6):672-7.

[26] Yu KK, Crew AB, Messingham KA, Fairley JA, Woodley DT. Omalizumab therapy for bullous pemphigoid. *J. Am. Acad. Dermatol.* 2014 Sep;71(3):468-74.

[27] Dimson OG, Giudice GJ, Fu CL, Van den Bergh F, Warren SJ, Janson MM, Fairley JA. Identification of a potential effector function for IgE autoantibodies in the organ-specific autoimmune disease bullous pemphigoid. *J. Invest. Dermatol.* 2003 May;120(5):784-8.

[28] Murrell DF, Daniel BS, Joly P, Borradori L, Amagai M, Hashimoto T, Caux F, Marinovic B, Sinha AA, Hertl M,Bernard P, Sirois D, Cianchini G, Fairley JA, Jonkman MF, Pandya AG, Rubenstein D, Zillikens D, Payne AS,Woodley D, Zambruno G, Aoki V, Pincelli C, Diaz L, Hall RP, Meurer M, Mascaro JM Jr, Schmidt E, Shimizu H,Zone J, Swerlick R, Mimouni D, Culton D, Lipozencic J, Bince B, Grando SA, Bystryn JC, Werth VP. *J. Am. Acad. Dermatol.* 2012 Mar;66(3):479-85.

In: Advances in Dermatology Research
Editor: James P. Vega

ISBN: 978-1-63482-226-8

Chapter 2

Bullous Pemphigoid: Broader Concepts

Ana Maria Abreu Velez, MD, PhD [*,1],
Enrique Velazquez Velez, MD [2]
and Michael S. Howard, MD [1]
[1]Georgia Dermatopathology Associates, Atlanta, Georgia, US
[2]HGM - Clinica CES - Clinica SOMER - Fundacion HUSVP, Rionegro and Medellin, Colombia, South America

Abstract

Bullous pemphigoid (BP) is a rare skin condition with tense, fluid-filled blisters, and urticarial or other lesions on areas of the lower abdomen, upper thighs or armpits (flexoral areas). BP has highest incidence in people older than 60. In BP, the immune system attacks the basement membrane zone (BMZ) of the skin at the junction of the epidermis and dermis; however, current data indicates that the BP autoimmune pathology may also attack dermal blood vessels, some stromal dermal areas, nerves, sweat glands and the BMZs of skin adnexal structures. The BP pathologic immune response that initially was thought to be predominately focused on IgG and Complement/C3 deposition at the cutaneous BMZ; however, recent data indicates that B and T lymphocytes, other immune system cells and inflammatory markers may be involved. In some cases, clinical lesions resembling classic BP can be triggered by taking medications; however, the immunopathogenesis of this disorder seems to be quite different. In BP, direct and indirect immunofluorescence of the skin usually shows reactivity in a linear pattern along the BMZ with IgG, Complement/C3 and sometimes IgE; other immunoglobulins and complement may also be present. Multiple markers have been also described in the BP blisters; however, the data is not always consistent. A number of immunoblotting (IB) analyses have indicated that two major antigenic proteins of epidermal extracts are targets in BP; specifically, the 230 kilodalton (kDa) BP antigen I (BP230 or BPAG1), and the 180-kDa BP antigen II (BP180, BPAG2 or Type XVII collagen). These antigenic proteins are detected by sera from patients with BP in various IB patterns; however, other

* Corresponding author: Ana Maria Abreu Velez, M.D., Ph.D., Georgia Dermatopathology Associates, 1534 North Decatur Rd., NE; Suite 206; Atlanta, Georgia 30307-1000, USA, Telephone: (404) 371-0077, Toll Free: (877) 371-0027, Fax: (404) 371-1900, E-mail: abreuvelez@yahoo.com.

putative antigens have also been documented. Including an 84 kDa protein and others. Enzyme-linked immunosorbent assays (ELISAs) have confirmed the immunoblotting assays. Some studies have shown that BPAGII has an extracellular domain; polyclonal rabbit antibodies raised against an extracellular, non-collagenous domain of the murine BP180 antigen were documented as pathogenic in a passive transfer model. Several investigators have suggested a relationship between clinical findings and laboratory data in BP. The clinical and pathologic BP differential diagnosis includes lichen planus pemphigoides, and pemphigus vegetans.

The treatment of BP usually includes corticosteroids such as prednisone, and other drugs that suppress the immune system. BP can be life-threatening, especially for older people who are already in poor health. The disease may have significant impact on the patient and their family, and have important economic consequences due to their disability and via complications in the immunosuppressive therapy. The diagnosis of BP is challenging for primary physicians, nurses and other health care providers, especially when they lack of the proper laboratory techniques for the diagnosis of BP. In vitro and *in vivo* animal models for BP are available, but many of them do not seem reproduce the *in vivo* clinical disease. The current medical literature offers an arsenal of biological medications, but none have therapeutically surpassed corticosteroids. The long term treatment of BP patients' needs to have a multidisciplinary and comprehensive approach, including therapists and nutritionists.

Keywords: bullous pemphigoid, antigens, mucous membrane pemphigoid, nerves, blood vessels, sweat glands, central and peripheral nervous system, lungs, heart

Declarations of conflicts of interest: None.

Funding: Georgia Dermatopathology Associates, Atlanta, Georgia, USA

Conflicts of interest: None.

Abbreviations and Acronyms

Bullous pemphigoid (BP)
blister fluid (BF)
lichen planus pemphigoides (LPP)
immunohistochemistry (IHC)
direct and indirect immunofluorescence (DIF and IIF)
hematoxylin and eosin (H&E)
basement membrane zone (BMZ)
sodium dodecyl sulfate (SDS)
SDS-PAGE (SDS polyacrylamide gel electrophoresis)
bullous pemphigoid antigen II (180 kDa) and I (230 kDa) (BP180 and BP230)
epidermolysis bullosa simplex (EBS)
intravenous immunoglobulin (IVIG)
kilodalton (kDa)
mast cells tryptase (MCT)

central nervous system (CNS)
immunoblotting (IB)
pemphigus vegetans (PEV)
enzyme-linked immunosorbent assay (ELISA)
epidermolysis bullosa aquisita (EBA)
molar (M)
phosphate buffered saline buffer (PBS)
eosinophil cationic protein (ECP)
tumor necrosis factor-alpha (TNF-alpha)
Airway, Breathing and Circulation (ABC)
drug induced bullous pemphigoid (DBP)

Introduction

The majority of autoimmune blistering diseases have blisters and/or vesicles, which are often pruritic, and manifest autoantibodies to diverse proteins. BP represents the most common autoimmune mucocutaneous subepidermal blistering disease worldwide [1-19]. Clinical history, hematoxylin and eosin (H&E) histology, direct and/or indirect immunofluorescence and salt split skin techniques are important diagnostic tools in BP. Other tools include immunoblotting (IB), enzyme-linked immunosorbent assays (ELISAs) and electron microscopy (EM) [1-18]. Corticosteroids remain the first-line systemic therapy for patients with moderate to severe bullous pemphigoid. However, steroid sparing agents are invaluable in inducing long-term remission while minimizing steroid associated side effects [1-18]. The BP treatment must be tailored to the individual patient's condition, and several other factors must be carefully considered in choosing appropriate therapy. In developing countries, challenges exist due to the lack of many diagnostic and therapeutic tools [1-18].

Historical Milestones: Years ago, most blistering diseases were called pemphigus and were classified as acute or chronic, and benign or malignant. These disorders were also classified by their sizes of blisters and by the presence of wheals or blebs [1-4]. The blisters could rupture and discharge puriform, bloody or milky exudate. (In the oldest descriptions found in books, monograms, and other publications, the epidermis was reported to “hang in shreds”. Sometimes crusts formed, with excoriated spots. Sometimes these diseases were described to be present in epidemics, usually in children, with symptoms such irritability, headache, lassitude, quick pulse, delirium, chills, rigor, irritability of the mucosae and occasional fevers [1-4] These descriptions show that entities such chicken pox, variola, autoimmune and non-autoimmune blistering diseases, and infections entities were often grouped as “blistering diseases” [1-4]. Most authors agree that itching or burning sensations were described by the patients. In several of the oldest publications, the authors described occasional cachectic conditions and death. In some cases, these authors reported skin fissures with secondary painful movement, alopecia, the eyelid ectropion and friable nails. Loss of appetite, diarrhea, Jarisch reactions, anemia, brain and lung edema, chronic degeneration of the liver, spleen and kidneys and weak muscles were also seen [1-4]. Selected early writers described pemphigus as contagious in some cases, and non-contagious in others. Some others noted maternal blisters after giving birth, insomnia, epiglottitic suffocations, and anatomic changes in the spinal cord. Early disease terms included pemphigus pruriginosus, pemphigus malignus, pemphigus cachecticus, pemphigus gangrenosum, chonic eczema vesiculosum, pemphigus syphiliticus, impetigo herpetiformis, pemphigoid eruptions and herpes iris [1-4]. Early treatments included recommendations of eating eggs, milk or cream; rest; and starch or gelatin gelatin baths [1-4]. Early autopsies on patients with blistering conditions included descriptions of fatty liver, enlarged adrenal glands, parechchimatous nephritis, hypersecretion of papillary dermal lymphatics and epidermal lymphedema among others [1-4]. The authors are now learning that these findings may reflect possible systemic immune compromise in patients with BP and other autoimmune blistering diseases. Although Civatte and others had noted that some bullous diseases were subepidermal and therefore distinct from pemphigus, Lever [5-7], in analyzing previous data and studying his own patients, clearly defined BP around 1953 as disease nosologically distinct from pemphigus and from dermatitis herpetiformis as defined by Duhring [8]. Later in 1965, Beutner *et al.* described that in BP patients, deposits of IgG and complement were directed against the basement membrane zone (BMZ) of the skin via indirect by direct immunofluorescence and indirect immunofluorescence (DIF, IIF) [9, 10]. These discoveries by Beutner, Lever, Jordon and others, provided the immunologic basis for differentiating pemphigoid from pemphigus. Skin organ culture and passive transfer models did not work well in BP. More complicated *in vitro* BP models indicated that more than IgG, complement and inflammatory cells were necessary for blister formation in BP [11]. Utilizing immunoblotting (IB) analysis and sodium dodecyl sulfate polyacrylamide gel electrophoresis (SDS-PAGE), two different BP antigens were identified and cloned. Specifically, these proteins were classified as BP230/BPAGI and BP180/BPAGII [11-15], according to their molecular weight in kilodaltons (kDa); several ELISAs have confirmed these findings. Mouse models of BP have indicated that BP180 is the pathogenic antigen, and that IgG, complement, and inflammatory cells are necessary for disease initiation; however, inconsistent data have also been reported. It also have been shown in experiments using passive transfer of experimental IgG (developed against the murine homolog of this determinant to neonatal BALB/c mice) that clinical, histologic, and immunopathologic alterations may occur, with similarities to those seen in patients with BP patients. However, no animal or cell culture study has been able to reproduce the chronicity of BP. Authors have reported multiple animal models with genetic manipulations; however, many of these studies lack proper controls.

Subepidermal Autoimmune Blisters: Recently, the traditional classification of subepidermal blistering diseases has been based on their patterns of inflammation [1-10]. Autoimmune blistering diseases are uncommon cutaneous disorders, characterized by varying presentations of mucosal and cutaneous bullae, blisters, plaques and wheals. However, some overlap occurs between the traditional categories, especially with subepidermal vesiculobullous diseases in which neutrophils or eosinophils represent the predominant infiltrating cell [1-10]. Special techniques, including electron microscopy, immunoelectron microscopy, immunoblotting, direct immunofluorescence(DIF), indirect immunofluorescence (IIF), IIF/salt split skin, and immunohistochemistry (IHC) have allowed many of the subepidermal blistering diseases to be characterized not only histologically on the basis of the anatomic split level within the BMZ, but also immunologically [16, 17]. Further, additional information helps to exclude viral blistering diseases, bullous allergic drug reactions and genodermatoses; this information may be provided via viral serology, viral culture, a history of previous intake of medications (including nonprescription medications) and possible genetic evaluation.

The total patient approach for a BP diagnosis. The epidemiologic history, family history, clinical history and physical examination, as well as the previously described laboratory studies are needed for a proper differentiation from other diseases.

Clinical History: Some important general points include age of onset, size, frequency and location of blisters, possible inciting factors (including trauma, sun exposure, foods, drugs, ongoing infections or neoplasms), prior diagnostic attempts, prior therapies, and extent of pain or pruritis [1-10, 18-20]. Review of systems should include looking for alterations of growth/development and mucosal involvement including oral, nasopharyngeal, ocular, genitotourinary, gastrointestinal or respiratory symptoms. Look for a family history of blistering diseases and for pertinent geographic/ethnic ancestries [1-10, 18-20].

Physical Examination: A complete physical examination should be performed, with an emphasis on inspection of all skin and mucosa. Evaluate the size, location and character of blisters and try to get an idea of the level of the splits in the lesions. Superficial blisters often manifest as crusted erosions; intraepidermal blisters are often flaccid, and may expand under pressure; intra-lamina lucida blisters are often tense and heal with no scarring(but sometimes atrophy); sub-lamina densa blisters usually heal with scarring, and milia are often present [1-10, 18-20].

BP Natural History: BP is the most common autoimmune skin blistering disease in the adult population in developed countries, with an estimated incidence that varies from 1 to 3 cases per 100,000 inhabitants per year to 1 in 40,000 [18-20]. In undeveloped countries, it seems to be the second most common autoimmune blistering disease; however, few relevant epidemiologic studies have been published [20-22]. A sex predisposition has not been clearly established. The course of this disease can be acute, chronic, or relapsing. BP usually manifests in the sixth or seventh decade of life; however, cases have been observed at other ages, including in children [20-22]. The most common clinical presentation includes scattered urticarial papules and plaques on the trunk, arms, and legs early in the disease. Later, blisters are often large, tense and located on an erythematous base. Occasionally the blisters are not clinically apparent, due to previous rupture. Acral sites may be involved. The most important symptom related by the patients is pruritis, which may be severe; in contradistinction, pemphigus patients often report a burning sensation [20-22]. In some BP patients, the pruritus seems not to be present. Overall, skin lesions are symmetrically distributed; the most common sites are consistently the flexor surfaces of the extremities, the groin, the axillae and the lower abdomen. The lesions generally heal without scarring, but in rare cases milia formation has been described. In some cases, BP is misdiagnosed as urticaria. The disease may initially present as tense vesicles and bullae on an urticarial base. The bullae can reach a size of several centimeters before rupturing [20-22] (See Table 1 and Figure 1). Blisters in the oral cavity are rare, may compromise the oropharynx and are classically non-scarring. Pemphigus vegetans (PEV) is considered a variant of BP. Occasionally, BP may be induced by medications such as furosemide, captopril, and penicillin; thus, classic BP needs to be differentiated from blistering allergic drug eruptions [17-22].

The physiopathologic aspects of BP include cutaneous deposition of autoantibodies, complement, fibrinogen, albumin and other products of proteases; this deposition results in the disruption of adhesive interactions between epidermal basal layer keratinocytes. The early dermatopathology studies in BP were led by Walter F. Lever, M.D [5-7]. On light microscopy, H&E staining classically reveals a subepidermal blister under an intact epidermis. When clinical blisters arise on erythematous skin, there is often a prominent cellular infiltrate in the papillary dermis consisting of numerous eosinophils, lymphocytes and neutrophils. Papillary dermal microabscesses of neutrophils and eosinophils are present in about 20% of BP cases [5-7], [see Figure 1].

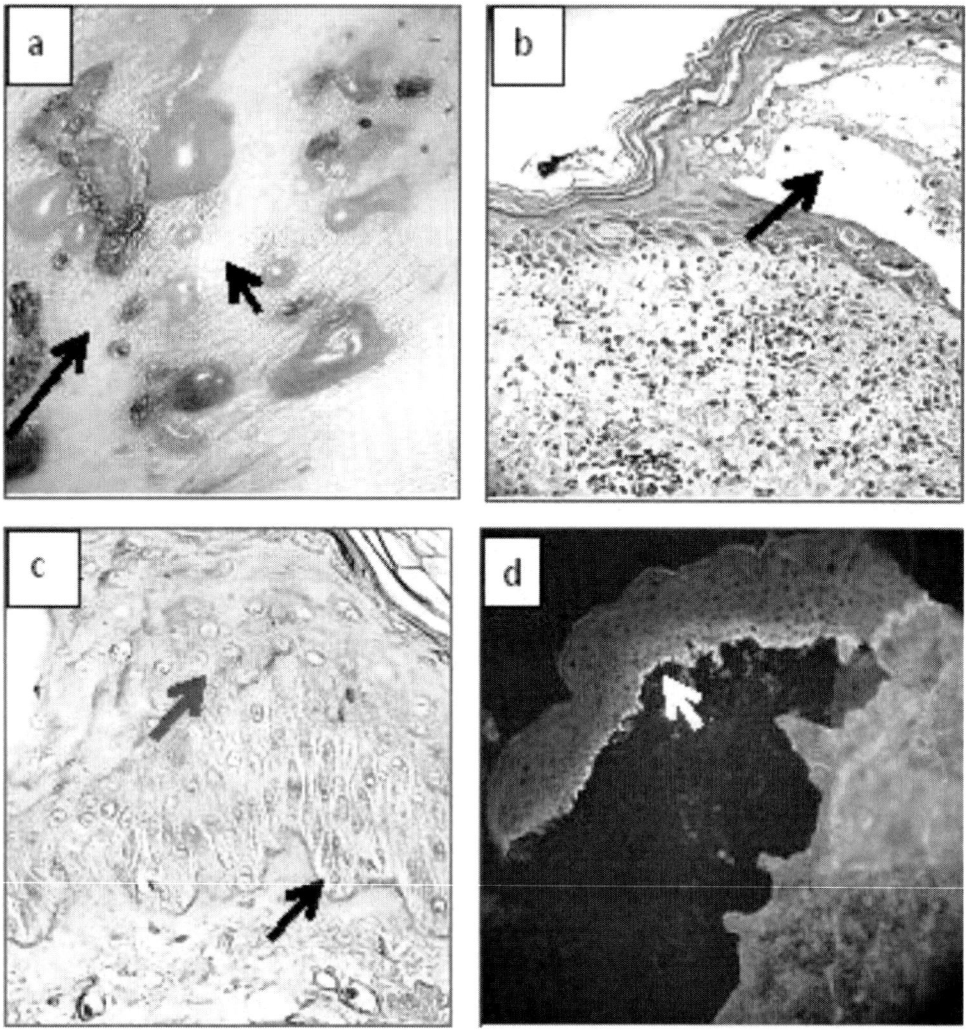

Figure 1. **a**. Shows a large blister, with erythema and crusts. **b.** An H&E stained section showing a subepidermal blister with inflammatory infiltrate; partial re-epithelialization of the blister base is present (black arrow). **c.** Shows a PAS stain, with positive thickening of the BMZ linear deposits (black arrow), and also some positivity in epidermal areas (red arrow). **d.** IIF. 1 M NaCl split skin shows positive staining using a FITC conjugated anti-human IgG antibody, and demonstrating linear reactivity on the epidermal/roof side of the split(yellow staining; white arrow).

Table 1. Summary of the main features in BP

Bullous Pemphigoid
BP clinical features: Usually presents in elderly patients (over 65 years). A sex predisposition has not been clearly established Most commonly affected areas are the trunk and extremities; head and mucous membranes are seldom affected. Large, fluid-filled, tense blisters and urticarial lesions on areas of the lower abdomen, upper thighs or armpits (flexoral areas). Pruritus is common, and lesions heal without scars.
H&E Staining: We highly encourage reviewing the H&E staining with any DIF and IIF, because many other disease produce pseudo-linear deposits of immunoglobulins and complement. Subepidermal bullae are present. Vacuolar degeneration of the epidermal basaloid layer may be noted. Eosinophils are present within the blister lumens, and also present within a superficial dermal infiltrate. The bases of the blisters re-epithelialize quickly, and the blister may thus appear intraepidermal.
DIF: We recommend contacting the immunofluorescence laboratory in advance to obtain the correct transport medium, and to coordinate shipping and for instructions on how to take the biopsy. Normal skin adjacent to a lesion is ideal for DIF. Classic findings include linear IgG and Complement/C3 at the BMZ. However, recent studies have also shown positive staining with IgD, IgM, Complement/C1q, c omplment/C3c, fibrinogen and albumin at the BMZ, around dermal blood vessels, neurovascular packages and eccrine sweat glands, and around BMZs of the sebaceous and the sweat glands.
Salt split skin/IIF: Positive staining is usually present along the blister roof; however, in some cases positive staining may be noted on both the blister roof and floor.
IHC staining: Reflects similar findings as DIF; however, it allows the pathologist to see many other patterns of reactivity.
Antigens detected by IB: (BP230/BPAGI), (BP180/BPAGII), P84, desmoplakins, and others to be identified.
ELISA: Commercially available against BP180/BPAGII NC16A, and BP230/BPAGI.
Electron microscopy: Ultrastructural alterations of superficial epidermal keratinocytes have been described using EM.
Cytokines and chemokines in lesional skin of patients with BP: IL-4, IL-13, IL10 CCL17, CCL18, IL-17, IL-6, tumor necrosis factor-alpha, IL-10 and Foxp3 have been reported.
Bullous Pemphigoid (please delete road)
Inflammatory markers, cell enzymes and their inhibitors detected in lesional skin of patients with BP: Mast cell tryptase, CD117/C-kit, S100, HAM56, CD1a, CD3, CD8, CD45, CD68, COX-2, HLA-DP, DQ, DR antigens and ribosomal protein s6-ps240 have been reported. Tissue inhibitor of metalloproteinase 1, matrix metalloproteinase 9, alpha-1 antitrypsin and metallothionein have also been found.
Blister fluid (BF) markers in patients with BP: TNF-alpha, IL-4, IL-10, IL17, CD200 and eosinophil cationic protein were present increased amounts in BF in patients with BP.

Table 1. (Continued)

Lungs, heart, cardiovascular system and kidney in BP: Vascular cell adhesion molecule-1, E-selectin, P-selectin, very late activation antigen-4, COX-2, HLA-DP, DQ, DR, many immunoglobins, complement factors, fibrinogen and other markers are present in these organs in multiple patients with BP.
Nerves and BP: BP230/BPAGI antigen is a plakin, and these molecules are expressed in the central as well as the peripheral neural system. Some isoforms have also described to be present in the neural system, and have putative clinical and pathologic implications.
Treatment: Local and systemic corticosteroids usually provides fast and effective control. Initial doses of oral prednisone are recommended at 0.5 to 1.0 mg/kg per day. The dose of prednisone can be tapered gradually over a period of months, to a maintenance dose between 5 and 10 mg/day. If lesions are intractable to prednisone at 10 mg/day, an additional immunosuppressive agent such as azathioprine or mycophenolate is warranted. If lesions are refractory to conventional therapy, intravenous immunoglobulin or rituximab are recommended. For moist cutaneous erosions, topical soaks with aluminum acetate for 10 minutes three times a day are often helpful. Recently, omalizumab has been added to BP treatment options due to its effect on IgE.
Differential diagnosis: Bullous amyloidosis, dermatitis herpetiformis, EBA, Linear IgA disease, chronic bullous disease of childhood, erythema multiforme, pemphigus vulgaris, cicatricial pemphigoid, toxic epidermal necrolysis, allergic contact dermatitis.
BP in animals: BP has been described in horses, and in Yucatan minature pigs.
BP variants: Lichen planus pemphigoides (LPP), pemphigoid vegetans (PEV) and drug induced bullous pemphigoid (DBP).

The dermal infiltrate in clinically non-inflamed skin lesions is sparse, perivascular, and primarily composed of lymphocytes and histiocytes. Multiple autoantibodies are directed against components of the BMZ [8, 9].

Direct immunofluorescence microscopy (DIF*)*: Initial studies demonstrating the autoimmune nature of BP were led by Ernst Beutner, Ph.D. and Robert Jordon, M.D. [9, 10]. These investigators demonstrated the increased diagnostic value of DIF biopsies taken from perilesional blister areas. Serologic studies, including indirect immunofluorescence/IIF can help to confirm the diagnosis, utilizing antigen sources such as normal human skin, monkey esophagus and/or guinea pig lips [9, 10]. It is recommended to contact the immunofluorescence lab beforehand to obtain the correct holding medium, and to coordinate shipping and biopsy instructions. In most laboratories, frozen sections of a DIF biopsy are incubated with antibodies against human IgG, IgA, IgM, Complement/C3, fibrinogen and albumin. In our laboratory, we routinely use these and also antibodies to IgD, IgE, Complement/C1q and Complement/C3c.

In rare laboratories, IgA and IgG subclasses are routinely performed; however, these subclasses are most often utilized in research applications [9, 10]. There are also variations in DIF methodology between different laboratories. Some laboratories routinely pre-incubate DIF biopsies in 1 molar (M) NaCl solution, to increase intra-lamina lucida dermal/epidermal separation prior to sectionin. The advantage of the former method is that the location of the antibody/complement deposits can be more easily determined. The salt split skin pre-incubation is especially useful in cases where epidermolysis bullosa acquisita (EBA) or BP is suspected. In EBA, the autoantibodies are found primarily on the dermal/floor side of the induced split, in contrast to BP, in which the antibodies are localized primarily to the epidermal/roof side [16, 17]. While the 1M NaCl DIF/IIF technique is most often used for differentiating BP from EBA, this technique can also be used to diagnose other less common autoimmune diseases [16, 17], (See Table 1).

Indirect immunofluorescence microscopy (IIF): Sera from patients with a positive DIF biopsy or patients who, for various reasons, have not had a skin biopsy performed can be analyzed via indirect immunofluorescence/IIF microscopy. In this procedure, frozen tissue sections are classically taken usually from healthy human skin (such as that obtained from plastic surgery reduction surgery, or infant penile foreskin), and are incubated with patient sera dilutions. Usually a serial dilution of the serum is utilized at 1:20 in phosphate buffered saline (PBS). The serum is then diluted to 1:40 and progressively further if positivity is found in initial sera, until the point when positive staining is no longer observed. The last dilution prior to the point where no more positive staining is observed is known as the patient's serum "titer". Knowing the serum titer in patients with BP is especially useful, because it has been shown to correlate with disease activity [9, 10].

Interestingly, sera from patients with a positive DIF biopsy are not always positive on IIF [8, 9, 16, 17]. In some instances, obtaining serum for IIF is obtained as an afterthought, after systemic therapy has already been initiated and can thus show negative results [8, 9, 16, 17]. Rather than human tissue, any laboratories routinely use primate esophagus as a substrate to test patient sera via IIF. The advantage of primate esophagus is that secondary antibodies which react with human skin are avoided and present a low background; in contrast, human skin contains normal immunoglobulin, located diffusely throughout the dermis that is recognized by anti-human secondary antibodies. The disadvantage with primate esophagus is that some human autoantibodies do not appear to cross-react well with primate tissue. The disadvantage with non-salt split human skin is that the background which appears in the dermis can sometimes make visualization of BMZ reactivity difficult [8, 9, 16, 17]. Separation of the epidermis from the dermis in 1 M NaCl split skin makes it easier to determine if reactivity is present on the epidermal or dermal side of the split. It is also possible that epitopes are exposed, or at least made more accessible for antibody binding after 1M NaCl splitting. For some or all of the reasons above, 1 M NaCl split skin yields a higher percentage of positive indirect IF results compared to either primate esophagus or non-salt split human skin at least in the cases of the diseases such cicatricial pemphigoid (CP) and linear IgA bullous dermatosis. Thus, 1 M NaCl split human skin should be ideally used as a substrate if these diseases are suspected [8, 9, 6, 17]. In our lab, we routinely use these methods: 1 M NaCl split normal human skin as a substrate for IIF, and non-split monkey esophagus for antibody titer determinations.

The DIF biopsies should be performed at the same time as the cutaneous H&E biopsies. We highly recommend reviewing the H&E stain with the DIF and IIF and correlating the findings in a single report because many other diseases produce pseudo-linear deposits of immunoglobulins and complement. In H&E biopsies, histopathologic findings may vary depending on whether the biopsy was taken from lesional skin, the lesional border or nonlesional skin [8, 9]. In BP, classic DIF of perilesional skin shows deposits of IgG and complement component C3 at the BMZ (see Figure 1). Classic IgG and Complement/C3 deposits are present in a continuous, fine linear pattern along the BMZ. In BP, linear deposits of IgG, Complement/C3, and often IgE are observed in the majority of the BP cases. The IgG4 subclass, and, to a lesser degree IgG1 are observed [8, 9]. Other immunoreactant classes are less frequently reported, because many laboratories worldwide do not perform extensive immunoreactant panels [19-21]. On IIF, 1 M NaCl split skin; autoantibodies are present predominantly on the blister roof in 90% of BP cases. IIF is usually performed on normal human or monkey esophagus substrate skin; the skin substrate separates through the lamina lucida on incubation in 1.0 M NaCl [16, 17]. Via non-salt split IIF, the majority of pertinent BP sera produce a consistent pattern of linear immunofluorescence at dilutions of 1:10 or higher. On 1 M NaCl split skin IIF, these same antibodies primarily bind to either the blister roof (epidermal pattern), blister floor (dermal pattern), or both the roof and floor (combined pattern). The binding patterns have been described in comparison with normal controls. Sera from patients with clinical and histologic features of EBA show a predominant dermal pattern. However, some sera from patients with BP and EBA show a combined pattern. Indirect immunoelectron microscopy of selected sera show antibodies producing the epidermal and combined patterns are anti-lamina lucida antibodies, and those producing the dermal pattern were anti-sublamina densa antibodies [16, 17]. These results show that IIF split skin is a dependable method for differentiating BP with anti-lamina lucida versus anti-sublamina densa antibodies, and that differentiating between these antibody patterns is essential for accurate diagnosis in some patients. The results also suggest that BP anti-lamina lucida antibodies may be of importance, but this data is not proven yet.

Immunoblotting (IB): IB analysis is usually performed by first separating solubilized epidermis and/or dermis or solubilized keratinocyte/fibroblast cell extracts, and then analyzing them via electrophoresis by SDS-PAGE. The separated proteins are then transferred onto nitrocellulose, and incubated first with patient sera, and then incubation with horseradish peroxidase (HRP) or alkaline phosphatase conjugated secondary antibodies. BP antigens which can be detected in this way include BP180, BP230 and others [11-15]. The primary autoantibodies detected in sera from patients with BP have been reported to primarily bind to two hemidesmosomal proteins, initially detected by IB and cDNA cloning as a 180-kD antigen (BPAG II; BP180; Collagen Type XVII), and a 230-kD antigen (BPAGI; BP230). BP230 is a plakin protein family member that promotes the association of hemidesmosomes with keratin intermediate filaments [11-15]. BP180 is a type II transmembrane collagen that is associated with hemidesmosome anchoring filament complexes, and is believed to harbor all or a portion of the primary pathogenic epitope responsible for the initiation of BP [11-15], (see Table 1). The extracellular domain of BP180 contains 15 interrupted collagenous domains. Rotary shadowing studies of purified BP180 reveal its intracytoplasmic region to be a globular head, and its ectodomain as a central rod joined to a flexible tail [11-15]. Some BP sera recognize both antigen proteins, while others detect only BP230 or BP180 or none. Recently, cDNAs for these antigens have been isolated, and the characteristics for these molecules have been investigated in more detail.

Other identified BP antigens: Some patients with bullous diseases have unusual BMZ autoantibodies, that react to antigens present in both the epidermal and dermal sides of salt split skin [29]. The combined staining pattern is due to antibodies directed in part to a 160-kDa BMZ antigen, present on the epidermal side of the split skin and to different antigen(s) present on the dermal side. The specific identity of these antigens (s) and the significance of this unusual type of combined staining antibody response are not known [29]. Sera of five patients with combined staining antibodies, 19 patients with single pattern BMZ staining (15 directed only to the epidermal, and four only to the dermal side of split skin) and 23 patients without BMZ antibody staining were tested for IB reactivity in 4% sodium dodecyl sulfate-PAGE (with 2 M urea) against proteins from both the dermal and epidermal sides of normal salt-split skin. Three (60%) of the combined staining sera had antibodies to an 82-84 kD antigen (p84), reproducibly present in dermal (but not epidermal) extracts of normal human skin. Antibodies to this antigen were absent in the 42 control sera [29]. IB affinity-purified antibody to p84 bound only to BMZ, on the dermal side of 1 M salt-split skin. By co-migration experiments, p84 differed from other BMZ proteins including the major and minor BP, cicatrizing pemphigoid, EBA antigens, Types III and IV collagen, laminin, and epiligrin. Thus, combined staining antibodies are directed in part to an 82-84 kD antigen (p84), a normal but previously undescribed component of the BMZ of human skin. The authors concluded that this antigen differs from the BMZ antigens recognized by autoantibodies in other subepidermal bullous diseases. The antibody response to p84 provides a specific marker for a novel autoimmune subepidermal blistering skin disease, and the significance of this finding remains to be elucidated [29].

Enzyme-linked immunosorbent assay (ELISA): The ELISA test is performed by coating small quantities of purified autoantigen onto 96-well plastic dishes, applying dilutions of patient sera, and visualizing with HRP or alkaline phosphatase conjugated secondary antibodies; the bound antibodies may then be quantified in a modified spectrophotometer, termed an ELISA reader [31-36]. This ELISA technique is currently limited by the availability of purified autoantigens, but several commercial ELISAs are available for BP. [31-36]. ELISAs for BP180 and BP230 (MCW2 and MCW1, respectively) were developed by a BP research group at the Medical College of Wisconsin [31-36]; ELISA development included data regarding a new antigen fragment titled NC16A. A recent study has shown that the BP180 ELISA is specific for the immunodominant NC16A domain of the BPAGII protein; however, the ELISA is exclusive of other parts of the NC16A domain [31-36]. The NC16A finding is consistent with the immunology concept that all conformational epitopes at least carry at least one or more linear epitopes [31-36].

Electron Microscopy and Immunoelectron Microscopy studies in BP: Transmission electron microscopy and immunoelectron microscopy data indicates that BP180 spans the lamina lucida, and inserts into the lamina densa. BP180 is targeted by autoantibodies from patients with BP, pemphigoid gestationis, CP and linear IgA dermatosis (LAD) [37-40]. Studies on non-inflamed skin lesions from BP patients reveal that dermal-epidermal cleavage occurs within the dermal-epidermal junction, i.e., through the lamina lucida [37-40].

Macrophage roles in BP: M2 macrophages play a critical role in the induction of T helper 2 (Th2) lymphocyte polarization [41-43]. Some authors have investigated the contribution of M2 macrophages to the pathogenesis of BP by using IHC staining for CD163 and CD206, as well as pSTAT1, pSTAT6, interleukin (IL)-4, IL-13, CCL17, CCL18 and Foxp3 from lesional skin of 10 cases of BP [41]. The authors reported that the numbers of CD163+ CD206+ M2 macrophages were higher in BP versus controls [43]. Further, pSTAT6+ cells, CCL17+ cells, CCL18+ cells and Foxp3+ regulatory T cells were prominent only in the lesional skin of BP. Other authors reported that HAM56, CD1a, CD68 and myeloid-histiocytic antigen were positive in the majority of BP patients in lesional skin [42, 43].

Mast cells proteases in BP: Several authors had described strong positivity for mast cell tryptase (MCT) and CD117/C-Kit in the majority of the skin biopsies with BP [44, 45].

Blister fluid in BP: Previous authors analyzed both the blister fluid (BF) and serum levels of IL-7 and TGF-beta1 in samples from 18 patients affected with BP. Eighteen sera from normal individuals were used as controls. These cytokines were present lower concentrations ($p<0.001$) in BF than in the sera [46]. In contrast, TNF-alpha, IL-10 and IL-4 present increased amounts in the BF, relative to the sera. In addition, the serum levels of these cytokines detected in BP patients were significantly correlated with disease intensity, determined via the number of blisters/erosions for each patient, peripheral B-lymphocyte counts and antibodies directed against the BMZ [46]. The authors concluded that a strong decrease of IL-7 production occurs in BP at the local level, and they believe the IL-7 reduction may have a biologic relevance in controlling a chronic, progressive disease [46].

Recently other authors studied BF from patients with BP for the presence of CD200. CD200 is a novel immunosuppressive molecule, existing both in cell membrane bound form and in a soluble form in serum (sCD200). CD200 acts to regulate inflammatory and acquired immune responses. The authors showed that sCD200 was found in serum and BF in a patient with BP, and that anti-IgE therapy impacted those levels [47]. These authors investigated 5 patients with BP, and 15 healthy controls. They performed clinical examinations; levels of anti-BP180 and soluble CD200 in the serum samples were quantified using ELISA kits [47]. The authors reported that serum soluble CD200 levels were observed to be statistically significantly higher in patients with BP, but also that no correlation was noted with other investigated metrics [47].

Other authors investigated whether the activation of eosinophils and coagulation are linked in BP. Authors evaluated the correlation between eosinophil cationic protein (ECP) levels and concentrations of the prothrombotic markers F1+2 and D-dimer in BF and blood samples of 30 BP patients, as well as in controls [48]. For both markers, the authors found higher levels in the serum as well as in the BF of the BP patients in comparison with the controls. The authors concluded that ECP levels were elevated in BF from BP patients, and correlated with markers of coagulation activation, supporting the concept that eosinophils initiate the coagulation cascade at the skin level [48].

Citokines in BP: Previous authors studied the serum levels of three cytokines, interleukin-6 (IL-6), tumor necrosis factor-alpha (TNF-alpha) and interleukin-10 (IL-10) in 15 patients with (BP compared with 20 healthy controls) to evaluate a possible involvement of these biological modulators in the clinical expression of this disease [49]. Determination of cytokine concentrations was obtained employing commercially available ELISA kits. The sera of BP patients showed increased levels of these three cytokines ($p < 0.01$) [49]. When the number of skin lesions (blisters and/or erosion) of each patient, employed as a marker of disease activity, were correlated with the serum levels of IL-6 and TNF-alpha, significant correlations were found (IL-6: $p < 0.01$ and TNF-alpha: $p < 0.01$, respectively), suggesting a possible role of these mediators in the development of BP blisters [49]. The authors also noted that Th17 lymphocytes seem to play crucial roles in the pathogenesis of BP; they studied the presence of lesional Th17 cells and Treg cells in BP, and correlated these molecules with BP disease severity [49]. IHC staining showed that both IL-17+ and Foxp3+ cells were present in higher numbers in BP lesions, compared with control skin [49].

***In situ* cellular infiltrate, and other inflammatory markers:** Eosinophils, neutrophils, and mast cells have all been implicated in the pathogenesis of BP. Previous authors did a comparative study, addressing the involvement of these cells in BP. Ten lesional skin biopsy specimens were identified retrospectively, and studied for tissue localization of eosinophil, neutrophil, and mast cell granule proteins. Subsequently, multiple skin biopsies of lesions in various BP developmental stages were obtained from 3 patients with untreated BP. Involved and uninvolved skin specimens were also obtained from 2 patients [50]. The authors used IIF, and identified lesions showing that eosinophils and extracellular granule protein deposition was very prominent in the areas of blistering.

The authors also reported that evolving lesions showed eosinophil granule protein deposition in all stages, but that the deposition was most marked in early erythematous and prebullous (urticarial) lesions and minimal in uninvolved skin [50]. Vascular cell adhesion molecule-1, E-selectin, and P-selectin were detected on BP dermal blood vessels, and very late activation antigen-4 was detected on mononuclear cells and eosinophils by IHC staining of the lesions. The authors reported that eosinophil granule proteins were increased in the peripheral blood, urine, and blister fluid (BF); and, that BF featured increased eosinophil survival that was inhibited by antibodies to interleukin-5 and interleukin-3 [50]. The authors further reported that although neutrophil and mast cell infiltration was observed in BP lesions, extracellular granule protein deposition from these cells was minimal except in two specimens. The authors concluded that eosinophil infiltration and deposition of granule proteins occur early in the development of BP lesions; that eosinophil-activating cytokines are present in BP BF, and that eosinophil-selective adhesion molecules are also present. These studies strongly support a specific role for eosinophils in blister formation in BP [50].

Recently we demonstrated that IHC staining is a good alternative to DIF for the diagnosis of BP, as well as other autoimmune blistering diseases [51]. We also showed that B and T lymphocytes [52], as well as other markers such cyclooxygenase-2 (COX-2) [53] and ribosomal protein s6-ps240 [54] are present in lesional skin of patients with BP. We have also shown that HLA-DP,DQ,DR antigen is highly expressed in the blisters in lesional skin of BP patients, as well as all dermal blood vessels that supply skin appendices [55]. We lately demonstrated that tissue inhibitor of metalloproteinase 1, matrix metalloproteinase 9, alpha-1 antitrypsin and metallothionein may play a pathophysiologic role in BP [56]. In addition to the BP immune response against the BMZ, we have documented that some reactivity occurs against eccrine glands, their ducts, and dermal blood vessels and nerves in BP; and that other immunoglobulins and complement factors seem to be part of BP pathobiology [57-60]. We have reported that vimentin may reflect areas of cutaneous involvement in BP [61], and that rouleaux and autoagglutination of erythrocytes associated with fibrin-like material are present in lesions from BP patients [62].

Lungs, heart, cardiovascular system and kidney in BP: In several cases of BP, an interstitial pneumonia associated with linear Immunoglobulin A/Immunoglobulin G bullous dermatosis has been documented [63]. These findings are not new to the pioneers that first investigated BP [63]. In addition, emphysematous and edematous lungs, pleural adhesions and pleural cavities containing bright red fluid have been documented in BP patient autopsies [65,68]. Right heart ventricle dilatation and thin right ventricle walls, as well as cardiac fatty degeneration have been documented in BP patient autopsies [64]. Fatty deposits outside the heart in the muscles and atheromatous aortic patches in the aorta has been also described in BP autopsies [64-68]. Thickened renal capsules, greasy liver surfaces and small spleens are also common findings in BP patient autopsies [64-68]. Other authors have reported BP associated with glomerulonephritis [70, 71].

Nerves and BP: It has been shown that sera of elderly BP patients with associated neurological disease recognizes BP antigens in the human brain [72]. Specific functions of alternative N-terminal isoforms of mouse BP neural antigens have also been documented [73]. Other authors have shown that the mouse dystonia musculorum gene is a neural isoform of BP antigen 1 [74]. Some authors have also recently reported that BP antigen 1 isoforms may represent a potential new target autoantigen in multiple sclerosis [75]. We have reported several cases of autoantibodies to nerves and neurovascular structures using DIF and IIF in BP patient lesional skin biopsies [58, 59].

Animal and *in vitro* models in BP: Several *in vitro* as well as *in vivo* models been developed to reproduce findings in human patients with BP. These models are classified as passive transfer models, active disease models, transfer of autoreactive lymphocyte models, transgenic models, humanized mouse models, and forced immunization models. An attempt at a passive model was made isolating IgG from patients with anti-laminin 332 mucous membrane pemphigoid or BP; the attempt failed to induce a pathogenic response in recipient neonatal mice [76-81]. The authors claimed that when rabbit IgG specific for human laminin 332 or murine type XVII collagen (BP180) was administered, the neonatal mice develop a blistering phenotype independent of complement and neutrophils.

In many other studies, immunocompromised animals were utilized; however, many authors claimed BP model success in these cases [76-81]. The authors recommend a careful approach when reading these articles, since many of these models do not reproduce the epidemiological and clinical features of BP in humans; they require a person well trained in genetics and immunology to properly interpret them.

Morbidity and Mortality associated with BP: Initial statistics on morbidity and mortality in BP was documented years ago, and was higher than current figures [21], possibly due to improvements in early diagnoses and therapeutic options. Previous reports that have addressed morbidity and mortality of BP in in different parts of the world. The overall mortality runs between 29% to-41% per year, but seems to be lower in the USA [83-85]. Many studies emphasize that the mobility and mortality is almost twice as high among residents of rural as urban areas, and in males and females of advanced age [83-85]. Primary comorbidities include cerebrovascular diseases (55%) and hypertension (39.36%); pre-existing conditions such as cardiopathy, diabetes and psoriasis are common. The authors believe that these preconditions and complications may actually represent partial sequelae of BP, and further research is needed to confirm these concepts. Multivariate analysis has revealed that increased age, bedridden condition, presence of cerebrovascular diseases at diagnosis, pre-existing cardiopathy and low serum albumin level were all associated with an elevated 1 year mortality rate [83-85].

Treatment of BP: The authors recommend the following general guidelines. 1) Do not rush. 2) When appropriate, follow the Airway, Breathing and Circulation (ABC) protocol. Airway, breathing, and circulation are vital for life, and many times we forget about this basic concept when treating patients with conditions such as BP. Many doctors try to immediately use the most expensive of the last immunosuppressant available in the market, where long-term studies do not reflect a greater efficacy of these medications versus better known therapeutic options, including steroids. [19, 20]. We need to ensure that the nurse and paramedical personal first work to stabilize the patient, especially those whom present clinically decompensated. 3) Check the complete clinical history of the patient, including any prescription and non-prescription medications. Review any contact with new substances, chemicals, fertilizers or other putative triggering factors [19, 20]. These factors may include ultraviolet radiation, thermal or electrical burns, surgical procedures, transplants, infections (in particular human herpes virus infections, cytomegalovirus, Epstein-Barr virus, HHV-6, hepatitis B and C viruses, Helicobacter pylori, and Toxoplasma gondii). 4) Request basic clinical workup tests, including a complete blood count (CBC). Request an electrolyte panel that measures serum levels of carbon dioxide, chloride, potassium, and sodium [19, 20]. Request a glucose test, because many immunosuppressant medications can alter the glucose levels. Request blood and skin cultures if the patient is hospitalized.

All the above tests should be repeated at least every two weeks, especially if immunosuppresants are therapeutically employed. Request an electrocardiogram, a TB test, a stool test and chest X Ray before initiating any strong or high dose immunosuppressants [19, 20]. We recommend sending these tests in the initial medical visit. Serum urea and creatinine are helpful because some patients will require decreases of immunosuppressant dosages if the patient has renal impairment associated with age. A urinalysis is also recommended [19, 20].

Patients with localized oral and /or skin involvement often respond to topical clobetasol gel or intralesional triamcinolone 3 times a day(5 to 10 mg/mL, injected sublesionally every 3 weeks as needed) [86, 89]. Patients with multiple skin and/or mucosal sites should be treated with systemic prednisone therapy. The systemic dosage classically ranges between 0.5 and 1 mg prednisone/kg/d [19, 20]. The dose of prednisone can be tapered slowly over a period of several months to a maintenance dose of a total of 5 to 10 mg/day. Methylprednisolone boluses are also recommended. Corticosteroids are often combined with other immunosuppressants in recalcitrant cases; electrolytic disorders often result from these treatments, especially in the elderly [19, 20]. Cyclophosphamide still has a place in the treatment of severe relapsing BP; continuous oral cyclophosphamide provides optimal immunosuppression, but it also produces the highest cumulative dose [90]. Therefore, pulsed cyclophosphamide regimens have been developed and are useful in severe forms of BP.

If the lesions are unresponsive, an additional immunosupressor should be considered in combination with prednisone. In some patients, mycophenolate mofetil is less myelosuppressive and hepatotoxic than corticosteroids [91]. Systemic adjuvant immunosuppressive therapy is necessary for patients with progressive disease. In spite of the advances in immunosuppressive medications and biologics, scarring is a significant complication in numerous cases [19, 20, 92]. Because BP affects many senior patients suffering from other medical problems, systemic corticosteriod complications may be severe in these cases. The personnel treating these patients need to be aware of secondary cutaneous infectious and other complications (e.g., erysipelas, lymphangitis, sepsis, phlegmons, cutaneous fistulas, atrophy and purpura) in patients treated with topical corticosteroids [92, 93]. Dapsone and sulfonamides, either alone in combination with topical or systemic corticosteroids may also be effective [94]. Specifically, dapsone at a dose of approximately 100 mg/ day is initiated at the same time as prednisone. The addition of dapsone often accelerates disease control, and thus allows a faster prednisone taper. Other researchers have describe the use of oral tetracycline, or a combination of tetracycline and niacinamide as successful treatments for BP. Intravenous immunoglobulin (IVIG), azathioprine, rituximab, and plasmapheresis have all been proposed as additional treatments [94-96] (see Table 1). In hospitalized patients, clinical isolation may help to avoid bacterial, fungal and/or viral secondary infections. In suspected infectious cases, we recommend cultures of cutaneous erosions, catheters, and serum cultures for early detection. If positive results are found, appropriate therapy should be quickly initiated. Counseling, psychological and nutritional support will assist in decreasing the morbidity and mortality associated with BP as well as stress within patient families.

A pitfall in comparing the safety versus the efficacy of steroid co-adjuvants use and/or biologics is found in the incidence and prevalence of BP. Only a few randomized, controlled studies are available; moreover, insufficient studies have been conducted to define optimal dose ranges and optimal durations of immunosuppressive treatments at different stages of BP.

Pemphigoid vegetans: (PVE) is a rare disease exhibiting clinical similarity to pemphigus vegetans, but with histologic and immunopathologic features of BP [97-102]. Only scarce cases have been reported; the precise relationship of PVE to BP is thus not clear. Clinically, pemphigoid vegetans classically presents with multiple, well-circumscribed, erythematous, erosive and vegetating plaques in the axillae, inframammary areas and neck [97-102]. Microscopic examination reveals epidermal hyperplasia, dermal/epidermal junctional separation, and prominent dermal eosinophilia [97-102]. By DIF, perilesional skin demonstrates linear deposits of IgG at the BMZ, primarily of the IgG4 subclass. On 1M NaCl split skin IIF, these antibodies are present on the blister roof of normal human skin [97-102]. By IB studies, the 230 kDa BPAGI antigen is one of the disease antigens in PVE [97-102]. Some authors have suggested that PVE is best classified as a BP variant, after reviewing a 57 year old man with intertriginous vegetating plaques. The histologic H&E examination and DIF of a biopsy specimen were identical to those of BP. IB studies and IIF of salt-split skin were negative [97-102]. Direct immunoelectron microscopy was consistent with BP. Based on a limited experience, previous authors have reported that PVE patients seem to improve with tetracycline and/or corticosteroids [97-102].

Drug induced bullous pemphigoid (DBP): Bullous pemphigoid (BP) is an acquired autoimmune disease characterized by subepidermal vesicles, with clinical macules and bullae. In contradistinction, DBP may be triggered by medications and other agents. However, similar disease lesions as BP may occur in DBP, with the formation of subepidermal blisters in the setting of allergic and/or other drug reactions [103-107]. A variety of drugs have been linked with the induction of DBP including captopril, ciprofloxacin, penicillamine, penicillins, phenacetin, sulfasalazine, galantamine hydrobromide, levetiracetam, enoxaparin, spironolactone chloroquine, furosemide, ibuprofen, phenacetin, mefenamic acid, nifedipine and others [103-107]. However, most authors do not report on the pathologic differentiation between classic BP and DBP. The medical literature reports that clinical DBP is very similar to idiopathic or classic clinical BP disease, although the clinical lesions often seem more polymorphic in BPD [103-107]. The clinical lesions of DBP may appear to look like drug-induced bullous dermatoses, bullous erythema multiforme, bullous eczematous dermatitis or bullous porphyria cutanea tarda [103-107]. The literature states that in DPB, the mucosal tissues are frequently involved. In DBP, epidermal and dermal edema is more common; however, acantholysis, vacuolar degeneration, and fibrin in the blister seem to be seen less than in classic BP. By DIF, DBP seems to be slightly different than classic BP. As examples, complement/C3c has been reported to be dotted and non-linear along the BMZ in DBP, in contrast to classic BP. In DBP, IgG has been reported to not be linear and continuous along the BMZ in contrast with autoimmune BP. Finally, fibrinogen seems to be negative at the BMZ in DBP, versus classic BP in which a linear BMZ pattern is often found.

Lichen planus pemphigoides (LPP) LPP, is an infrequent skin disorder, has been generally considered to represent a mixture of the clinical, histopathologic and immunologic patterns of lichen planus (LP) and BP [19, 20, 108-111]. LPP is characterized by the development of tense blisters, often located on the extremities, in a patient with lichen planus. LPP is predominantly idiopathic; however, in rare cases, it has been associated with drug administration. One pertinent example was development of the disease after the use of captopril [19, 20, 108-111]. Histologic changes include a subepidermal blister and a mild, perivascular dermal infiltrate of lymphocytes. Sometimes, there are a few eosinophils and neutrophils beneath the blister and a lichenoid, lymphohistiocytic infiltrate at the BMZ. Occasionally, Civatte bodies are present in the basilar epidermis at the margins of the blister. LPP needs to be distinguished from vesiculobullous dermatomyositis, in which a subepidermal blister occurs with a weak infiltrate of lymphocytes in the upper dermis. Interface changes are usually very mild in this condition, in contrast to LPP [19, 20, 108-111].

Spontaneous BP in animals: BP has been reported as a spontaneous disorder in horses and Yucatan minature pigs [112-113].

Conclusion

BP is the most common autoimmune, subepidermal blistering disease. However, given 1) an aging population with multiple medications and 2) widespread exposure to chemical agents, the overall population now often presents many blistering disorders due to allergies and drug reactions [1-17].

When approaching a patient with possible BP, many factors must be considered in choosing appropriate therapy: 1) the precise diagnosis, 2) severity of the condition and body site affected, 3) presence of comorbidities, and 4) ability to tolerate systemic therapy. For diagnostic clues, we must take into the account the location and chronicity of the blisters, and the presence or absence of oral, ocular and/or mucosal involvement. Variants of BP have been described, including pemphigoid vegetans; however, this disease is not well characterized. The diagnosis of BP requires clinical data; skin biopsies (in 10% buffered formalin) for H&E examination, and skin biopsies (in Michel's transport medium) for DIF, IIF, immunoblotting and ELISA assays [1-17].

Topical and systemic corticosteroids remain mainstays of therapy in BP; however, multiple other immunosupressors and/or "steroid sparing agents" such as azathioprine have been demonstrated to be of great therapeutic value [1-17].

The prognosis depends on each case; rapid diagnosis avoids complications, and assists in maintaining a good quality of life for each patient. We encourage an multidisciplinary collaboration for the diagnosis and correct treatment of difficult cases of BP. Current *in vivo* and *in vitro* models to study BP are difficult to correlate to the *in vivo* disease. In general, relapse episodes are not common; systemic corticosteroids represent the most common therapy for generalized BP.

References

[1] A practical treatise of the skin diseases. Shoemaker JB. New York D Apleton and company. 1890.

[2] A practical treatise of the skin diseases. Louis Adolphus Duhring, Second edition, philadelphia. J.B lippincott & company 1881.

[3] A treatise on diseases of the skin by T McCall Anderson, London, Charles Griffin & Co., 1987.

[4] Vassileva S, Drenovska K, Manuelyan K. Autoimmune blistering dermatoses as systemic diseases. *Clin Dermatol*. 2014;32:364-75.

[5] Lever WF. Pemphigus and pemphigoid. Charles C. Thomas, Springfield,1965.

[6] Lever WF. Pemphigus and pemphigoid: a review of the advances made since 1964. *J Am Acad Dermatol,* 1979;1:1-31.

[7] Lever WF. Differential diagnosis of pemphigus vulgaris, bullous pemphigoid and dermatitis herpetiformis. *Med Klin*. 1967;62:1173-86.

[8] Civatte A Diagnostic histopathologique de la dermatite polymorphe douloureuse ou maladie de Duhring-Brocq. *Ann Dermatol Syph.* 1943. 3:1–30.

[9] Jordon RE, Sams WM Jr, Beutner EH. Complement immunofluorescent staining in bullous pemphigoid. *J Lab Clin Med*. 1969;74:548-56.

[10] Jordon RE, Beutner EH, Witebsky E, Blumental G, Hale WL, Lever WF. Basement zone antibodies in bullous pemphigoid. *JAMA*. 1967; 29:751-56.

[11] Gammon WR, Merritt CC, Lewis DM, Sams WM Jr, Carlo JR, Wheeler CE Jr. An in vitro model of immune complex-mediated basement membrane zone separation caused by pemphigoid antibodies, leukocytes, and complement. *J Invest Dermatol.* 1982;78:285-90.

[12] Stanley JR, Tanaka T, Mueller S, Klaus-Kovtun V, Roop D. Isolation of a complementary DNA for bullous pemphigoid antigen by use of patients' autoantibodies. *J Clin Invest*. 1988;82:1864-70.

[13] Stanley JR, Hawley-Nelson P, Yuspa SH, Shevach EM, Katz SI. Characterization of bullous pemphigoid antigen: a unique basement membrane protein of stratified epithelia. *Cell.*1981;24:897-03.

[14] Labib RS, Anhalt GJ, Patel HP, Mutasim DF, Diaz LA. Molecular heterogeneity of the bullous pemphigoid antigens as detected by immunoblotting. *J Immunol.* 1986;136:1231-35.

[15] Giudice GJ, Emery DJ, Diaz LA. Cloning and primary structural analysis of the bullous pemphigoid autoantigen, BP180. *J Invest Dermatol*. 1992;99:243-50.

[16] Gammon WR, Briggaman RA, Inman AO 3rd, Queen LL, Wheeler CE. Differentiating anti-lamina lucida and anti-sublamina densa anti-BMZ antibodies by indirect immunofluorescence on 1.0 M sodium chloride-separated skin. *J Invest Dermatol.* 1984;82:139-44.

[17] Gammon WR, Kowaleski C, Chorzelski TP, Kumar V, Briggaman RA, Beutner EH. Direct immunofluorescestudies of sodium chloride-separated skin in the differential diagnosis of bullous pemphigoid and epidermolysis bullosa acquisita. *J Am Acad Dermatol*. 1990;22:664-60.

[18] Tanaka M, Hashimoto T, Dykes PJ, Nishikawa T. Clinical manifestations in 100 Japanese bullous pemphigoid cases in relation to autoantigen profiles. *Clin Exp Dermatol.* 1996;21:23-27.

[19] Abreu Velez AM, Vasquez-Hincapie DA, Howard MS. Autoimmune basement membrane and subepidermal blistering diseases. *Our Dermatol Online*. 2013; 4(Suppl.3): 647-62.

[20] Calle-Isaza J, Avila IC, Abreu Velez AM. Enfermedades ampollosas autoinmunes de la piel. Parte 1, enfermedades del grupo de los pénfigos. *Iatreia*. 2014;27: 309-19.

[21] Korman N. Bullous pemphigoid. *J Am Acad Dermatol.* 1987;16,907-24.
[22] Bernard P, Vaillant L, Labeille B. Incidence and distribution of subepidermal autoimmune bullous skin disease in three French regions. *Arch Dermatol.*1995;31:48-52.
[23] Zillikens D, Wever S, Roth A, Weidenthaler-Barth B, Hashimoto T, Bricker EB. Incidence of autoimmune subepidermal blistering diseases in a region of central Germany. *Arch Dermatol.* 1995;131:957-58.
[24] Wong SN, Chua SH. Spectrum of subepidermal immunobullous disorders seen at the National Skin Centre, Singapore: a 2-year review. *Br J Dermatol.* 2002;147:476-80.
[25] Daneshpazhooh M, Chams-Davatchi C, Payandemehr P, Nassiri S, Valikhani M, Safai-Naraghi Z. Spectrum of autoimmune bullous diseases in Iran: a 10-year review. *Int J Dermatol.* 2012;51:35-41.
[26] Zaraa I, Kerkeni N, Ishak F, Zribi H, El Euch D, Mokni M, et al. Spectrum of autoimmune blistering dermatoses in Tunisia: an 11-year study and a review of the literature. *Int J Dermatol.* 2011;50:939-44.
[27] Nanda A, Dvorak R, Al-Saeed K, Al-Sabah H, Alsaleh QA. Spectrum of autoimmune bullous diseases in Kuwait. *Int J Dermatol.* 2004;43:876-81.
[28] McCuin JB, Hanlon T, Mutasim DF. Autoimmune bullous diseases: Diagnosis and management. *Dermatol Nurs.* 2006;18:20-25.
[29] Gao SQ, Bystryn JC. Identification of a novel basement membrane antigen (p84) defined by sera with antibodies to both the epidermal and dermal side of split skin. *J Invest Dermatol.* 1994;102:236-40.
[30] Niimi Y, Zhu ZX, Bystryn JC. Identification of basement membrane zone antigens defined by antibodies that react to both the epidermal and dermal side of 1 M sodium chloride split skin. *J Invest Dermatol.* 1991;97:312-17.
[31] Giudice GJ, Wilske KC, Anhalt GJ, Fairley JA, Taylor AF, Emery DJ, et al. Development of an ELISA to detect anti-BP180 autoantibodies in bullous pemphigoid and herpes gestationis. *J Invest Dermatol.* 1994;102:878-81.
[32] Yang B, Wang C, Chen S, Chen X, Lu X, Tian H, et al. Evaluation of the combination of BP180-NC16a enzyme-linked immunosorbent assay and BP230 enzyme-linked immunosorbent assay in the diagnosis of bullous pemphigoid. *Indian J Dermatol Venereol Leprol.* 2012;78:722-27.
[33] Zillikens D, Mascaro JM, Rose PA, Liu Z, Ewing SM, Caux F, et al. highly sensitive enzyme-linked immunosorbent assay for the detection of circulating anti-BP180 autoantibodies in patients with bullous pemphigoid. *J Invest Dermatol.* 1997;109:679-83.
[34] Döpp R, Schmidt E, Chimanovitch I, Leverkus M, Bröcker EB, Zillikens D. IgG4 and IgE are the major immunoglobulins targeting the NC16A domain of BP180 in Bullous pemphigoid: serum levels of these immunoglobulins reflect disease activity. *J Am Acad Dermatol.* 2000;42:577-83.
[35] Mariotti F, Grosso F, Terracina M, Ruffelli M, Cordiali-Fei P, Sera F, et al. Development of a novel ELISA system for detection of anti-BP180 IgG and characterization of autoantibody profile in bullous pemphigoid patients. *Br J Dermatol.* 2004;151:1004-10.

[36] Fairley JA, Bream M, Fullenkamp C, Syrbu S, Chen M, Messingham KN. Missing the target: characterization of bullous pemphigoid patients who are negative using the BP180 enzyme-linked immunosorbant assay. *J Am Acad Dermatol.* 2013;68:395-03.

[37] Schaumburg-Lever G, Rule A, Schmidt-Ullrich R, Lever WF. Ultrastructural localization of in vivo bound immunoglobulins in bullous pemphigoid--a preliminary report. *J Invest Dermatol.* 1975;64:47-49.

[38] Ishikura T. [A comparative ultrastructural study of blister formation in bullous pemphigoid, dermatitis herpetiformis and erythema multiforme. *Nihon Hifuka Gakkai Zasshi.* 1974;84:453-72.

[39] Schaumburg-Lever G, Orfanos CE, Lever WP. Electron microscopic study of bullous pemphigoid. *Arch Dermatol.* 1972;106:662-67.

[40] Lever WF. Differential diagnosis of pemphigus vulgaris, bullous pemphigoid and dermatitis herpetiformis. *Med Klin.* 1967;62:1173-76.

[41] Furudate S, Fujimura T, Kambayashi Y, Kakizaki A, Aiba S.Comparison of CD163+ CD206+ M2 Macrophages in the Lesional Skin of Bullous Pemphigoid and Pemphigus Vulgaris: The Possible Pathogenesis of Bullous Pemphigoid. *Dermatology.* 2014 2014;229:369-78

[42] Abreu Velez AM, Brown VM, Howard MS. Cytotoxic and antigen presenting cells present and non-basement membrane zone pathology in a case of bullous pemphigoid. *Our Dermatol Online*, 2012;3:93-99.

[43] Abreu Velez AM, Calle-Isaza J, Howard MS. CD1a, HAM56, CD68 and S-100 are present in lesional skin biopsies from patients affected by autoimmune blistering diseases. *Our Dermatol Online.* 2014; 5:113-17.

[44] Zebrowska A, Wagrowska-Danilewicz M, Danilewicz M, Stasikowska-Kanicka O, Kulczycka-Siennicka L, Wozniacka A, Waszczykowska E. Mediators of mast cells in bullous pemphigoid and dermatitis herpetiformis. *Mediators Inflamm.* 2014;936545.

[45] Abreu-Velez AM, Roselino AM, Howard MS. Mast cells, Mast/Stem Cell Growth Factor receptor (c-kit/cd117) and IgE may be integral to the pathogenesis of endemic pemphigus foliaceus. *Our Dermatol Online.* 2013; 4 (Suppl.3): 596-00.

[46] Giacalone B, D'Auria L, Bonifati C, Ferraro C, Riccardi E, Mussi A, D'Agosto G, Cordiali-Fei P, Ameglio F. Decreased interleukin-7 and transforming growth factor-beta1 levels in blister fluids as compared to the respective serum levels in patients with bullous pemphigoid. Opposite behavior of TNF-alpha, interleukin-4 and interleukin-10. *Exp Dermatol.* 1998;7:157-61.

[47] Akman-Karakaş A, Yalcin AD, Koç S, Gumuslu S, Ergun E, Genc GE, Ongut G, Uzun S, Alpsoy E. Serum soluble CD200 level was higher in patients with bullous pemphigoid during the active phase of the disease than for healthy individuals. *Clin Lab.* 2014;60:1237-40.

[48] Arakawa M, Dainichi T, Ishii N, Hamada T, Karashima T, Nakama T, Yasumoto S, Tsuruta D, Hashimoto T. Lesional Th17 cells and regulatory T cells in bullous pemphigoid. *Exp Dermatol.* 2011;20:1022-44.

[49] Tedeschi A, Marzano AV, Lorini M, Balice Y, Cugno M. Eosinophil cationic protein levels parallel coagulation activation in the blister fluid of patients with bullous pemphigoid. *J Eur Acad Dermatol Venereol.* 2014 Mar 20.

[50] Borrego L, Maynard B, Peterson EA, George T, Iglesias L, Peters MS, Newman W, Gleich GJ, Leiferman KM. Deposition of eosinophil granule proteins precedes blister

formation in bullous pemphigoid. Comparison with neutrophil and mast cell granule proteins. *Am J Pathol.* 1996;148:897-09.

[51] Abreu Velez AM, Googe PB, Howard MS. Immunohistochemistry versus immunofluoresence in the diagnosis of autoimmune blistering diseases. *Our Dermatol Online.* 2013; 4(Suppl.3): 627-30.

[52] Abreu Velez AM, Googe PB, Howard MS. *In situ* immune response in skin biopsies from patients affected by autoimmune blistering diseases. Our Dermatol Online. 2013; 4(Suppl.3): 606-12.

[53] Abreu Velez AM, Calle-Isaza J, Howard MS. Cyclo-oxygenase 2 is present in the majority of lesional skin from patients with autoimmune blistering diseases. Our Dermatol Online. 2013; 4:476-78.

[54] Abreu Velez AM, Googe PB, Howard MS. Ribosomal protein s6-ps240 is expressed in lesional skin from patients with autoimmune skin diseases. *North Am J Med Sci.* 2013; 5:604-08.

[55] Abreu Velez AM, Calle-Isaza J, Howard MS. HLA-DP, DQ, DR is expressed in all lesional skin from patients with autoimmune skin diseases. *Our Dermatol Online.* 2014; 5:125-28.

[56] Abreu Velez AM, Yepes-Naranjo MM, Avila IC, Londoño ML, Googe PB, Velásquez-Velez JE, Velez ID, Upegui YA, Jimenez-Echavarria A, Mesa-Herrera NR, Yi H, Calle-Isaza J, Howard MS. Tissue inhibitor of metalloproteinase 1, matrix metalloproteinase 9, αlpha-1 antitrypsin, metallothionein and urokinase type plasminogen activator receptor in skin biopsies from patients affected by autoimmune blistering diseases. *Our Dermatol Online.* 2013; 4: 275-80.

[57] Abreu-Velez AM, Smith JG Jr, Howard MS. IgG/IgE bullous pemphigoid with CD45 lymphocytic reactivity to dermal blood vessels, nerves and eccrine sweat glands. *N Am J Med Sci.* 2010;2: 540-43.

[58] Abreu Velez AM, Calle-Isaza J, Howard MS. A case of bullous pemphigoid with immunoreactivty to blood vessels and sweat glands. *Our Dermatol Online.* 2013; 4(Suppl.3): 621-24.

[59] Abreu Velez AM, Howard MS. Neural reactivity detected by immunofluorescence in a patient with a localized blistering disease. *Our Dermatol Online,* 2013;4: 91-94.

[60] Abreu Velez AM, Girard JG, Howard MS. IgG bullous pemphigoid with antibodies to IgD, dermal blood vessels, eccrine glands and the endomysium of monkey esophagus. *Our Dermatol Online.* 2011;2:48-51.

[61] Abreu Velez AM, Smoller BR, Howard MS. Rouleaux and autoagglutination of erythrocytes associated with fibrin-like material in skin biopsies form patients with autoimmune blistering diseases. *Our Dermatol Online.* 2013; 4(Suppl.3): 613-15.

[62] Abreu Velez AM, Vásquez-Hincapié DA, Howard MS. Vimentin may reflect areas of cutaneous involvement in biopsies from patients with autoimmune skin diseases. *Our Dermatol Online.* 2014; 5:140-43.

[63] Kakugawa T, Tomimura S, Hayashi T, Sakamoto N, Ishimatsu Y, Mukae H, Kohno S. *Respiration.* 2013;86:347-351.

[64] No authors. In memory of Professor Dr. Felix von Bärensprung by Otto Veit. 1865. *Am J Dermatopathol.* 1982;4:45-85.

[65] Bonifazi M, Zuccatosta L, Poidomani G, Ranaldi R, Gasparini S. Bullous pemphigoid with the unusual complication of tracheobronchial involvement. *Chest*. 2013;143:236-38.

[66] Oshikawa K, Sugiyama Y, Kitamura S.Yoshioka D, Ishii H, Uchida T, Fujiwara S, Umeki K, Sakamoto N, Kadota J. Interstitial pneumonia associated with bullous pemphigoid. *Chest*. 2012;141:795-97.

[67] Oshikawa K, Sugiyama Y, Kitamura S. Diffuse panbronchioliltis associated with bullous pemphigoid. *Nihon Kyobu Shikkan Gakkai Zasshi*. 1995;33:1019-23.

[68] Baum T, Shropshire AT. Interaction of cardiopulmonary chemoreceptor (Bezold-Jarisch) and somatosympathetic reflexes. *Arch Int Pharmacodyn Ther*. 1979;239:99-08.

[69] Gammon WR, Lewis DM, Carlo JR, Sams WM Jr, Wheeler CE Jr. Pemphigoid antibody mediated attachment of peripheral blood leukocytes at the dermal-epidermal junction of human skin. *J Invest Dermatol*. 1980; 75:334–39.

[70] Ghohestani RF, Rotunda SL, Hudson B, Gaughan WJ, Farber JL, Webster G, Uitto J. Crescentic glomerulonephritis and subepidermal blisters with autoantibodies to alpha5 and alpha6 chains of type IV collagen. *Lab Invest*. 2003 May;83:605-11.

[71] Barnadas MA, Gelpí C, Rocamora V, Baró E, Ballarín J, Nadal C, Bielsa A, Aróstegui J, Alomar A. Bullous pemphigoid associated with acute glomerulonephritis. *Br J Dermatol. 1998* May;138:867-71.

[72] Chen J, Li L, Chen J, Zeng Y, Xu H, Song Y, Wang B. Sera of elderly bullous pemphigoid patients with associated neurological diseases recognize bullous pemphigoid antigens in the human brain. *Gerontology*. 2011;57:211-16.

[73] Jefferson JJ, Leung CL, Liem RK. Dissecting the sequence specific functions of alternative N-terminal isoforms of mouse bullous pemphigoid antigen 1. *Exp Cell Res*. 2006;312:2712-25.

[74] Brown A, Bernier G, Mathieu M, Rossant J, Kothary R. The mouse dystonia musculorum gene is a neural isoform of bullous pemphigoid antigen 1. *Nat Genet*. 1995;10:301-06.

[75] Laffitte E, Burkhard PR, Fontao L, Jaunin F, Saurat JH, Chofflon M, Borradori L. Bullous pemphigoid antigen 1 isoforms: potential new target autoantigens in multiple sclerosis? *Br J Dermatol*. 2005;152:537-40.

[76] Sams W M Jr, Gleich G J. Failure to transfer bullous pemphigoid with serum from patients. *Proc Soc Exp Biol Med* 1971: 136: 1027–31.

[77] Anhalt G J, Bahn C F, Labib R S, Voorhees J J, Sugar A, Diaz L A. Pathogenic effects of bullous pemphigoid autoantibodies on rabbit corneal epithelium. *J Clin Invest* 1981: 68: 1097–01.

[78] Liu Z, Diaz L A, Troy J L et al. A passive transfer model of the organ-specific autoimmune disease, bullous pemphigoid, using antibodies generated against the hemidesmosomal antigen, BP180. *J Clin Invest* 1993: 92: 2480–88.

[79] Zhao M, Trimbeger M E, Li N, Diaz L A, Shapiro S D, Liu Z. Role of FcRs in animal model of autoimmune bullous pemphigoid. *J Immunol* 2006: 177: 3398– 05.

[80] Chen R, Fairley J A, Zhao M L et al. Macrophages, but not T and B lymphocytes, are critical for subepidermal blister formation in experimental bullous pemphigoid: macrophage-mediated neutrophil infiltration depends on mast cell activation. *J Immunol* 2002: 169: 3987–92.

[81] Fairley J A, Burnett C T, Fu C L, Larson D L, Fleming M G, Giudice G J. A pathogenic role for IgE in autoimmunity: bullous pemphigoid IgE reproduces the early phase of lesion development in human skin grafted to nu/nu mice. *J Invest Dermatol* 2007: 127: 2605–11.

[82] Zone J J, Taylor T, Hull C, Schmidt L, Meyer L. IgE basement membrane zone antibodies induce eosinophil infiltration and histological blisters in engrafted human skin on SCID mice. *J Invest Dermatol* 2007:127: 1167–74.

[83] Serwin AB, Musialkowska E, Piascik M. Incidence and mortality of bullous pemphigoid in north-east Poland (Podlaskie Province), 1999-2012: a retrospective bicentric cohort study. *Int J Dermatol.* 2014;53:e432-37.

[84] Bernard P. Mortality of bullous pemphigoid in Asia: the same as in Europe? *Br J Dermatol.* 2014,170:1216-17.

[85] Lee JH, Kim SC. Mortality of patients with bullous pemphigoid in Korea. J Am Acad Dermatol. 2014;71:676-83.

[86] Walsh SR, Hogg D, Mydlarski PR. Bullous pemphigoid: From bench to bedside. Drugs 2005;65:905-26.

[87] Westerhof W. Treatment of bullous pemphigoid with topical clobetasol propionate. J Am Acad Dermatol. 1989;20:458-61.

[88] Spivey J, Nye AM. Bullous pemphigoid: corticosteroid treatment and adverse effects in long-term care patients. Consult Pharm. 2013;28:455-62.

[89] Stockman A, Beele H, Vanderhaeghen Y, Naeyaert JM. Topical class I corticosteroids in 10 patients with bullous pemphigoid: correlation of the outcome with the severity degree of the disease and review of the literature. *J Eur Acad Dermatol Venereol.* 2004;18:164-68.

[90] Gual A, Iranzo P, Mascaró Jr JM. Treatment of bullous pemphigoid with low-dose oral cyclophosphamide: a case series of 20 patients. *J Eur Acad Dermatol Venereol.* 2014;28:814-18.

[91] Beissert S, Werfel T, Frieling U, Böhm M, Sticherling M, Stadler R, Zillikens D, Rzany B, Hunzelmann N, Meurer M, Gollnick H, Ruzicka T, Pillekamp H, Junghans V, Bonsmann G, Luger TA. A comparison of oral methylprednisolone plus azathioprine or mycophenolate mofetil for the treatment of bullous pemphigoid. Arch Dermatol. 2007;143:1536-42.

[92] McCuin JB, Hanlon T, Mutasim DF. Autoimmune bullous diseases: Diagnosis and management. Dermatol Nurs. 2006;18:20-25.

[93] Boughrara Z, Ingen-Housz-Oro S, Legrand P, Duong TA, Roujeau JC. Cutaneous infections in bullous pemphigoid patients treated with topical corticosteroids. *Ann Dermatol Venereol.* 2010;137:345-51.

[94] Venning VA, Millard PR, Wojnarowska F. Dapsone as first line therapy for bullous pemphigoid. *Br J Dermatol.* 1989;120:83-92.

[95] Meurer M. Immunosuppressive therapy for autoimmune bullous diseases. Clin Dermatol. 2012;30:78-83.

[96] Schmidt E, Hunzelmann N, Zillikens D, Bröcker EB, Goebeler M. Rituximab in refractory autoimmune bullous diseases. Clin Exp Dermatol 2006;31:503-08.

[97] Winkelmann RK, Su WP. Pemphigoid vegetans. *Arch Dermatol.* 1979;115:446-448.

[98] Ueda Y, Nashiro K, Seki Y, Otsuka F, Tamaki K, Ishibashi Y. Pemphigoid vegetans. *Br J Dermatol.* 1989;120:449-53.

[99] Kim J, Chavel S, Girardi M, McNiff JM. Pemphigoid vegetans: a case report and review of the literature. *J Cutan Pathol.* 2008;35:1144-47.

[100] Chan LS, Dorman MA, Agha A, Suzuki T, Cooper KD, Hashimoto K. Pemphigoid vegetans represents a bullous pemphigoid variant. Patient's IgG autoantibodies identify the major bullous pemphigoid antigen. *J Am Acad Dermatol.* 1993;28:331-35.

[101] Ahn BK, Kim SC. Pyodermatitis-pyostomatitis vegetans with circulating autoantibodies to bullous pemphigoid antigen 230. *J Am Acad Dermatol.* 2004;50:785-88.

[102] Delpuget-Bertin N, Bernard P, Bedane C, Boulinguez S, Garnier A, Bonnetblanc JM. Pemphigoid vegetans. An immunoelectron microscopic study. *Ann Dermatol Venereol.* 1997;124:467-69.

[103] Lloyd-Lavery A, Chi CC, Wojnarowska F, Taghipour K. The associations between bullous pemphigoid and drug use: a UK case-control study. *JAMA Dermatol.* 2013;149:58-52.

[104] Warner C, Kwak Y, Glover MH, Davis LS. Bullous pemphigoid induced by hydrochlorothiazide therapy. *J Drugs Dermatol.*2014;13:360-62.

[105] Karadag AS, Bilgili SG, Calka O, Onder S, Kosem M, Burakgazi-Dalkilic E. A case of levetiracetam induced bullous pemphigoid. *Cutan Ocul Toxicol.* 2013,32:176-78.

[106] Kashihara M, Danno K, Miyachi Y, Horiguchi Y, Imamura S. Bullous pemphigoid-like lesions induced by phenacetin. Report of a case and an immunopathologic study. *Arch Dermatol.*1984,120:1196-99.

[107] Lee JJ, Downham TF II. Furosemide-induced bullous pemphigoid: case report and review of literature. *J Drugs Dermatol.* 2006;5:562-64.

[108] Diab M, Coloe J, Bechtel MA. Bullous pemphigoid precipitated by galantamine hydrobromide. *Cutis.* 2009;83:139-40.

[109] Ludgate MW, Greig DE. Bullous systemic lupus erythematosus responding to dapsone. *Australas J Dermatol.* 2008;49:91-93.

[110] Stingl G, Holubar K. Coexistence of lichen planus and bullous pemphigoid. A immunopathological study. *Br J Dermatol.* 1975;93:313-20.

[111] Saurat JH, Guinepain MT, Didierjean L, Sohier J, Puissant A. Coexistence of lichen planus and bullous pemphigoid (an immunofluorescence study of a lichen pemphigoides"). *Ann Dermatol Venereol.* 1977;104:368-74.

[112] Willsteed E, Bhogal BS, Das AK, Wojnarowska F, Black MM, McKee PH. Lichen planus pemphigoides: a clinicopathological study of nine cases. *Histopathology.* 1991;19:147-54.

[113] Olivry T, Mirsky M L, Singleton W et al. A spontaneously arising porcine model of bullous pemphigoid. *Arch Dermatol Res* 2000: 292: 37–45.

[114] Olivry T, Borrillo A K, Xu L et al. Equine bullous pemphigoid IgG autoantibodies target linear epitopes in the NC16A ectodomain of collagen XVII (BP180, BPAG2). *Vet Immunol Immunopathol* 2000: 73: 45–52.

In: Advances in Dermatology Research
Editor: James P. Vega
ISBN: 978-1-63482-226-8

Chapter 3

Dermal Neurovascular Structures Demonstrate Autoimmune Reactivity in Lesional Skin of a Patient with Bullous Pemphigoid

Ana Maria Abreu Velez, MD, PhD[*,1],
Jorge Enrique Velazquez Velez, MD[2]
and Michael S. Howard, MD[1]
[1]Georgia Dermatopathology Associates, Atlanta, Georgia, US
[2]*HGM - Clinica CES - Clinica SOMER - Fundacion HUSVP, Rionegro and* Medellin, Colombia, South America

Abstract

Bullous pemphigoid (BP) is a bullous disease of autoimmune origin. These disorders are the result of an inflammatory process that causes skin lesions, with local increases of pro-inflammatory mediators. Alterations of the vessels, nerves or/or neurovascular structures have been previously described in BP. Here we aim to confirm reactivity to vessels and nerves in a case of BP.

Case report: A 68 year old Caucasian male presented with a sudden appearance of erythematous papules, plaques and few blisters on the abdomen, back, arms, and thighs; focal excoriations were present, with some itching and burning sensations.

Materials and Methods: Skin biopsies were taken for hematoxylin and eosin (H&E) staining and immunohistochemistry (IHC), and for direct and indirect immunofluorescence (DIF, IIF) with 1 M NaCl split skin studies.

Results: The H&E staining demonstrated a subepidermal blister with luminal cells including eosinophils, lymphocytes, some monocytes and rare neutrophils. Partial re-epithelialization of the blister base was appreciated. A mild, superficial, perivascular dermal infiltrate was present, with similar cells as those present within the blister lumen. Some dermal blood vessels seemed be damaged and/or dilated. DIF and IIF showed

* E-mail: abreuvelez@yahoo.com, Tel.: (404) 371-0077, Toll Free: (877) 371-0027, Fax: (404) 371-1900.

positivity for anti-human IgG, IgA, IgE, Complement/C1q, fibrinogen and albumin. These same antibodies were positive against the dermal blood vessels and some neurovascular structures as well as at the BMZ of sebaceous and eccrine sweat glands. IgM and complement/C3 were negative. IHC demonstrated thrombomodulin, von Willembrand factor, vascular endothelial growth factor, Complement/C5b-9/MAC, HLA-DP, DQ, DR, antigen, HLA-ABC, BCL-2, cyclo-oxygenase 2, and CD8 to be positive around dermal blood vessels and on the basement membranes of some skin appendices.

Discussion: Although the reactivity to vessels and/or neurovascular structures and the BMZs of skin appendices has not been extensively studied in BP, our case and other cases indicate that these BP positive autoantibodies colocalizing with neurovascular markers could explain the clinical skin burning, pain and/ or itching sensations described in BP patients with BP, as well as also some neurovascular structural alterations in patients with BP.

Case report: A 68 year old Caucasian male presented with a sudden appearance of erythematous papules, plaques and few blisters on the abdomen, back, arms, and thighs; focal excoriations were also noted. Some of the lesions were violaceous and itchy. The patient was taking only vitamin supplements.

Keywords: bullous pemphigoid, nerves, vessels, stromal cell junctions, BCL2, sebaceous gland basement membranes

Abbreviations and Acronyms

Bullous pemphigoid (BP)
immunohistochemistry (IHC)
direct and indirect immunofluorescence (DIF, IIF)
hematoxylin and eosin (H&E)
basement membrane zone (BMZ)
B-cell lymphoma 2 gene (BCL2)
tissue inhibitor of metalloproteinases 1 (TIMP-1)
4',6-diamidino-2-phenylindole) (DAPI)
cyclooxygenase-2 (COX-2)
vascular endothelial growth factor (VEGF)
optimal cutting temperature (OCT)
molar (M)

Introduction

Bullous pemphigoid (BP) is an autoimmune skin disease for which the etiology is idiopathic and unknown, with the highest incidence in elderly patients [1-3]. BP is often characterized by linear IgG and Complement/C3 deposits along the skin basement membrane zone (BMZ) on direct immunofluorescence (DIF). On indirect immunofluorescence (IIF), in the majority of patients the BMZ antibodies bind to the epidermal (roof) side of salt split skin sections. However, in many patients it is possible to find BMZ antibodies on both sides of the split [1-3]. In addition, Western immunoblotting has demonstrated that BP antibodies usually react with both the 230 kD BPAGI and 180 kD BPAGII bullous pemphigoid antigens [1-3]. Passive transfer into animals of human BP IgG or IgE antibodies against type XVII collagen has shown that these antibodies are putatively antigenic. However, there are also secondary BP immune responses, including complement activation, mast cell degranulation, and infiltration of neutrophils and/or eosinophils [1].

Materials and Methods

Lesional skin was biopsied and studied utilizing hematoxylin and eosin (H&E) staining, as well as via 1) IHC, 2) direct immunofluorescence (DIF) and 3) indirect immunofluorescence (IIF) with 1 molar (M) NaCl split skin.

Direct immunofluoresence (DIF): In brief, for DIF we incubated 4 micron thickness sections on slides with secondary antibodies as previously described [4-18]. We utilized FITC conjugated rabbit anti-total IgG, IgA, IgM, complement/C1q and complement/C3. These antibodies were used at a 1:25 dilution; we also utilized fibrinogen and albumin, at a 1:50 dilution. All of the preceding antibodies were obtained from Dako (Carpinteria, California, USA). In addition, anti-human IgE antiserum (Epsilon chain) was obtained from Kent Laboratories (Bellingham, Washington, USA) and anti-human IgD antibodies from Southern Biotechnology (Birmingham, Alabama, USA); these antibodies were utilized at 1:25 dilutions. We also utilized a rhodamine conjugated antibody to *Ulex europaeus agglutinin* 1 from Vector Laboratories (Burlingame, California USA). We also use rabbit anti-human IGMA FITCI conjugated from Rockland laboratories (Limerick, PA). The DIF slides were counterstained with 4',6-diamidino-2-phenylindole (Dapi)(Pierce, Rockford, Illinois, USA). The samples were consistently run with positive and negative controls. We classified our findings as negative (-), weakly positive (+), positive (+++) and strongly positive (++++).

Salt-split normal human skin for IIF. Adult fresh normal skin, obtained from healthy patients undergoing cosmetic reduction surgery, was cut into fragments 1.0 cm x 1.0 cm and washed with PBS. The fragments were then incubated in 1 M NaCl solution for 48-72 h at 4°C. The split skin was then imbedded in optimal cutting temperature (OCT) compound for frozen-section IIF diagnosis.

Indirect immunofluorescence on sodium chloride-split skin. IIF was performed on 4-μm cryostat sections of salt-split normal human skin, as described previously [4-18]. The serum samples were serially diluted to 1:10 and added onto the slides with the split skin. The sections were incubated for 30 min at room temperature in a moist chamber. After washing three times with PBS, the sections were incubated with FITC-conjugated goat anti-human IgG (Dako, Denmark) for 30 min at room temperature. The sections were viewed utilizing a fluorescent microscope.

Immunohistochemistry (IHC): We performed IHC utilizing multiple monoclonal and polyclonal antibodies from Dako (Carpinteria, California, USA). We utilized 1) mouse anti-human B-cell lymphoma-2 (BCL2) oncoprotein, clone 124; 2) cyclooxygenase 2 (COX-2), clone CX-294; 3) monoclonal mouse HLA-DP, DQ, DR antigen, Clone CR3/43; 4) von Willembrand factor; 5) HLA-ABC antigen, Clone W6/32; 6) metallothionein, clone E9; 7) tissue inhibitor of metalloproteinases 1, clone VT7; 8) vascular endothelial growth factor (VEGF), clone VG1 (of the 6 different isoforms of VEGF, this antibody labels the VEGF-

121, VEGF-165, and VEGF-189 isoforms); 9) CD4, clone 4B12; 10) CD8, Clone C8/144B; 11) CD15, Clone Carb-3 and 12) thrombomodulin, clone 1009. For our IHC testing, we utilized a dual endogenous peroxidase blockage, with the addition of a Dako Envision dual link (to assist in chromogen attachment). We then applied the chromogen 3,3-diaminobenzidine (DAB), and counterstained with hematoxylin. The samples were run in a Dako Autostainer Universal Staining System. Positive and negative controls were consistently performed. The staining was performed as previously described [4-18].

IHC double staining: These were performed utilizing a Leica (Buffalo Grove, Illinois, USA) double staining system. Specifically, for primary staining we utilized a Bond Max platform autostainer with bond polymer refined Red detection DS9390, an alkaline phosphatase linker polymer and fast red chromogen (red staining). For our secondary staining, we utilized bond polymer refined detection DS9800, a horseradish peroxidase linker polymer and DAB chromogen (brown staining).

Results

Microscopic description: Examination of the H&E tissue sections demonstrates a subepidermal blistering disorder. Within the blister lumen, occasional eosinophils were seen,

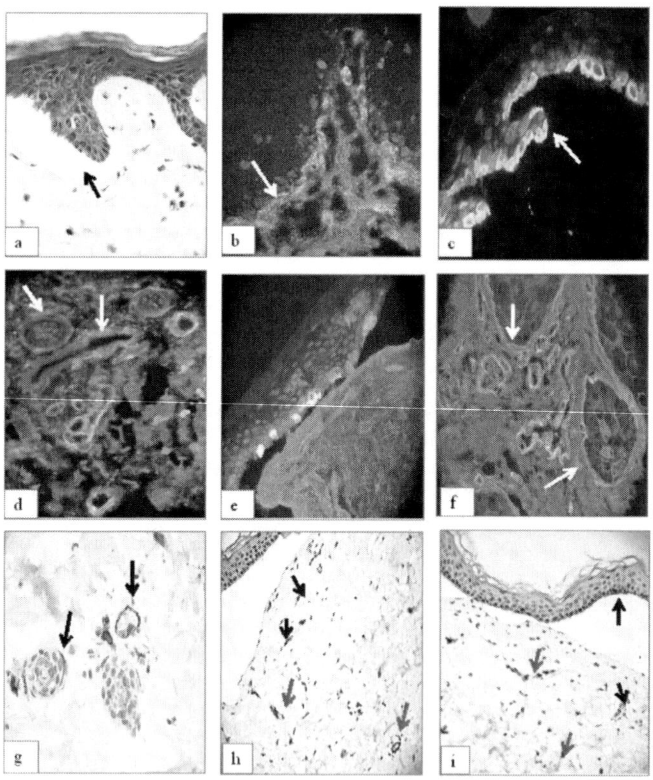

Figure 1 a. H&E stain showing a subepidermal blister (black arrow), with a few inflammatory cells (black arrow). b. DIF with positive linear BMZ staining using FITC conjugated anti-human fibrinogen (green staining; white arrow).

Also, note the colocalizing positive staining with collagen IV antibody (yellow staining; white arrow). The epidermal keratinocyte nuclei were counterstained with DAPI (blue) (200X). c. IIF on 1 M NaCl split skin, showing positive BMZ staining on the epidermal(roof) side of the blister split using FITC conjugated anti-human IgG (green staining, white arrow); also note the colocalizing positive staining for collagen IV (yellow staining; white arrow). The epidermal keratinocyte nuclei were counterstained with DAPI in blue (200X). d. DIF positive staining, using FITC conjugated anti-human IgG in the upper and intermediate dermal blood vessels and around some nerves(yellow staining; white arrows) that colocalizes with collagen IV (orange staining; white arrows). e. IIF, using 1 M NaCl split skin showing positive BMZ staining along the epidermal/roof side of the blister split, especially in some individual cells using FITC conjugated anti-human IgG (white staining, red arrows). f. DIF positive staining, using FITC conjugated anti-human I-GMA against the BMZs of sebaceous glands (green staining; white arrows). Colocalization is noted with Collagen IV (orange staining; white arrows). g. IHC positive staining, with HLA-DP, DQ, DR antigen was positive against the upper and intermediate dermal blood vessels, and in some areas of the sweat ducts (brown staining, black arrows). h. IHC positive double staining with von Willembrand factor (brown staining, red arrows), positive on dermal blood vessels, and Factor XIIIa positive on dermal dendrocytes close to these vessels (black arrows, red dots). i. IHC positive double staining for COX-2, in a linear arrangement at the BMZ and on several dermal blood vessels (red staining; black arrows) and for CD68 in individual cells, especially around dermal blood vessels (brown staining, red arrows).

Discussion

Bullous pemphigoid (BP) is a skin disorder presenting with tense, fluid-filled blisters, and urticarial or other lesions concentrated on the lower abdomen, upper thighs or armpits (flexoral areas) [1-3]. BP is most common in people older than 60. In BP, the immune system attacks the cutaneous basement membrane zone (BMZ). Previously, minimal attention has been focused on the roles of dermal blood vessels and the basement membrane zones of the sebaceous glands and other appendageal structures in BP [1-3]. Our group has previously documented BP autoreactivity to nerves, blood vessels and eccrine sweat glands [4-18]. We had reported the presence of several inflammatory markers to be positive in and/or around dermal vessels in BP including COX-2, proteases and protease inhibitors. We have also reported rouleaux phenomena in dermal blood vessels in BP [4-18]. The BP involvement of dermal blood vessels includes those feeding the skin appendices [4-18]. We have described positive staining for many antigen presenting cells, such as CD68, around dermal blood vessels.

Our previous data indicates that dermal blood vessels and some stromal/dermal blood vessel areas, nerves, eccrine glands and the BMZs of hair follicular units may also be involved in BP [4-18]. In the current case, we also reported positive staining to dermal blood vessels and nerves, with the antibodies also fixing complement. We noted important reactivity in the dermal blood vessels and nerves for anti-HLA-ABC antigens, as well as with HLA-DP, DQ, DR; these findings indicate an active antigen presenting cell phenomenon, involving dermal blood vessels.

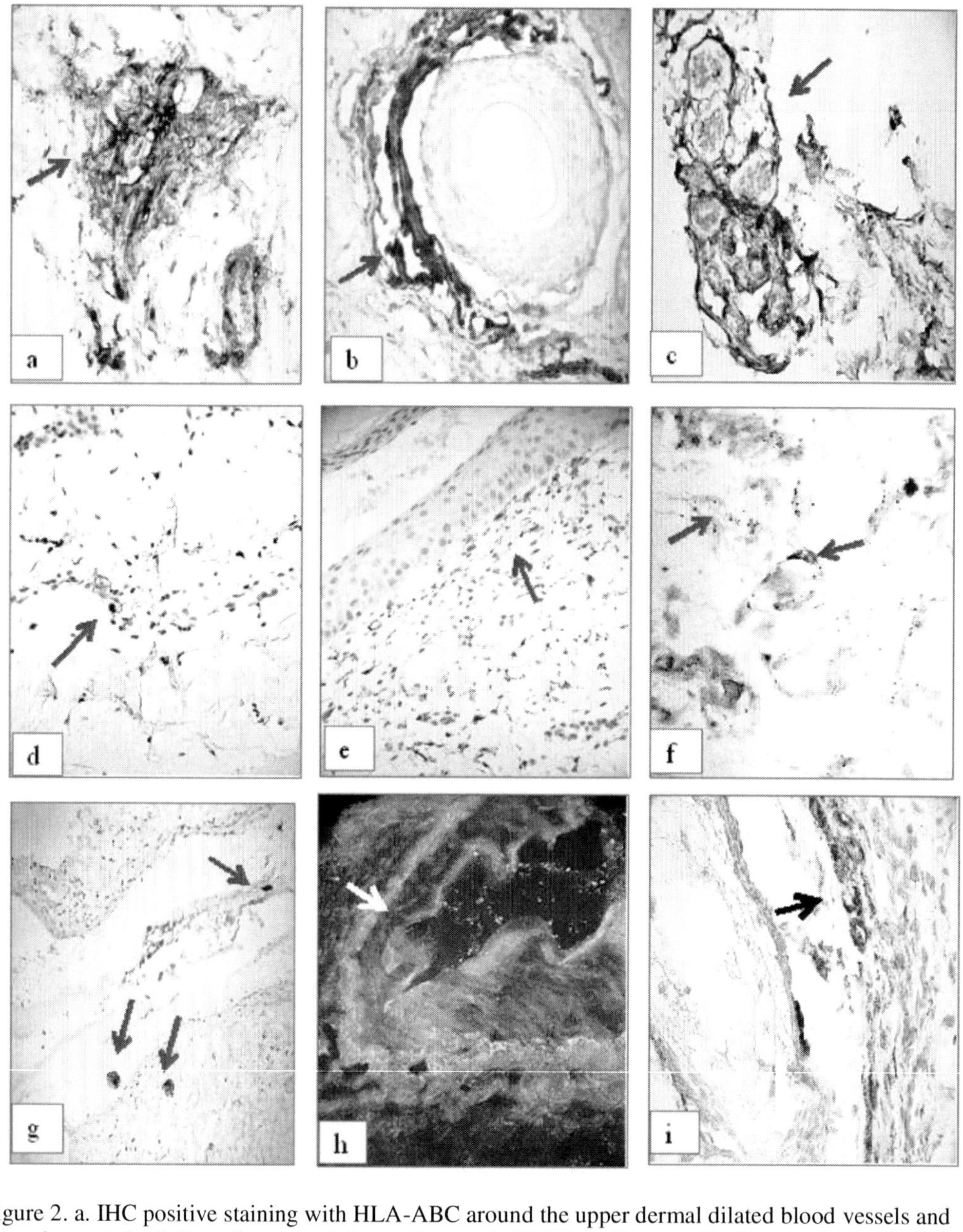

Figure 2. a. IHC positive staining with HLA-ABC around the upper dermal dilated blood vessels and around sweat gland ducts (brown staining, red arrows) (100X). b. Same antibody as a, demonstrating positive staining of blood vessels around a hair follicle (brown staining, red arrow) (200X). c. Same antibody as a and b, staining blood vessels around eccrine sweat glands (brown staining; red arrow). d. IHC staining for TIMP1, showing positivity in junctional areas between small dermal blood vessels and dermal stromal cells (brown staining; red arrow) (200X). e. IHC, with positive metallothionein in the junctional areas between small dermal blood vessels and dermal stromal cells (brown staining; red arrow) (200X). f. Thrombomodulin, demonstrating some type of fragmentation in some dermal vascular cells (brown dots, red arrows). g. Positive staining for VEGF, that seems to be extruding from the dermis into the blisters (brown staining; red arrows) (100X). h. IIF using 1 M NACL split skin, showing positivity around the upper dilated dermal vessels using FITC conjugated anti-human fibrinogen(yellow staining, white arrow) (200X). i. IHC positive staining for using complement/C5b-9/MAC on dermal blood vessels close to a sebaceous gland BMZ (brown staining; black arrow).

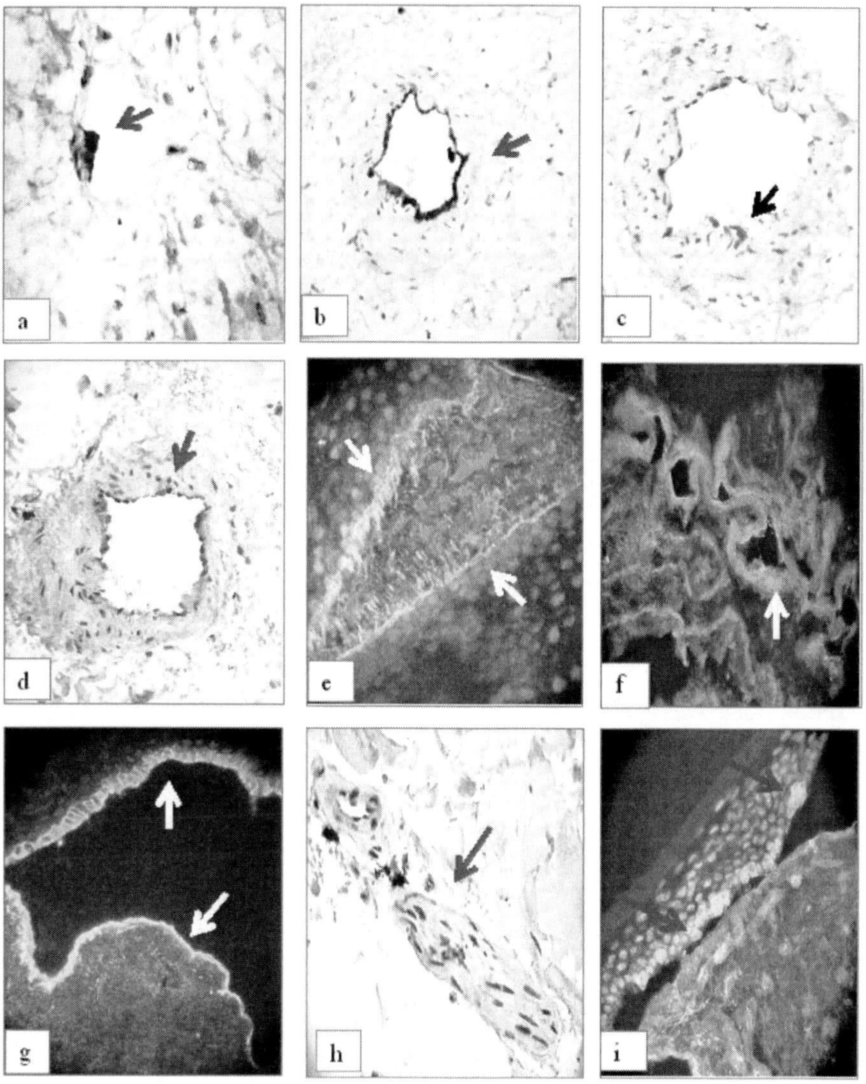

Figure 3. a. IHC positive staining for VEGF, showing a large dark brown structure extruding from what seemed to be a damaged dermal blood vessel (brown staining; red arrow) (400X). b. IHC stain using von Willembrand factor, positive in a dilated dermal blood vessel (brown staining; red arrow) (400X). c. Cox-2, positive in a dilated dermal blood vessel (red staining, black arrow). d. The same dermal blood vessel as in c, also positive for HLA-DP, DQ, DR antigen (brown staining, red arrow) (400X). e. DIF positive staining using FITC conjugated anti-human IgG in the upper and intermediate dermal blood vessels(yellow staining; white arrows) and some nerves that colocalized with collagen IV (orange staining, white arrows) (400X). f. DIF positive on upper dermal dilated blood vessels using FITC conjugated anti-human fibrinogen (green staining, white arrow) (200X). g. DIF using 1 M NaCl split skin, shows positivity on both sides(roof and floor) of the skin split using FITC conjugated anti-human Complment/C3c(green staining, white arrows) (200X). h. IHC positive staining for HLA-DP, DQ, DR antigen against some structures inside a nerve (possibly blood vessels feeding the nerve (brown staining; red arrow). i. IIF using 1 M NaCl split skin, showing positive staining for FITC conjugated anti-human IgA. Note the staining along the BMZ on the epidermal side of the blister split, especially in some individual cells (green/white staining; red arrows). The nearby orange staining is Texas red conjugated anti-collagen IV; the nuclei of nearby epidermal keratinocytes were counterstained with TOPRO3(blue/violet).

We also detected fragmentation of some dermal blood vessels using antibodies to vascular endothelial growth factor (VEGF) and to thrombomodulin, indicating possible vascular fragmentation and damage as a result of the immune response. We speculate that damage to epidermal nerves in BP may occur because intraepidermal nerves exist in proximity to desmosomes; blistering, acantholysis, and separation could occur in these areas, potentially exposing neural antigens to autoreactivity. Thrombomodulin is an endothelial cell transmembrane glycoprotein and is an anticoagulation cofactor. The normal distribution of thrombomodulin includes the lining of blood and lymphatic vessels, mesothelial cells and some macrophages of the lung, meningeal lining cells, synovial cells, syncytiotrophoblasts, megakaryocytes and platelets [19].

VEGF is a key regulator of physiological angiogenesis during embryogenesis, skeletal growth and reproductive functions [20]. Some authors have used IHC staining to investigate the expression of thrombomodulin in the epidermis. The authors reported the expression of thrombomodulin in Malpighian layer keratinocytes [19]. These authors also investigated the expression of thrombomodulin in some BP patients, and found that in contrast to what occurs in the skin of patients with pemphigus vulgaris and/or foliaceus, in BP thrombomodulin is present outside the blister [19].

Other authors have analyzed the serum levels of VEGF, soluble E-selectin (sE-selectin, an isoform of the cell membrane E-selectin, an adhesion molecule synthesized only by endothelial cells), and TNF-alpha in 8 patients with BP versus a control group [20]. In addition, serum sE-selectin levels were measured over time and compared with the serum anti-epithelium antibody titers [20]. The authors reported a significantly increased in these three markers (VEGF, sE-selectin and TNF-alpha) in the sera of patients with BP (p at least < 0.01), in comparison to the controls. In addition, the authors reported all three variables were also significantly correlated with the number of clinical lesions (p at least < 0.01) [20]. In our case, we noted dotted staining with VEGF and formation of rounded structures that likely represented debris from damaged blood vessels.

Regarding the role of dermal blood vessels in the pathogenesis on BP, other studies have been reported [21]. Previous authors also studied the serum levels of three cytokines, interleukin-6 (IL-6), tumor necrosis factor-alpha (TNF-alpha) and interleukin-10 (IL-10) in 15 patients with BP (compared with 20 healthy controls), and evaluated any involvement of these biological modulators in the clinical expression of this disease. The sera of BP patients showed increased levels of these three cytokines ($p < 0.01$). When the number of skin lesions (blisters and/or erosions) of each patient, were correlated with the serum levels of IL-6 and TNF-alpha, significant correlations were found (IL-6, $p < 0.01$ and TNF-alpha, $p < 0.01$, respectively), suggesting a possible role of these mediators in the development of BP blisters [21].

On the basis of this data, the authors suggested that at least IL-6 and TNF-alpha were associated with the clinical expression of BP; the authors also suggested that endothelial activation (possibly induced by the TNF-alpha activity), seemed to be an important phase of BP development [21].

BPAGI is a 230 kD protein and a plakin; it has been shown that plakins are important in embryonic development, affecting integrity of the the heart, neuroepithelium, skin and vasculature.

Previous authors reported that sera from a patient with BP with neurological changes recognized BP antigens by immunoblotting (IB) in skin and brain tissue [22]. In mice lacking the BPAG1 gene, neurons exhibited perturbations in their intermediate filaments and microtubules, leading to swellings and changes in the axons [23]. Indeed, we also have shown that patients affected by endemic pemphigus foliaceus in El Bagre, Colombia, South America had compromise of the nerves in the central neural system as well as the peripheral sympathetic and parasympathetic nerves [24].

In regard to our observed positivity with TIMP and metallothionein, we had previously found similar positivity in other BP cases [25-26]. Regarding our observed positive staining in junctional areas between dermal blood vessels and the surrounding mesenchymal tissue, the significance of this finding is not known.

In summary, in our current and previous studies we have noted several BP patients with autoimmune disease alterations in neurovascular structures. Based on our data and that of other authors we suggest further investigation of autoimmune pathologic damage at the cutaneous BMZs of skin appendices, as well as in dermal neurovascular structures in BP.

Acknowledgment

Jonathan S. Jones, HT(ASCP) at Georgia Dermatopathology Associates provided excellent technical assistance.

Conflicts of Interest

None.

Funding

Georgia Dermatopathology Associates, Atlanta, Georgia, USA.

References

[1] Sitaru C. Bullous pemphigoid: a prototypical antibody-mediated organ-specific autoimmune disease. *J. Invest. Dermatol.*, 2009; 129:822-24.

[2] Abreu Velez A. M., Vasquez-Hincapie D. A., Howard M. S. Autoimmune basement membrane and subepidermal blistering diseases. *Our Dermatol. Online*, 2013; 4(Suppl.3): 647-642.

[3] Calle-Isaza J., Avila I. C., Abreu Velez A. M. Enfermedades ampollosas autoinmunes de la piel. Parte 1, enfermedades del grupo de los pénfigos. *Iatreia*, 27: 309-19.

[4] Abreu Velez A. M., Calle-Isaza J., Howard M. S. A case of bullous pemphigoid with immunoreactivty to blood vessels and sweat glands. *Our Dermatol. Online*, 2013; 4(Suppl.3): 621-24.

[5] Abreu Velez A. M., Smith J. G. Jr., Howard M. S. IgG/IgE bullous pemphigoid with CD45 lymphocytic reactivity to dermal blood vessels, nerves and eccrine sweat glands. *North Am. J. Med. Sci.*, 2010; 2: 538-41.

[6] Abreu Velez A. M., Howard M. S.. Collagen I. V. in normal skin and in pathologic processes. *North Am. J. Med. Sci.,* 2012; 4:1-8.
[7] Abreu Velez A. M., Brown V. M., Howard M. S. Cytotoxic and antigen presenting cells present and non-basement membrane zone pathology in a case of bullous pemphigoid. *Our Dermatol. Online,* 2012; 3: 93-99.
[8] Abreu Velez A. M., Girard J. G., Howard M. S. IgG bullous pemphigoid with antibodies to IgD, dermal blood vessels, eccrine glands and the endomysium of monkey esophagus. *Our Dermatol. Online,* 2011; 2: 48-51.
[9] Abreu Velez A. M., Googe P. B., Howard M. S. Ribosomal protein s6-ps240 is expressed in lesional skin from patients with autoimmune skin diseases. *North Am. J. Med. Sci.*, 2013; 5:604-08.
[10] Abreu Velez A. M., Googe P. B., Howard M. S. *In situ* immune response in skin biopsies from patients affected by autoimmune blistering diseases. *Our Dermatol. Online*, 2013; 4(Suppl.3): 606-12.
[11] Abreu Velez A. M., Calle-Isaza J., Howard M. S. Cyclo-oxygenase 2 is present in the majority of lesional skin from patients with autoimmune blistering diseases. *Our Dermatol. Online*, 2013; 4:476-78.
[12] Abreu Velez A. M., Yepes-Naranjo M. M., Avila I. C., Londoño M. L., Googe P. B., Velásquez-Velez J. E., Velez I. D., Upegui Y. A., Jimenez-Echavarria A., Mesa-Herrera N. R., Yi H., Calle-Isaza J., Howard M. S. Tissue inhibitor of metalloproteinase 1, matrix metalloproteinase 9, αlpha-1 antitrypsin, metallothionein and urokinase type plasminogen activator receptor in skin biopsies from patients affected by autoimmune blistering diseases. *Our Dermatol. Online,* 2013; 4: 275-80.
[13] Abreu Velez A. M., Calle-Isaza J., Howard M. S. CD1a, HAM56, CD68 and S-100 are present in lesional skin biopsies from patients affected by autoimmune blistering diseases. *Our Dermatol. Online*, 2014; 5:113-17.
[14] Abreu Velez A. M., Calle-Isaza J., Howard M. S. HLA-DP, DQ, DR is expressed in all lesional skin from patients with autoimmune skin diseases. *Our Dermatol. Online*, 2014;5:125-28.
[15] Abreu Velez A. M., Howard M. S. Neural reactivity detected by immunofluorescence in a patient with a localized blistering disease. *Our Dermatol. Online,* 2013;4: 91-94.
[16] Abreu Velez A. M., Girard J. G., Howard M. S. IgG bullous pemphigoid with antibodies to IgD, dermal blood vessels, eccrine glands and the endomysium of monkey esophagus. *Our Dermatol. Online*, 2011; 2: 48-51.
[17] Abreu Velez A. M., Smoller B. R., Howard M. S. Rouleaux and autoagglutination of erythrocytes associated with fibrin-like material in skin biopsies form patients with autoimmune blistering diseases. *Our Dermatol. Online*, 2013;4(Suppl.3): 613-15.
[18] Abreu Velez A. M., Vásquez-Hincapié D. A., Howard M. S. Vimentin may reflect areas of cutaneous involvement in biopsies from patients with autoimmune skin diseases. *Our Dermatol. Online*, 2014; 5:140-43.
[19] Mizutani H., Ohyanagi S., Nouchi N., Inachi S., Shimizu M. Tissue factor and thrombomodulin expression on keratinocytes as coagulation/anti-coagulation cofactor and differentiation marker. *Australas J. Dermatol.*, 1996 May; 37 Suppl. 1:S48-49.
[20] Ameglio F., D'Auria L., Cordiali-Fei P., Mussi A., Valenzano L., D'Agosto G., Ferraro C., Bonifati C., Giacalone B. Bullous pemphigoid and pemphigus vulgaris: correlated

behaviour of serum VEGF, sE-selectin and TNF-alpha levels. *J. Biol. Regul. Homeost. Agents,* 1997;11: 148-53.

[21] D'Auria L., Mussi A., Bonifati C., Mastroianni A., Giacalone B., Ameglio F. Increased serum IL-6, TNF-alpha and IL-10 levels in patients with bullous pemphigoid: relationships with disease activity. *J. Eur. Acad. Dermatol. Venereol.,* 1999;12:11-15.

[22] Vu T. N., Lee T. X., Ndoye A., Shultz L. D., Pittelkow M. R., Dahl M. V., et al. The pathophysiological significance of nondesmoglein targets of pemphigus autoimmunity. Development of antibodies against keratinocyte cholinergic receptors in patients with pemphigus vulgaris and pemphigus foliaceus. *Arch. Dermatol.*, 1998; 134:971–80.

[23] Miyakawa T., Deshimaru M., Sumiyoshi S., Teraoka A., Tatetsu S. Experimental organic mercury poisoning; pathological changes in peripheral nerves. *Acta. Neuropathol.*, 1970; 15:45–55.

[24] Abreu Velez A. M., Howard M. S., Grossniklaus H. E., Gao W., Hashimoto T. Neural system antigens are recognized by autoantibodies from patients affected by a new variant of endemic pemphigus foliaceus in Colombia. *Clin. Immunol.*, 2011;31:356-68.

[25] Abreu Velez A. M., Howard M. S., Smoller B. R. Antibodies to pilosebaceous units, in a new variant of pemphigus foliaceus. *Eur. J. Dermatol.*, 2011; 21:371-375.

[26] Abreu Velez A. M., Googe P. B., Howard M. S. Immunohistochemistry versus immunofluoresence in the diagnosis of autoimmune blistering diseases. *Our Dermatol. Online,* 2013; 4(Suppl.3): 627-30.

In: Advances in Dermatology Research
Editor: James P. Vega
ISBN: 978-1-63482-226-8

Chapter 4

Expression of Immunologic Markers Varies between Intact Blister and Traumatized Blister Areas in a Patient with Bullous Pemphigoid

Ana Maria Abreu Velez, MD, PhD*[*,1]*,
***Billie L. Jackson, MD*[2]**
***and Michael S. Howard, MD*[1]**
[1] Georgia Dermatopathology Associates, Atlanta, Georgia, US
[2] Dermatologist, Macon, Georgia, US

Abstract

Background: The clinical presentation of bullous pemphigoid (BP) is variable; blistering skin lesions may be present, but an urticarial or erythematous rash may also precede the appearance of the blisters. The patients themselves may also traumatize blister lesions, and spontaneous ulceration of the skin may occur.

Aim: We sought to compare the immune changes in intact bullous pemphigoid lesions, versus ulcerated lesions. Here we aim to describe these changes, utilizing a skin biopsy containing both intact and ulcerated bullous pemphigoid lesional areas via hematoxylin and eosin histology (H&E), as well as direct immunofluorescence (DIF) and immunohistochemistry (IHC).

Results: The findings in these areas demonstrated distinctly different patterns of the immune response. In the intact blister areas, markers such as HLA-DP, DQ, DR antigen, cyclooxygenase-2 (COX-2), B-cell lymphoma 2(BCL2), CD3, CD68, alpha-1 antitrypsin, mast cell tryptase, von Willembrand factor and Factor XIIIa demonstrated positive staining in some areas of the blister and around adjacent dermal blood vessels. However, in ulcerated areas, most of these markers primarily compartmentalized in a linear manner

[*] Corresponding author: Ana Maria Abreu Velez, M.D., Ph.D., Georgia Dermatopathology Associates, 1534 North Decatur Rd., NE; Suite 206; Atlanta, Georgia 30307-1000, USA, Telephone: (404) 371-0077, Toll Free: (877) 371-0027, Fax: (404) 371-1900, E-mail: abreuvelez@yahoo.com.

at the base of the ulcer. We interpreted the ulcerated area pattern as evidence of the immune system attempting to phagocytose or extrude the ulcerated tissue. P53 demonstrated positive staining in nascent blister areas, but negative staining within the ulcer. CD4, CD20 and GFAP demonstrated negative staining in intact blister areas and in ulcerated areas.

Conclusion: We suggest that the immune response that is present around the ulcerated areas is acting as a secondary immune response, for the purpose of removing damaged tissue. Thus, we suggest the primary bullous pemphigoid immune response creates the blisters, and the secondary immune response forms as a result of ulceration of the tissue. Further studies are warranted to confirm these immunologic possibilities.

Keywords: bullous pemphigoid, eosinophils, HLA-DP, DQ, DR antigen, COX-2, BCL2, blister, ulcers, immune response

Abbreviations and Acronyms

BP	Bullous pemphigoid
IHC	immunohistochemistry
DIF, IIF	direct and indirect immunofluorescence
H&E	hematoxylin and eosin
BMZ	basement membrane zone
MCT	mast cell tryptase
BCL2	B-cell lymphoma-2
COX-2	cyclooxygenase-2
Dapi	4',6-diamidino-2-phenylindole

Introduction

Bullous pemphigoid (BP) is a cutaneous autoimmune blistering disease. These disorders are characterized by autoantibodies formed against epidermal proteins. Clinically, these disorders often present with blisters and erosions on the skin and/or mucous membranes [1-5]. BP primarily affects elderly patients [1-5]. Clinical criteria and histopathologic characteristics are not sufficient for a precise diagnosis. Additional testing, such as a biopsy for direct immunofluorescence (DIF), serologic tests for autoantibodies titers either by ELISA and or by indirect immunofluorescence (IIF) and immunoblotting may be needed to confirm a diagnosis [1-5]. In many cutaneous autoimmune blistering diseases, the detection of serum autoantibodies have been shown to correlate with disease activity and may be helpful in deciding treatment options for the patients. We recently demonstrated that immunohistochemistry (IHC) is a valuable alternative to DIF in the diagnosis of BP, as well as other autoimmune blistering diseases [6]. We also reported that B and T lymphocytic markers, as well as other markers including cyclooxygenase-2 (COX-2) and ribosomal protein S6-ps240 are present in the lesional skin of BP patients [7-11]. We have previously shown that mast cell tryptase (MCT), c-kit/CD117 and IgE are also present in the lesional skin of these patients [12]. Further, we recently demonstrated that tissue inhibitor of metalloproteinase 1, matrix metalloproteinase 9, alpha-1 antitrypsin, metallothionein and urokinase type plasminogen activator receptor may play specific roles in BP [13]. We reported the presence of CD1a, HAM56, CD68, S-100 and HLA-DP, DQ, DR antigen in lesional skin of patients with BP [14, 15]. In addition to the immune response against the basement membrane zone (BMZ) of the skin, we noted that some BP reactivity occurs against patient dermal sweat glands and ducts, and their associated blood vessels and nerves [16-18]. Finally, we have previously reported that vimentin may reflect areas of cutaneous dermal BP involvement, and rouleaux and autoagglutination of erythrocytes associated with fibrin-like material are presented in BP lesions. [6-15].

Case Report

A 58 year old female consulted her dermatologist for the sudden onset of pruritic blisters. These blisters would come and go, primarily on the lower back, abdomen, and legs. A physical examination revealed several small, tense blisters on an erythematous base. Some lesions were ulcerated. A skin biopsy for hematoxylin and eosin (H&E) and IHC staining was taken in formalin, as well a second biopsy in Michel's transport medium for DIF. The patient's diagnosis was confirmed as BP, and oral and topical steroids were provided with clinical improvement.

Materials and Methods

Lesional skin was biopsied and studied utilizing hematoxylin and eosin (H&E) staining, as well as via IHC and DIF. In brief, for DIF we incubated 4 micron thickness sections on slides with secondary antibodies as previously described [6-18]. We utilized FITC conjugated rabbit anti-total IgG, IgA, IgM, Complement/C1q and Complement/C3. These antibodies were used at a 1:25 dilution; we also utilized fibrinogen and albumin, at a 1:50 dilution. All of the preceding antibodies were obtained from Dako (Carpinteria, California, USA). In addition, anti-human IgE antiserum (Epsilon chain) was obtained from Kent Laboratories (Bellingham, Washington, USA) and anti-human IgD antibodies from Southern Biotechnology, Birmingham, Alabama, USA; these antibodies were uutilized at 1:25 dilutions. We also utilized a rhodamine conjugated antibody to Ulex europaeus agglutinin 1 from Vector Laboratories (Burlingame, California USA). The DIF slides were counterstained with 4',6-diamidino-2-phenylindole (Dapi)(Pierce, Rockford, Illinois, USA). The samples were run with positive and negative controls.

Immunohistochemistry (IHC)

We performed IHC utilizing multiple monoclonal and polyclonal antibodies from Dako (Carpinteria, California, USA). We utilized polyclonal rabbit anti-human myeloperoxidase; monoclonal mouse anti-human B-cell lymphoma-2 (BCL2), oncoprotein, Clone 124; anti-human cyclooxygenase 2 (COX-2), Clone CX-294; anti-human HLA-DP, DQ, DR antigen,

Clone CR3/43; anti-human mast cell tryptase (MCT); von Willebrand Factor, Clone F8/86; p53 protein, Clone DO-7; CD20, Clone L26; anti-human CD4 and polyclonal rabbit anti-human alpha-1-antitrypsin. For our IHC testing, we utilized a dual endogenous peroxidase blockage with the addition of a Dako Envision dual link (to assist in chromogen attachment). We then applied the chromogen 3,3-diaminobenzidine(DAB), and counterstained with hematoxylin. The samples were run in a Dako Autostainer Universal Staining System. Positive and negative controls were consistently performed. The staining was performed as previously described [10-17].

IHC Double Staining

These were performed utilizing a Leica (Buffalo Grove, Illinois, USA) double staining system. Specifically, for primary staining we utilized a Bond Max platform autostainer with bond polymer refined Red detection DS9390, alkaline phosphatase linker polymer and fast red chromogen. For the secondary staining, we utilized bond polymer refine detection DS9800 horseradish peroxidase linker polymer and DAB chromogen (brown staining).

The following antibodies were utilized from Leica/Novocastra: monoclonal mouse anti-human podoplanin/D2-40, polyclonal rabbit anti-human CD3, Monoclonal mouse anti-human CD8, anti-human CD20, anti-human CD68, anti-human glial fibrillary acidic protein (GFAP) and Factor XIIIa.

Results

H&E

Examination of the H&E tissue sections demonstrated a subepidermal blistering disorder, with one nascent blister and one older blister. Focal re-epithelialization of one of the blister bases was seen. Focal epidermal cytoid bodies were appreciated.

Within the intact blister lumen, numerous eosinophils are present, with occasional lymphocytes also seen. Neutrophils were rare. Within the dermis, a mild, superficial, perivascular infiltrate of lymphocytes, histiocytes and many eosinophils were identified. An ulcer filled with fibrinous material was present adjacent to the blisters (see Figures 1 and 2). The adjacent ulcerated area showed necrotic and apoptotic material on the ulcer.

DIF

Displayed the following results: IgG (++, positive deposition around lesional blister roof and negative on the basement membrane zone (BMZ); also some positive ANCAs (IgG within the epidermis and around dermal blood vessels); IgA (++, positive on the lesional blister roof); IgM (++, positive on the lesional blister roof and negative on the BMZ); IgD (+, focal and punctate, epidermal stratum corneum); IgE (-); complement/ C1q (++, positive on lesional blister roof and negative on the BMZ); Complement/C3 (++, Positive on lesional blister roof and negative on BMZ; positive around dermal blood vessels); Kappa light chains (++, positive on lesional blister roof and negative on the BMZ); Lambda light chains (++, Positive on lesional blister roof and negative on the BMZ); albumin (++, positive under the BMZ and around dermal blood vessels) and fibrinogen (++, positive under BMZ and around dermal blood vessels) (see Figures 1 and 2). The DIF biopsy only contained a perilesional and lesional blister, and contained only one part of the ulcerated area.

During the DIF testing, we observed under darkfield microscopy excretion of an unknown, dark material on the skin surface (see Figure 2 e and f). DIF in the ulcerated lesions showed loss of the linear patterns of deposition of immunoglobulins and complement normally seen at the BMZ; instead, deposits of these antibodies were noted in the subjacent vessels (see Figure 2 g).

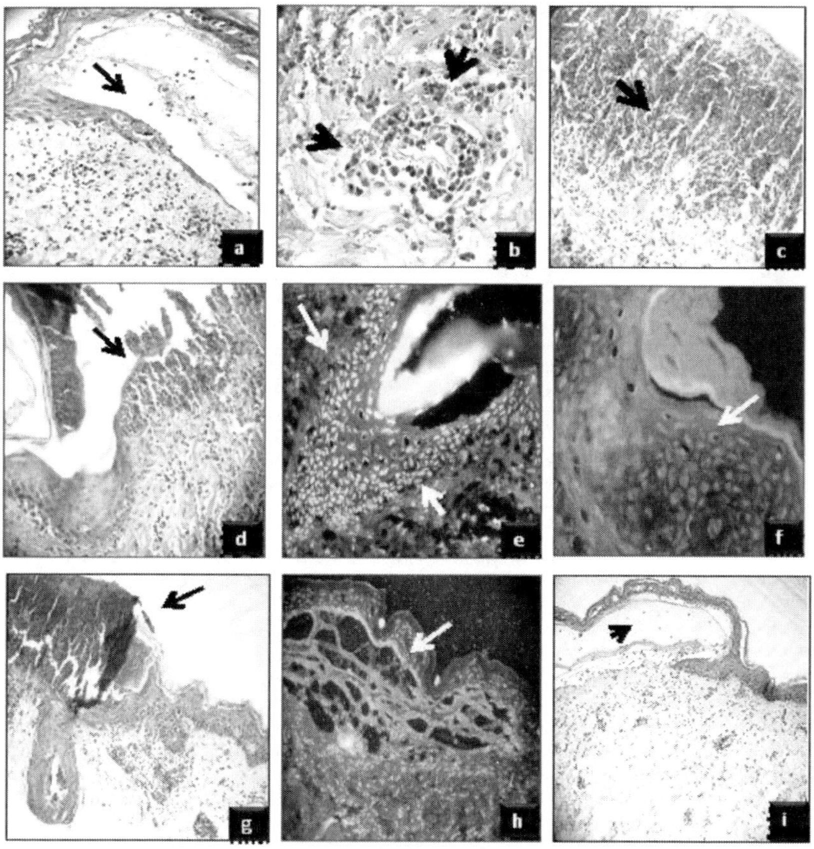

Figure 1 H&E, DIF and other stains comparing the intact blister versus the ulcerated area. a through d, H & E stains. a, shows a subepidermal intact blister (black arrow) (100X). b, Shows an infiltrate with eosinophils around the upper dermal blood vessels under the blister (400X) (black arrows). c and d, Show the ulcerated area (black arrows) (200X). e and f, DIF showing in e, positive staining along the BMZ of a hair follicle with FITC conjugated anti-human albumin (green staining; white arrows). The follicle stains with rhodamine conjugated Ulex Europaeous agglutinnin 1(red staining). The cell nuclei were counterstained with DAPI (blue). f, Positive staining against some epidermal keratinocyte nuclear structures, using FITC conjugated anti-human IgD(white arrow). g. PAS staining shows the ulcerated area (black arrow) (100X). h. DIF using FITC conjugated anti-human IgM show positive staining in the blister (green staining; white arrow). i. PAS staining highlights the ulcerated area (black arrow) (40X).

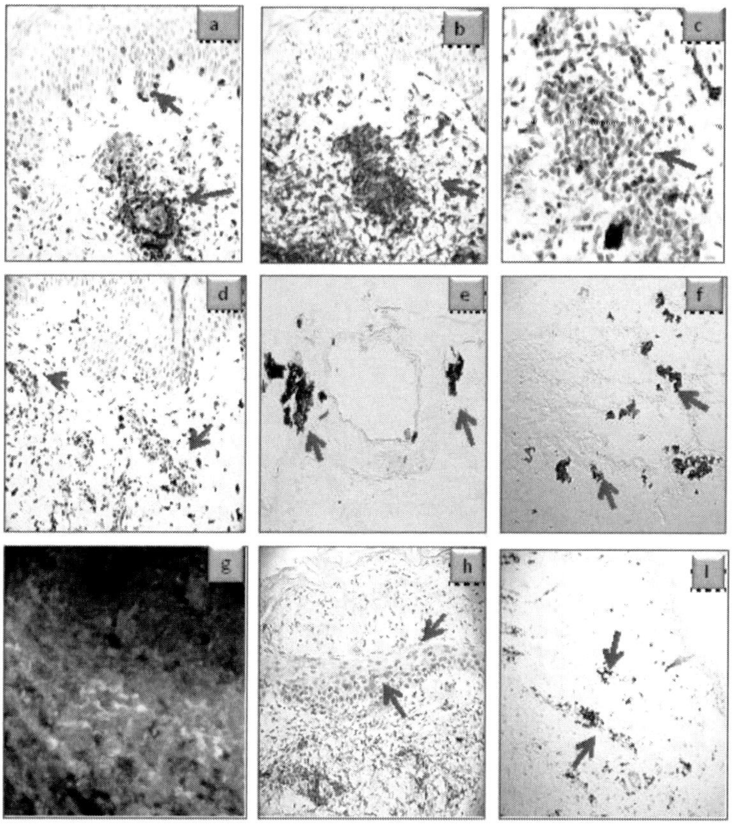

Figure 2. IHC and DIF comparison between the blister and the ulcerated area. a through d, IHC. a. IHC staining, using a double staining system with the Leica Bond-Max and fast red chromogen (red staining) against von Willembrand factor antibody. In brown, the stain was against BCL2 using DAB chromogen (red arrows). b. Same technique, with red staining for von Willembrand factor brown staining against HLA-DP, DQ, DR. The red arrow shows a perfect overlapping of both antibodies. c. In this case, the red staining is for von Willembrand factor and the brown is to podophilin (D2-40). Please notice that the inflammatory infiltrate (blue cells) are present around both the blood vessels and the lymphatics (red arrow). d. In red, von Willembrand factor and in brown, Factor XIIIa (red arrows). e and f. Dark field microscopy shows a dark material that seemed to be extruded from the dermis in proximity to the blister (red arrows). g, DIF, showing positivity around dermal blood vessels under the ulcerated area, using FITC conjugated antihuman IgG antibodies (green staining; red arrow). h. IHC staining with von Willembrand factor in red and with Factor XIIIa in brown, showing positivity in a "linear fashion under the ulcer"(red arrows). i. IHC positive staining with CD3 around the vessels surrounding the intact blister (brown staining; red arrows).

Immunohistochemistry (IHC) Staining

In the intact blister, markers such as HLA-DP, DQ, DR antigen, cyclooxygenase-2 (COX-2), B-cell lymphoma 2, CD3, CD68, von Willembrand factor, alpha-1 antitrypsin and mast cell tryptase were noted as being positive in some areas of the blister itself and the subjacent vessels, and in inflammatory cells surrounding the intact blister. However, in the ulcerated areas, most of these markers seemed to be compartmentalized, primarily in "linear fashion" at the base of the ulcer (see Figures 1 through 3). Strong staining with HLA-DP, DQ,

DR antigen was seen near non-ulcerated areas, specifically around most of the upper dermal blood vessels under and surrounding the blister, around dermal sweat duct blood vessels, and in the epidermis in proximity to the blister. COX-2, HLA-DP, DQ, DR antigen, and BCL2 demonstrated similar patterns. P53 was positive in the "normal skin" around the blisters along the BMZ, and completely negative under the ulcer. P53 was also positive in a newly formed blister along the BMZ. CD4, CD20 and GFAP were negative in both intact blister and ulcerated areas. Using darkfield microscopy, we also observed extrusion of an unknown, dark material onto the skin surface (Figure 2).

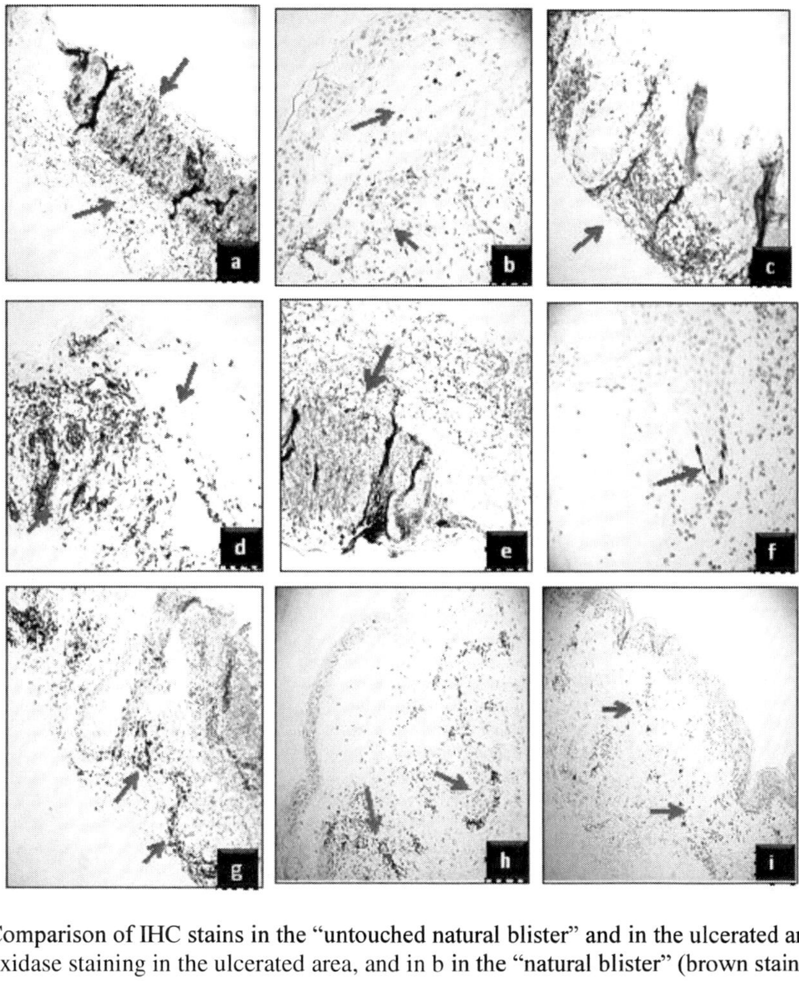

Figure 3. Comparison of IHC stains in the "untouched natural blister" and in the ulcerated area. a. Myeloperoxidase staining in the ulcerated area, and in b in the "natural blister" (brown staining; red arrows). c and d. IHC staining with HLA-DP, DQ, DR in the ulcerated area in c versus the "blister" in d (brown staining; red arrows). e and f. Show staining with COX-2 stains in the in the ulcerated area in e, versus the "natural blister" in f. g and h IHC staining with BCL2 in the ulcerated area in g, versus the "natural blister" in h. i. Positive staining for mast cell tryptase in some cells around the dermal blood vessels of the dermis (red arrows).

In Figure 3, we show the differences in IHC expression in the ulcerated areas, and in the blistered areas. Von Willembrand factor was positive around the blood vessels, and did co-localize with BCL2 and with HLA-DP, DQ, DR antigen (see Figure 3). The eosinophils colocalized perfectly with HLA-DP, DQ, DR antigen. CD3 and CD8 were positive in the upper dermal infiltrate under the blister and around the blood vessels; however, CD4, CD20 and GFAP were negative. MCT was positive around the upper dermal blood vessels. In Figure 3, we summarize the results of a comparison of IHC staining data of the ulcerated and blistered areas. Figure 3 a and b. IHC staining with myeloperoxidase shows strong staining in the ulcerated area in a, relative to the blistered area in b. c and d IHC staining with HLA-DP, DQ, DR antigen in an ulcerated area, versus a blistered area. We observed that the primary immune response was via intact blood vessel-like structures; these can be clearly noted in the blistered areas, whereas in the ulcerated areas we noted destruction of these skin anatomical structures. In e and f, we show staining with COX-2 to be very strong in the ulcerated area, versus some type of partial linear staining on the BMZ in the blistered areas. In g and h, we show a similar pattern of staining with BCL2 in the ulcerated area versus the blistered area; specifically, stain compartmentalization was noted around the dermal blood vessels. MCT was positive around the upper vessels of the dermis in both categories.

Discussion

The initial presentation of pemphigoid is very variable, as blistering skin lesions may be present; however, an urticarial or erythematous rash may precede the appearance of the blisters. The patient may cause accidental or deliberate rubbing; spontaneous denudation and ulceration of the lesions may also occur [1-5]. Comparing the presence of several biological markers in the blistered and ulcerated areas, we were able to see two different patterns of reactivity. In the intact blister areas, we found an immune response as previously described by us in several publications [6-16]. This reactivity seems to be part of the "natural history" of the disease. However, we could not find evidence of previous documentation of the immune response in the ulcerated areas.

In the intact blister areas, we were able to demonstrate overlapping staining with von Willembrand Factor, HLA-DP, DQ, DR antigen and the eosinophils; thus, the dermal blood vessels are expressing these markers, and the eosinophils are playing an active role in the immune response. Some authors have also described the co-cololization between eosinophils and HLA-DP, DQ, DR antigen molecules [21]. We also were able to demonstrate that the inflammatory infiltrate is present around both blood vessels and lymphatics in proximity to the intact blister. We also demonstrated positive staining with Factor XIIIa that labels dermal dendrocytes, a specific population of bone marrow derived dendritic cells in the skin distinct from Langerhans cells and which share some features common to mononuclear phagocytes. The majority of cells that were Factor XIIIa positive were also positive to CD68 using double IHC staining. However, some cells that were Factor XIIIa positive were not double stained with CD68, indicating a modified dendritic antigen presentation. To our surprise, BCL2 was very positive in the majority of the inflammatory cells around the blister and the inflammatory infiltrate. BCL2 is specifically considered as an important anti-apoptotic protein, and is thus classified as an oncogene; two isoforms has been described [22]. P53 is also a proapototic marker, and this was present around some edges of the blister and not seen in the ulcerated area. Damage to the BCL2 gene has been identified as a cause of a number of malignancies, including melanoma, breast and prostate cancer, chronic lymphocytic leukemia and lung cancer; it has also been associated with schizophrenia and autoimmunity [22]. BCL2 is also related to resistance to cancer treatments. Simultaneous over-expression of BCL2 and the proto-oncogene myc may produce aggressive B-cell malignancies, including lymphoma.

The BCL2 pathway is largely present in all eukaryotic cells, as a modulator of survival [22, 23]. However, recently discoveries have demonstrated that BCL2 molecules are indispensable for activation and maturation of T lymphocytes after antigen presentation [23-24]. Regulated apoptosis is vital for both the development and the subsequent maintenance of the immune system. Interleukins, including IL-2, IL-4, IL-7 and IL-15, profoundly influence lymphocyte survival during the vulnerable stages of VDJ rearrangement and later in ensuring cellular homeostasis, but the genes specifically accountable for the development and maintenance of the lymphocytes have not been identified [23-24]. Our work suggests some type of immune response in the cells expressing BCL2, the exact nature of which is unknown.

Another interesting finding was the presence of positive staining against some nuclear structures in the epidermis by using DIF and FITC conjugated anti-human IgD. The significance of this finding warrants further investigation.

We were not able to determine the nature of the unknown material on lesional skin when using darkfield microscopy. We will watch for this phenomenon in other cases to see if this was a unique finding in this case, or if is expressed in the disease.

Conclusion

We conclude that even in the same patient a non-damaged blister seems to have quite different immunologic and pathologic changes from an ulcerated blister area. These findings may reflect the diversity of clinical lesions we often see in patients with BP. We interpreted multiple changes in the ulcerated areas as the immune system attempting to extrude the entire ulcerated tissue.

Acknowledgments

Mr. Jonathan S. Jones at Georgia Dermatopathology Associates provided excellent technical assistance.

Declarations of conflict of interest: None.

Funding: Georgia Dermatopathology Associates, Atlanta, Georgia, USA.

References

[1] Jordon RE, Sams WM Jr, Beutner EH. Complement immunofluorescent staining in bullous pemphigoid. *J Lab Clin Med.* 1969;74:548-556

[2] Wick G, Beutner EH. Quantitative studies of immunofluorescent staining. 3. Comparison of different antigens in an indirect immunofluorescent staining system for

human IgG using the basement zone antibodies of bullous pemphigoid. *Immunology.* 1969;16:149-156.

[3] Beutner EH, Jordon RE, Chorzelski TP. The immunopathology of pemphigus and bullous pemphigoid. *J Invest Dermatol.* 1968;51:63-80.

[4] Abreu Velez AM, Vasquez-Hincapie DA, Howard MS. Autoimmune basement membrane and subepidermal blistering diseases. *Our Dermatol Online.* 2013; 4(Suppl.3): 647-662.

[5] Calle-Isaza J, Avila IC, Abreu Velez AM. Enfermedades ampollosas autoinmunes de la piel. Parte 1, enfermedades del grupo de los pénfigos. *Iatreia.* 2014;27: 309-319.

[6] Abreu Velez AM, Googe PB, Howard MS. Immunohistochemistry versus immunofluoresence in the diagnosis of autoimmune blistering diseases. *Our Dermatol Online.* 2013; 4(Suppl.3): 627-630.

[7] Abreu-Velez AM, Smith JG Jr, Howard MS. IgG/IgE bullous pemphigoid with CD45 lymphocytic reactivity to dermal blood vessels, nerves and eccrine sweat glands. *N Am J Med Sci.* 2010;2:540-543.

[8] Abreu Velez AM, Googe PB, Howard MS. Ribosomal protein s6-ps240 is expressed in lesional skin from patients with autoimmune skin diseases. *North Am J Med Sci.* 2013; 5:604-608.

[9] Abreu Velez AM, Googe PB, Howard MS. *In situ* immune response in skin biopsies from patients affected by autoimmune blistering diseases. Our Dermatol Online. 2013; 4(Suppl.3): 606-612.

[10] Abreu Velez AM, Calle-Isaza J, Howard MS. Cyclo-oxygenase 2 is present in the majority of lesional skin from patients with autoimmune blistering diseases. Our Dermatol Online. 2013; 4(4):476-478. DOI: 10.7241/ourd.20134.120

[11] Abreu Velez AM, Brown VM, Howard MS. Cytotoxic and antigen presenting cells present and non-basement membrane zone pathology in a case of bullous pemphigoid. *Our Dermatol Online*, 2012; 3: 93-99.

[12] Abreu-Velez AM, Roselino AM, Howard MS. Mast cells, Mast/Stem Cell Growth Factor receptor (c-kit/cd117) and IgE may be integral to the pathogenesis of endemic pemphigus foliaceus. *Our Dermatol Online.* 2013; 4(Suppl.3): 596-600.

[13] Abreu Velez AM, Yepes-Naranjo MM, Avila IC, Londoño ML, Googe PB, Velásquez-Velez JE, Velez ID, Upegui YA, Jimenez-Echavarria A, Mesa-Herrera NR, Yi H, Calle-Isaza J, Howard MS. Tissue inhibitor of metalloproteinase 1, matrix metalloproteinase 9, αlpha-1 antitrypsin, metallothionein and urokinase type plasminogen activator receptor in skin biopsies from patients affected by autoimmune blistering diseases. *Our Dermatol Online.* 2013; 4: 275-280.

[14] Abreu Velez AM, Calle-Isaza J, Howard MS. CD1a, HAM56, CD68 and S-100 are present in lesional skin biopsies from patients affected by autoimmune blistering diseases. *Our Dermatol Online.* 2014; 5: 113-117.

[15] Abreu Velez AM, Calle-Isaza J, Howard MS. HLA-DPDQDR is expressed in all lesional skin from patients with autoimmune skin diseases. *Our Dermatol Online.* 2014; 5:125-128.

[16] Abreu Velez AM, Calle-Isaza J, Howard MS. A case of bullous pemphigoid with immunoreactivty to blood vessels and sweat glands. *Our Dermatol Online.* 2013; 4(Suppl.3): 621-624.

[17] Abreu Velez AM, Howard MS. Neural reactivity detected by immunofluorescence in a patient with a localized blistering disease. *Our Dermatol Online,* 2013;4: 91-94.

[18] Abreu Velez AM, Girard JG, Howard MS. IgG bullous pemphigoid with antibodies to IgD, dermal blood vessels, eccrine glands and the endomysium of monkey esophagus. *Our Dermatol Online.* 2011; 2: 48-51.

[19] Abreu Velez AM, Smoller BR, Howard MS. Rouleaux and autoagglutination of erythrocytes associated with fibrin-like material in skin biopsies form patients with autoimmune blistering diseases. *Our Dermatol Online.* 2013; 4(Suppl.3): 613-615.

[20] Abreu Velez AM, Vásquez-Hincapié DA, Howard MS. Vimentin may reflect areas of cutaneous involvement in biopsies from patients with autoimmune skin diseases. *Our Dermatol Online.* 2014; 5: 140-143.

[21] Günther C[1], Wozel G, Meurer M, Pfeiffer C. Up-regulation of CCL11 and CCL26 is associated with activated eosinophils in bullous pemphigoid. *Clin Exp Immunol.* 2011;166:145-153.

[22] Droin NM, Green DR. Role of BCL2 family members in immunity and disease. *Biochimica et Biophysica Acta.* 2004; 1644:179– 188.

[23] Farsaci B, Sabzevari H, Higgins JP, Di Bari MG, Takai S, Schlom J, Hodge JW. Effect of a small molecule BCL2 inhibitor on immune function and use with a recombinant vaccine. *Int. J. Cancer*: 2010;127, 1603–1613.

[24] Opferman JT, Letai A, Beard C, Sorcinelli MD, Ong CC, Korsmeyer SJ. Development and maintenance of B and T lymphocytes requires antiapoptotic MCL-1. *Nature* 2003;426:671–6.

In: Advances in Dermatology Research
Editor: James P. Vega
ISBN: 978-1-63482-226-8

Chapter 5

A Bullous Pemphigoid-Like Allergic Drug Reaction, with Clues for Differentiation versus Classic Bullous Pemphigoid

Ana Maria Abreu Velez, MD, PhD[*,1]
Vickie M. Brown, MD[2] *and Michael S. Howard, MD*[1]
[1]Georgia Dermatopathology Associates, Atlanta, Georgia, US
[2]Dermatology, Milledgeville, Georgia, US

Abstract

Background: Bullous pemphigoid (BP) is an acquired autoimmune disease characterized by subepidermal vesicles, with clinical macules and bullae. In contradistinction, drug induced bullous pemphigoid (DBP) may be triggered by medications and other agents. Presently, minimal pathologic differences have been documented to differentiate between these two entities. We present a case of a drug-induced bullous pemphigoid-like reaction, and review critical aspects that seem to differentiate these entities.

Case report: A 68 year old male was consulted for the presence of erythematosus plaques, papules and tense blisters on the abdomen and thighs, after the intake of multiple medications.

Materials and Methods: Skin biopsies were taken for hematoxylin and eosin review and immunohistochemistry, and for direct immunofluorescence studies.

Results: The H&E histology showed small subepidermal blisters with minimal fibrin and some eosinophils within the blister lumens; no epidermal vacuolar degeneration or acantholysis were noted. Not significant edema was noted in the epidermis or dermis. Direct immunofluorescence revealed dotted Complement/C3c and linear, discontinuous

* Corresponding author: Ana Maria Abreu Velez, M.D., Ph.D., Georgia Dermatopathology Associates, 1534 North Decatur Road., NE; Suite 206; Atlanta, Georgia 30307-1000 USA, Telephone: (404) 371-0077, Toll Free: (877) 371-0027, Fax: (404) 371-1900, E-mail: abreuvelez@yahoo.com.

IgG deposits along the basement membrane zone (BMZ). In addition, cells strongly positive for CD20 and BCL-2 were noted within the lesional inflammation.

Conclusion: Some histologic clues favoring a bullous pemphigoid-like allergic drug reaction may include absence of epidermal vacuolar degeneration, edema, fibrin deposits, blister festoons and a significant luminal eosinophilic infiltrate. In addition to these findings, CD20 cells are normally not found in most cases of classic BP; in classical BP, HLA-DPDQDR is often strongly expressed in the lesions, which was not the case here. In addition, in contrast to classic BP, we noted discontinuous staining at the BMZ with immunoglobulins and complement.

Keywords: bullous pemphigoid, drug induced bullous pemphigoid, BCL-2

Abbreviations and Acronyms

BP	Bullous pemphigoid
DBP	Drug induced bullous pemphigoid
IHC	immunohistochemistry
DIF, IIF	direct and indirect immunofluorescence
H&E	hematoxylin and eosin
BMZ	basement membrane zone
BCL-2	B-cell lymphoma 2 gene
TIMP-1	tissue inhibitor of metalloproteinases 1
LAT	linker for activation of T cells

Case Report

A 68 year old Caucasian male presented with a sudden appearance of erythematous papules, plaques and few blisters on the abdomen, back, arms, and thighs; focal excoriations were also noted. Some of the lesions were violaceous. The patient was taking Lisinopril angiotensin converting enzyme(ACE inhibitor), Glyburide (micronase), Metformin, over the counter cinnamon, Aleve, *ProAir*® HFA (albuterol sulfate), Symbicort® (budesonide/formoterol fumarate dihydrate), *Cartia XT* (Diltiazem Hydrochloride Extended Release), Aciphex (rabeprazole sodium), *Spiriva*®**,** HandiHaler® (tiotropium bromide inhalation powder), Tacrolimus cream and ciprofloxacin. The patient presented a clinical history of chronic obstructive pulmonary disease (COPD), hay fever and allergies, diabetes and arthritis. A skin biopsy for hematoxylin and eosin stain (H&E) and immunohistochemistry (IHC) was taken, as well as a biopsy for direct immunofluorescence (DIF) studies.

Introduction

Autoimmune bullous pemphigoid (BP) is a skin disease for which the etiology is idiopathic and unknown, with the highest occurrence in elderly patients [1]. However, similar disease lesions may occur with the formation of subepidermal blisters in the setting of an allergic drug reaction [2-7]. Minimal data is available regarding subtle pathologic differences between BP and drug induced BP. Drug-induced BP variants are often characterized by linear IgG and C3 along the basement membrane zone (BMZ) on direct immunofluorescence (DIF); on indirect immunofluorescence, the antibodies bind to the epidermal side (roof) of salt split skin. In addition, Western immunoblotting has demonstrated that DBP antibodies react with both the 230 kD and 180 kD bullous pemphigoid (BP) antigens [2-7]. Histologically, is also accepted that drug-induced BP often seems to be similar to typical BP, demonstrating an eosinophil-rich subepidermal blister. We report a case of drug induced BP with several subtle differences from classic autoimmune BP that have not been previously described.

Materials and Methods

Hematoxylin and eosin (H&E) staining, immunohistochemistry (IHC) and direct immunofluroresence (DIF) studies were performed as previously described [8-14]. We utilized the following antibodies: monoclonal mouse anti-human linker for activation of T cells (LAT) protein, HLA-ABC, HLA-DPDQDR, CD4, CD8, CD20, CD45, Complement/C5b-9/MAC, monoclonal mouse anti-human B-cell lymphoma 2 (BCL-2) oncoprotein clone 124, CD20y, Complement/C3c and C3d, CD99, tissue inhibitor of metalloproteinases 1(TIMP-1), monoclonal mouse anti-human myeloid/histiocyte antigen (Clone MAC 387), metallothionein, polyclonal rabbit anti-human myeloperoxidase(all from Dako, Carpinteria, California, USA), and HAM-56 from Cell Marque.

Direct Immunofluorescence (DIF)

For DIF, we incubated 4 micron glass slides with our secondary antibodies as previously described [8-14]. We utilized FITC conjugated rabbit anti-total IgG (Dako, Carpinteria, California, USA) at a 1:25 dilution. The samples were run with positive and negative controls. We also utilized FITC conjugated rabbit antisera to human IgG, IgA, IgM, Complement/C1q, complement/C3, fibrinogen and albumin.

Anti-human IgA antiserum (alpha chain) and anti-human IgM antiserum (mu chain) were obtained from Dako. Anti-human IgE antiserum (epsilon chain) was obtained from Vector Laboratories (Burlingame, California, USA). Anti-human IgD FITC-conjugated antibodies were obtained from Southern Biotechnology (Birmingham, Alabama, USA). The slides were counterstained with 4',6-diamidino-2-phenylindole(DAPI) (Pierce, Rockford, Illinois, USA). A mouse anti-collagen IV monoclonal antibody (Invitrogen, Carlsbad, California, USA) was also utilized, with secondary donkey anti-mouse IgG antisera (heavy and light chains) conjugated with Alexa Fluor 555 (Invitrogen).

Results

Microscopic Description

Examination of the H&E tissue sections demonstrates an early subepidermal blistering disorder. Within the blister lumen, several eosinophils were present, with occasional lymphocytes. Neutrophils were rare. Dermal papillary festoons were not observed. Within the dermis, a mild, superficial, perivascular infiltrate of lymphocytes, histiocytes and eosinophils is identified. No significant edema or fibrin were seen in the lesions (see Figure 1).

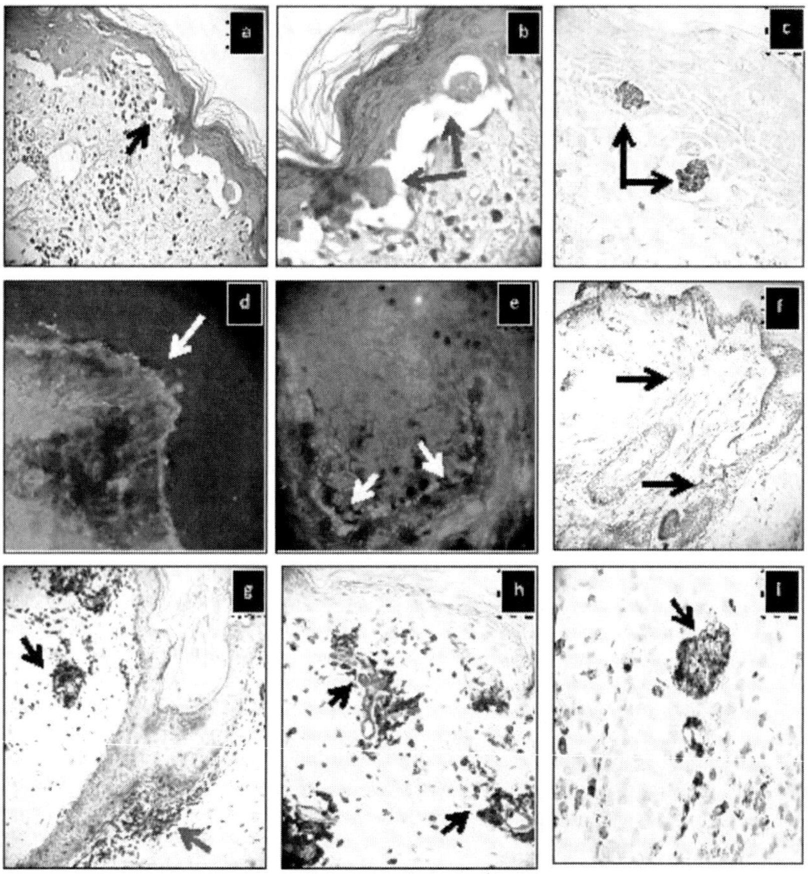

Figure 1. a. H&E staining shows a subepidermal blister (black arrow) with upper dermal perivascular infiltrate featuring lymphohistiocytic cells and few eosinophils and rare neutrophils (100X). b. H&E staining at 400X shows eosinophilic round bodies, present in the blister areas (red arrows). In c, IHC staining with anti-human Complement/C3d, showing positivity to the bodies in b. The same reactivity is seen around upper dermal blood vessels, suggesting that these structures may be the source of Complement in the blister (black arrows). d. DIF, featuring FITC conjugated IgG in a pseudo-linear BMZ pattern, in contrast to that regularly seen in autoimmune bullous pemphigoid (yellow staining; white arrow). e. DIF with FITC conjugated anti-human Complement/C3c "dotted staining" along the BMZ (green staining; white arrow). f. IHC stain showing C5b-9/MAC positive around skin appendix supply blood vessels (brown staining; black arrows). g. Double IHC staining, utilizing CD45 in brown and HLA-DP, DQ, DR in red is seen around dermal blood vessels (black arrow), as well around vessels near a sebaceous gland(lower red arrow). Please note that the BMZ of the sebaceous glands stains

positive for HLA-DP, DQ, DR. h. Identical markers and colors as in g, with higher magnification showing the positive blood vessel staining for HLA-DPDQDR(red staining; black arrows) and the cells around them positive for CD45(brown staining; black arrows) (200X). i. IHC, showing positive staining with myeloperoxidase around a sebaceous gland, and also inside a hair follicle (brown staining; black arrow).

Direct Immunofluorescence(DIF)

We observed the following results: IgG (+; focally linear at BMZ; focal positivity around superficial and deep dermal blood vessels); IgA(-); IgM(-); IgD (-); IgE (-); complement/C3 (+; focal, microgranular deposits in dots at the basement membrane zone of the skin, (BMZ); focal positivity around dermal blood vessels); Kappa light chains (+; focal positivity around upper dermal blood vessels and on dermal eccrine glands); Lambda light chains (+; focal linear BMZ and focal positivity around dermal blood vessels); albumin (+; focal linear at the BMZ; focal positivity around superficial and deep dermal blood vessels) and fibrinogen (+; focal linear BMZ; focally around superficial and deep dermal blood vessels) (see Figures 1 and 2).

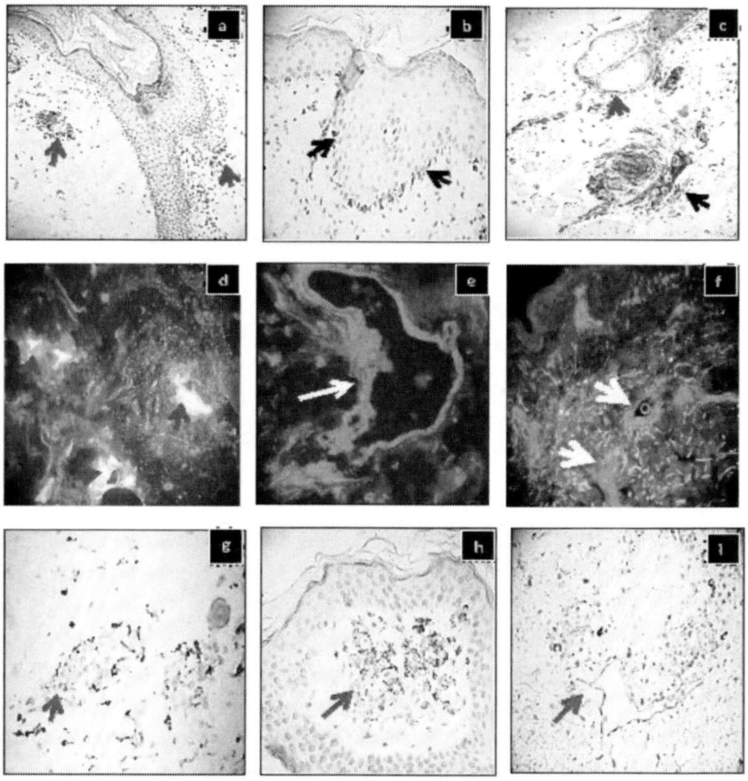

Figure 2. The dermal blood vessels exhibit significant involvement in this disease. a. Double staining IHC, showing positive cells with CD4 in brown and CD8 in red colocalizing around upper dermal blood vessels(especially near hair follicles) (red arrows). b. IHC, demonstrating positive staining with BCL-2 at the base of a hair follicle (brown staining; red arrow). c. Double IHC staining, showing positive CD45 in brown and positive HLA-DP, DQ, DR in red around the BMZs of a sebaceous gland

(red arrow), as well as around deep dermal neurovascular complexes (black arrow). d. DIF, showing positivity using FITC conjugated anti-human fibrinogen around upper and intermediate depth dermal blood vessels (green-white staining; red arrows). The nuclei of nearby cells were counterstained with Dapi (light blue). e. DIF, showing positivity for FITC conjugated anti-human lambda light chains around dermal blood vessels (green staining; white arrow). f. DIF, showing positive staining for FITC conjugated anti-human IgE to upper and intermediate dermal blood vessels (green staining; white arrows) as well as some uneven staining in dermal papillary areas of the BMZ (red arrows) g. IHC staining, using anti-human HAM-56 and positive around dermal blood vessels (brown staining; red arrow). h. IHC staining, positive for LAT around upper dermal blood vessels (brown staining; red arrow). i. IHC with LAT positive staining around dermal blood vessels (brown staining; red arrow); thus, T lymphocyte activation is occurring near the vessels.

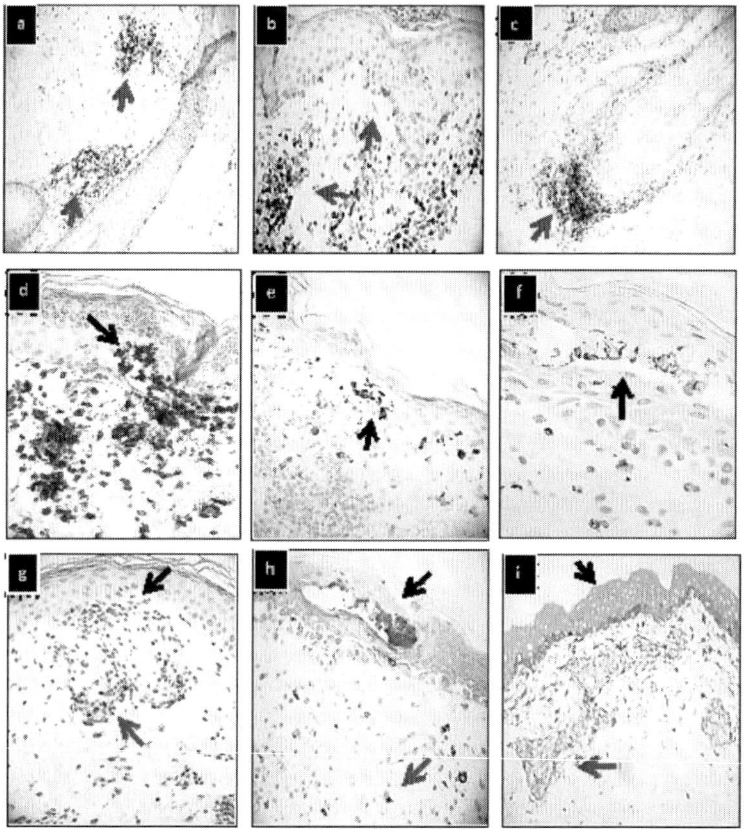

Figure 3. a, b and c. IHC positive staining with BCL-2. In a, against inflammatory cells around a hair follicle (100X). In b, against an inflammatory infiltrate around upper dermal blood vessels as well as along the BMZ (brown staining; red arrows). c. At the base of a hair follicle (brown staining; red arrow). d. Double staining with IHC, showing positive cells with CD45 in brown and HLA-DPDQDR in red in the area of the blister. Please note that the CD45 positive cells are present in an area where the HLA-DP, DQ, DR expression is diminished(black arrow). e. IHC staining with CD68, positive in the blister area (brown staining; black arrow). f. Positive staining with HAM-56 in the blister and under the blister (brown staining, black arrow). g. Double staining with IHC, showing positive cells for CD4 in brown and for CD8 in red, colocalizing around dermal blood vessels (red arrow) and at the BMZ (black arrow). h. IHC staining for TIMP-1 shows positive staining in the epidermis and inside the blister (brown staining; black arrow), as well as in several areas in the dermis that seem to be some type of cell junction between small blood vessels and dermal stromal cells (brown staining; red arrow). i. IHC staining for metallothionein, positive within the epidermis (brown staining; black arrow) and also around dermal blood vessels and on selected dermal cells(brown staining; red arrow).

Immunohistochemistry

HLA-ABC was positive in the epidermis, as well as in the upper vessels and dermal infiltrate. C-5b-9/MAC was positive in some patches at the BMZ, in several dermal vessels, between dermal collagen fibers and around the sweat glands. CD20y, CD4, CD8, BCL-2 and LAT were positive around the upper dermal blood vessels in the infiltrate. CD45 was also positive around those vessels, and also within the infiltrate around focal hair follicles.

BCL-2 was also positive at the base of some hair follicles, along with CD20y. HAM-56 and myeloid/histiocyte antigen were positive in the blister, and in the vessels under the blister. TIMP-1 was positive in the epidermis, and around dermal blood vessels in the inflamatory infiltrate. Metallothionein was positive along the epidermal BMZ, around dermal blood vessels and on selected other dermal cells. No strong expression of HLA-DP, DQ, DR was noted in the blisters; a fibrin was noted in the blisters. No linear, well-defined IgG or Complement/C3 was noted along the BMZ. No vacuolar degeneration was noted along the BMZ. Only a few infiltrate cells around upper dermal blood vessels were positive for CD15(See Figures 1 through 3). Of further interest, myeloperoxidase positive cells amalgamated with HLADRDPDQ and CD45 positive cells along the BMZ, forming rounded bodies (Figures 1 a through c).

Discussion

A diversity of drugs have been associated with the induction of DBP including captopril, ciprofloxacin, penicillamine, penicillins, phenacetin, sulfasalazine, galantamine hydrobromide, levetiracetam, enoxaparin, spironolactone chloroquine, furosemide, ibuprofen, phenacetin, mefenamic acid, nifedipine and others [1-5]. However, most authors do not place much emphasis on pathologic differentiation between classical BP and DBP. The medical literature reports that clinical BPD is very similar to idiopathic or classic clinical BP disease, although the clinical lesions seem to often be polymorphic in BPD [2-5]. The clinical lesions of BPD seem to resemble drug-induced bullous dermatoses, erythema multiforme, eczematous dermatitis or porphyria cutanea tarda [2-5]. The literature states that in DPB, the mucous membranes are often involved; however, in our case no mucosal lesions were noticed. In Table 1, we noted the main differences we were able to find in this DBP case, versus our classic BP cases. In DBP, epidermal and dermal edema were lacking; further, the acantholysis, vacuolar degeneration, and fibrin in the blister were not seen as in classic BP. In our case DIF, we also noticed that our findings seemed to be a slightly different that in classic BP. For examples, in our DBP case, C3C was dotted and non-linear along the BMZ, in contrast to classic BP. Our DBP IgG was also not completely linear and continuous along the BMZ. Our DBP fibrinogen was negative at the BMZ, versus classic BP in which a linear BMZ pattern may be found. For more details, please see Table 1.

Table 1. Comparison and contrast between classic BP and our DBP case, including histopathologic findings and IHC and DIF staining

Disease feature	BP	DBP
Overall H&E	The subepidermal blister contains substantial fibrin, eosinophils and afew dendritic cells within its lumen. Epidermal spongiosis and acantholysis, and vacuolar degeneration of the BMZ are noted. Intraepidermal eosinophilic abscesses may be seen. Dermal edema is noted in the area around the blisters. Some inflammatory cells are noted among dermal cell junctions.	The blister contains little or no fibrin or dendritic cells. Minimal spongiosis, lack of intraepidermal eosinophilic abscesses, and lack of both acantholysis and vacuolar degeneration of the BMZ. Minimal dermal edema around the blisters. Lack of inflammatory cells among dermal cell junctions. No dermal festoons.
Eosinophils	Strong infiltrate around the upper dermal blood vessels, and inside subepidermal blisters.	A few cells within the subepidermal blister lumen, along with perivascular and interstitial infiltrates.
Neutrophils	Usually present with the eosinophils within dermal papillae. Sometimes small numbers are present within the subepidermal blisters.	Often present in significant numbers, especially under the BMZ as well as around upper dermal blood vessels.
Lymphohistiocytic infiltrate	Primarily around the upper dermal blood vessels.	Around upper and intermediate dermal blood vessels, as well as around skin adnexal structures(including hair follicles and eccrine glands).
Myeloperoxidase (IHC)	Positive around the upper dermal blood vessels.	Significantly positive around upper dermal blood vessels and under the BMZ, and/or present within the blister.
CD15 (IHC)	Significantly positive under the BMZ, and around upper dermal blood vessels.	Minimally positive.
CD4 (IHC)	Minimally seen around upper dermal blood vessels, and/or close to the blisters.	Commonly seen around upper dermal blood vessels, and/or close to the blisters.
CD8 (IHC)	Commonly seen around upper dermal blood vessels, and/or the blisters.	Commonly seen around upper dermal blood vessels, and/or the blisters.
CD20(IHC)	Negative.	Positive around the upper dermal blood vessels
CD45 (IHC)	Commonly seen around upper dermal blood vessels.	Commonly seen around upper dermal blood vessels, and/or the blisters.
IgG(DIF)	Linear at the BMZ, as well as on dermal eccrine glands.	Dotted BMZ and/or irregular linear, not complete linear pattern.
Fibrinogen (DIF)	Negative.	Linear pattern at the BMZ.
IgM (DIF)	Linear BMZ pattern, as well as on eccrine glands.	Basically negative.
IgD (DIF)	Similar to patterns of the other immunoglobulins and complement components.	Negative.
IgE (DIF)	Tendency to be linear positive at the BMZ, as well as present around upper dermal blood vessels.	Scattered cells positive in the dermis; spot positivity in the papillary dermis, and around some upper and intermediate dermal blood vessels.
Complement/C3c (DIF).	Linear pattern at the BMZ, as well as on eccrine glands.	Dotted and/or irregular pattern at the BMZ, not completely linear.
Complement/C3d (DIF)	Positive in some upper dermal blood vessels, subjacent to the blisters.	Positive around the upper dermal blood vessels.

In our case, we initially suspected BP; however, following a review of the immune response we rendered a diagnosis of DBP. Many alleged drug reactions are single case reports, particularly with patients taking multiple medications. It is often thus difficult to determine which associations are coincidental, and which are genuine. In occasional reports, recrudescence following re-exposure to the offending agent has been documented. The precise mechanism of drug-induced blistering is unknown, although multiple factors have been suggested, including direct toxicity to BMZ constituents or intercellular junctions with resultant autoantibody production. Thus, the offending drug may function as a hapten, or have similar antigenicity to BMZ components. In our case, serum was not available for study and we could not perform indirect immunofluoresence.

Some histologic features of DBP that have been documented include linear IgG and C3 along the BMZ on DIF. On indirect immunofluorescence, the pertinent antibodies bind to the epidermal side (roof) of salt split skin. In addition, Western immunoblotting has demonstrated that pertinent antibodies react with both the 230 kD BPAGI and 180 kD BP BPAGII antigens. In our case, serum was not available for indirect immunofluoresence. Histologically, drug-induced variants are similar to typical bullous pemphigoid, being characterized by an eosinophil-rich subepidermal blister. Based on the fact that in our practice we routinely test for IgG, IgM, IgA, IgD, IgE, fibrinogen, albumin, complement/C1q and C3c, in most cases of autoimmune BP we have noted that most of our immunoglobulins and complement are positive in a similar pattern along the BMZ and involving dermal eccrine glands. In our case, IgD and IgM were completely negative, contrary what we have occasionally seen in classical BP. Also, in our case, sweat gland reactivity was very weak, and instead most of the reactive markers were noted in the sweat gland ducts. Of interest, we found that cells expressing CD4, CD20 and CD45 were colocalizing with BCL-2; BCL-2 is considered an important anti-apoptotic protein; its gene is classified as an oncogene, and two isoforms has been described [14,15]. However, recent discoveries have noted that BCL-2 molecules are indispensable for activation and maturation of T lymphocytes after antigen presentation [14, 15]. In our case, the colocalization of and B and T cell markers with BCL-2 is consistent with this data and warrants further studies in immunity.

Conclusion

Obtaining a thorough medication history is important when considering a BP diagnosis, as a number of pharmacological agents have been reported to trigger similar phenomena.

Acknowledgments

Mr. Jonathan S. Jones at Georgia Dermatopathology Associates provided excellent technical assistance.

Conflicts of interest: None.

Funding: Georgia Dermatopathology Associates, Atlanta, Georgia, USA

References

[1] Abreu Velez AM, Vasquez-Hincapie DA, Howard MS. Autoimmune basement membrane and subepidermal blistering diseases. *Our Dermatol Online*. 2013; 4(Suppl.3): 647-2.

[2] Lloyd-Lavery A, Chi CC, Wojnarowska F, Taghipour K. The associations between bullous pemphigoid and drug use: a UK case-control study. *JAMA Dermatol.* 2013;149:58-2.

[3] Warner C, Kwak Y, Glover MH, Davis LS. Bullous pemphigoid induced by hydrochlorothiazide therapy. *J Drugs Dermatol.*2014;13:360-2.

[4] Karadag AS, Bilgili SG, Calka O, Onder S, Kosem M, Burakgazi-Dalkilic E. A case of levetiracetam induced bullous pemphigoid. *Cutan Ocul Toxicol*. 2013,32:176-8.

[5] Kashihara M, Danno K, Miyachi Y, Horiguchi Y, Imamura S. Bullous pemphigoid-like lesions induced by phenacetin. Report of a case and an immunopathologic study. *Arch Dermatol.*1984,120:1196-9.

[6] Lee JJ, Downham TF II. Furosemide-induced bullous pemphigoid: case report and review of literature. *J Drugs Dermatol*. 2006;5:562-4.

[7] Diab M, Coloe J, Bechtel MA. Bullous pemphigoid precipitated by galantamine hydrobromide. *Cutis*. 2009;83:139-0.

[8] Abreu Velez AM, Calle-Isaza J, Howard MS. A case of bullous pemphigoid with immunoreactivty to blood vessels and sweat glands. *Our Dermatol Online*. 2013; 4(Suppl.3): 621-4.

[9] Abreu Velez, AM, Barth G, Howard MS. Thrombomodulin overexpression surrounding a subepidermal bullous allergic drug. *Our Dermatol Online*. 2013; 4: 514-6.

[10] Abreu Velez AM, Smith JG Jr, Howard MS. IgG/IgE bullous pemphigoid with CD45 lymphocytic reactivity to dermal blood vessels, nerves and eccrine sweat glands. *North Am J Med Sci*. 2010**;** 2: 538-1.

[11] Abreu Velez AM, Howard MS. Collagen IV in normal skin and in pathologic processes. North Am J Med Sci. 2012; 4:1-8.

[12] Abreu Velez AM, Brown VM, Howard MS. Cytotoxic and antigen presenting cells present and non-basement membrane zone pathology in a case of bullous pemphigoid. *Our Dermatol Online,* 2012; 3(2): 93-99. DOI: 10.7241/ourd.20122.19

[13] Abreu Velez AM, Girard JG, Howard MS. IgG bullous pemphigoid with antibodies to IgD, dermal blood vessels, eccrine glands and the endomysium of monkey esophagus. *Our Dermatol Online.* 2011; 2(2): 48-51.

[14] Droin NM, Green DR. Role of Bcl-2 family members in immunity and disease. *Biochimica et Biophysica Acta.* 2004; 1644:179– 188.

[15] Farsaci B, Sabzevari H, Higgins JP, Di Bari MG, Takai S, Schlom J, Hodge JW. Effect of a small molecule BCL-2 inhibitor on immune function and use with a recombinant vaccine. *Int. J. Cancer*: 2010;127, 1603–1613.

In: Advances in Dermatology Research
Editor: James P. Vega
ISBN: 978-1-63482-226-8

Chapter 6

Bullous Pemphigoid due to Anti-TNFalpha

Vincenzo Bettoli, Stefania Zauli, Michela Ricci and Annarosa Virgili*
Department of Medical Sciences, Section of Dermatology,
University of Ferrara, Arcispedale S. Anna, Ferrara, Italy

Abstract

Anti-tumor necrosis factor-α (TNFα) agents are increasingly being used for rapidly expanding number of autoimmune diseases, principally cutaneous, rheumatic and gastroenterological. With this use and longer follow-up periods of treatment, there are a growing number of reports of the development of autoimmune processes related to the use of anti-TNFα (cutaneous vasculitis, lupus-like syndrome, systemic lupus erythematosus and interstitial lung disease). Despite anti-TNFα can be used to treat severe forms of autoimmune bullous skin diseases, few cases of pemphigus vulgaris and bullous pemphigoid occurring under anti-TNFα therapy have been described. The triggering role of anti-TNFα blockers remains unclear but it can not be excluded that they could be an immunologic trigger for autoimmune conditions in predisposed individuals. These drugs may act as triggers by either modifying the immune response or altering the antigenic properties of the cutaneous antigens. Based on authors' experience it seems that different type of anti-TNFα blockers influences the immune response in different way.

The authors propose our personal experience and a review of the cases of autoimmune bullous skin diseases induced by anti-TNFα agents reported in literature.

* Correspondence to: Dr. Stefania Zauli MD, Department of Medical Sciences, Section of Dermatology, Azienda Ospedaliera Universitaria di Ferrara, Arcispedale Sant'Anna, Ferrara, Via Aldo Moro 8, 44124 Cona [FE], Italy, Tel: +39 0532 688129; Fax: +39 0532 206791, E-mail: stefania.zauli@libero.it

Introduction

Tumour necrosis factor-alpha (TNFα) is a cytokine that plays a crucial role in causing inflammation by means of predominantly T-cell-mediated tissue damage. TNFα have been clearly identified as having a pivotal role in different kinds of autoimmune/inflammatory diseases. For this reason anti-TNFα agents have increasingly being used for rapidly expanding number of diseases principally cutaneous, rheumatic and gastroenterological. The autoimmune bullous skin diseases, pemphigus vulgaris and bullous pemphigoid, are included in the list of diseases that benefiting from the treatment with TNFα blockers.

In particular, in bullous pemphigoid the mast cell are responsible for the secretion of TNFα. The serum level of TNFα are reported to be correlated with both the severity and number of lesions, and also blister fluid contains high level of this cytokine [1].

Etanercept, Infliximab, and Adalimumab are the anti-TNFα agents developed to date.

Etanercept is an artificially engineered dimeric fusion protein that mimics the inhibitory effects of naturally occurring soluble TNFα receptors.

Infliximab and Adalimumab are monoclonal antibodies that work by binding to TNF-α thus preventing it from activating TNF receptors. Infliximab is a genetically engineered antibody consisting of 25% murine sequences in the variable region of the antibody, while Adalimumab is a human antibody.

Probably these drugs with different mechanism of action and biosimilarity, influence the immune system in different ways [2].

Despite the anti-TNFα drugs have been used successfully in the treatment of different types of autoimmune/inflammatory diseases, with these use and longer follow-up periods of treatment, unexpectedly there are a growing number of reports of the development of autoimmune processes related to the use of anti-TNFα agents. These autoimmune adverse processes mainly include cutaneous vasculitis, lupus-like syndrome, systemic lupus erythematosus and interstitial lung disease [3] but only a few cases of pemphigus vulgaris and bullous pemphigoid occurring under therapy have also been described (Table 1) [4-8].

In 2008, Ramos-Casals et al. reviewed 379 cases of autoimmune diseases secondary to anti-TNFα agents through a baseline Medline search of articles published between January 1990 and May 2008. Among those cases, there were no reports of autoimmune bullous skin disease [3].

In 2008, Daulat et al. first described a case of pemphigus vulgaris occurring during anti-TNFα therapy (Etanercept) [4]. In 2009, Stausbol-Gron et al. first described a case of bullous pemphigoid occurring during Adalimumab administration [5]. A further case of bullous pemphigoid due to Etanercept has been described in 2009 by Bordignon et al. in a patient with rheumatoid arthritis [6].

In 2010, Boussemart et al. described two cases of autoimmune bullous skin diseases occurring during anti-TNFα therapy: one case of bullous pemphigoid under Adalimumab treatment and one of pemphigus fogliaceus under Infliximab treatment [7]. A further case of bullous pemphigoid related to Etanercept in a psoriatic patient has been reported by Kluk et al, in 2011 [8]. All patients improved after discontinuation of the suspect drug and administration of systemic corticosteroid treatment [4-8]. A case of pemphigus in a patient with pustular psoriasis treated with Infliximab has been also reported, but this patient had also a high malignant non Hodgkin lymphoma. Therefore in this case the pemphigus could be defined as paraneoplastic [9]. The latency period between drug beginning and the onset of skin manifestations seems variable, from 2 months [short-time] to 3 years [long-time] [4-8].

Recently, the authors have been described a further case of bullous pemphigoid occurring in a patient undergoing Infliximab (5 mg/kg) for Ulcerative Colitis. Twenty days after the second infusion [during the induction phase] she developed an itching urticarial eruption located on her trunk and limbs.

Table 1. Revision of the cases of autoimmune bullous disease reported in literature [4-8]

Authors, years of pubblication	Disease	Anti-TNFα drug [dosage]	Latency	Bullous disease
Daulat et al, 2008	Psoriasis	Etanercept [50 mg sc 1 or 2 weekly]	2 years	Pemphigus vulgaris
Stausbol-Gron et al, 2009	Psoriatic arthritis	Adalimumab [40 mg sc every 2 weeks]	12 weeks	Bullous pemphigoid
Bordignon et al, 2009	Rheumatoid arthritis	Etanercept [25 mg sc twice weekly]	2 years	Bullous pemphigoid
Boussemart et al, 2010	Rheumatoid arthritis	Adalimumab [40 mg sc every 2 weeks]	3 years	Bullous pemphigoid
Boussemart et al, 2010	Rheumatoid arthritis	Infliximab [3 mg/Kg]	7 months	Pemphigus vulgaris
Kluk et al, 2011	Psoriasis	Etanercept [25 mg sc twice weekly]	2 months	Bullous pemphigoid

Over several days this eruption developed into blisters on erythematous skin. Nikolsky's sign was negative. The mucosae were not involved. Histological examination of skin biopsy revealed a superficial dermal inflammation consisting of lymphocytes. Deposition of IgG and C3 along the basement membrane was detected by direct immunofluorescence, confirming the clinical suspect of bullous pemphigoid. In the absence of any other known cause, the authors considered the chimeric anti-TNFα drug as a possible inducing factor.

For this reason Infliximab was stopped while systemic corticosteroids were started to keep both dermatologic and gastrointestinal disease under control.

After the resolution of the skin eruption, the patient started another anti-TNFα [Adalimumab, 40 mg s.c. every other week after the induction phase] obtaining clinical improvement of Ulcerative Colitis in one month [10]. After five months the patient still maintains complete clinical remission. Surprisingly vesicular-bullous lesions did not appear during the treatment with this human anti-TNFα, confirming as probably the two drugs influence the immune system in different ways [2].

Pemphigus and the pemphigoid group are autoimmune conditions in which autoantibodies cause skin blistering secondary to loss of connections between skin cells. Pemphigus is characterized by intraepidermal blister due to antibodies that recognize cell adhesion molecules, the desmogleins. A small group of patients can develop pemphigus after certain medications, principally penicillamine and captopril [6]. In the bullous pemphigoid autoantibodies are specific for the hemidesmosomal bullous pemphigoid antigens BP230 and collagen type XVII, so the blister detachment is subepidermal. Bullous pemphigoid can be induced by systemic ingestion or local use of certain drugs. Two main types of drug-induced bullous pemphigoid may be distinguished: an acute, self-limited variety showing definitive resolution after the withdrawal of the culprit drug [drug-induced bullous pemphigoid] and a chronic type that seems merely to precipitate by drug administration. In the long run it assumes the characteristics of the classic disease [drug-triggered bullous pemphigoid] [11].

In predisposed individuals, drugs may act as triggers by either modifying the immune response or altering the antigenic properties of the cutaneous antigens [12].

The triggering role of anti-TNFα blockers remains unclear. It seems that the ability of an anti-TNFα agent to induce or to cure an autoimmune disease is associated with the immunological profile of each patient, and, more specifically, it depends on the level of INFγ and IL-4 [1].

To conclude, the possibility of an autoimmune cutaneous bullous disease should be considered when managing patients who are under treatment with biological agents. Conversely, TNFα antagonist can be an effective alternative therapy for these diseases.

Further studies need to establish the efficacy of anti-TNFα in the treatment of autoimmune bullous disorders and to solve this controversy.

References

[1] Stavropoulos PG, Soura E, Antoniou C. Drug-induced pemphigoid: a review of the literature. *J. Eur. Acad. Dermatol. Venereol* 2014;doi:10.1111/jdv.12366.

[2] Sands BE, Blank MA, Patel K, van Deventer SJ. Long-term treatment of rectovaginal fistulas in Crohn's disease: response to infliximab in the ACCENT II Study. *Clin. Gastroenterol. Hepatol.* 2004;2:912-920.

[3] Ramos-Casals M, Brito-Zerón P, Soto MJ, Cuadrado MJ, Khamashta MA. Autoimmune diseases induced by TNF-targeted therapies. *Best Pract. Res. Clin. Rheumatol.* 2008;22:847-861.

[4] Daulat S, Detweiler JG, Pandya AG. Development of pemphigus vulgaris in a patient with psoriasis treated with etanercept. *J. Eur. Acad. Dermatol. Venereol* 2009;23:483-484.

[5] Stausbøl-Grøn B, Deleuran M, Sommer Hansen E, Kragballe K. Development of bullous pemphigoid during treatment of psoriasis with adalimumab. *Clin. Exp. Dermatol.* 2009;34:285-286.

[6] Bordignon M, Belloni-Fortina A, Pigozzi B, Tarantello M, Alaibac M. Bullous pemphigoid during long-term TNF-alpha blocker therapy. *Dermatology* 2009;219:357-358.

[7] Boussemart L, Jacobelli S, Batteux F, et al. Autoimmune bullous skin diseases occurring under anti-tumor necrosis factor therapy: two case reports. *Dermatology* 2010;221:201-205.

[8] Kluk J, Goulding JM, Bhat J, Finch TM. Drug-induced bullous pemphigoid: cases triggered by intravenous iodine and etanercept. *Clin. Exp. Dermatol.* 2011;36:871-873.

[9] Scholberl A, Allmacher C, Flegl N, Krahl B, Krahl D, Amon U. Paraneoplastic pemphigus due to high malignant non Hodgkin lymphoma in a patient with pustular psoriasis treated with infliximab. *Aktuelle Dermatologie* 2010;36:129-132.

[10] Ricci M, Zauli S, Zelante A, Trevisani L, Virgili A, Bettoli V. Bullous pemphigoid occurring under anti-tumor necrosis factor-α therapy. *Int. J. Colorectal. Dis.* 2014;29:1573-1574.

[11] Ruocco V, Sacerdoti G. Pemphigus and bullous pemphigoid due to drugs. *Int. J. Dermatol.* 1991;30:307-312.

[12] Lo Schiavo A, Ruocco E, Brancaccio G, Caccavale S, Ruocco V, Wolf R. Bullous pemphigoid: etiology, pathogenesis, and inducing factors: facts and controversies. *Clin. Dermatol.* 2013;31:391-399.

In: Advances in Dermatology Research
Editor: James P. Vega
ISBN: 978-1-63482-226-8

Chapter 7

Desquamative Gingivitis as an Oral Manifestation of Mucous Membrane Pemphigoid: Diagnosis and Treatment

Hiroyasu Endo[*,1], *Terry D. Rees*[2], *Hideo Niwa*[3], *Kayo Kuyama*[4], *Hirotsugu Yamamoto*[4] *and Takanori Ito*[1]

[1]Department of Oral Diagnosis, Nihon University, School of Dentistry at Matsudo, Japan
[2]Department of Periodontics, Texas A&M University Baylor College of Dentistry, Dallas, TX, US
[3]Department of Head and Neck Surgery, Nihon University, School of Dentistry at Matsudo, Japan
[4]Department of Oral Pathology, Nihon University, School of Dentistry at Matsudo, Japan

Abstract

Mucous membrane pemphigoid (MMP) is one of a group of autoimmune, subepithelial blistering diseases that predominantly affect mucous membranes. Desquamative gingivitis (DG) is a common manifestation of MMP. Both histopathological examination and direct immunofluorescence testing are essential to establish a final diagnosis. Early recognition and treatment of MMP can improve the prognosis, but diagnostic delays are common in DG because obtaining a diagnostic biopsy is technically challenging. The stab-and-roll biopsy technique is designed to prevent the epithelium from being removed from the biopsy specimen. The complications caused by scarring and associated loss of function often require surgical intervention in MMP patients. Early diagnosis of MMP is critical, and immunosuppressive treatment may prevent serious complications in mucous membranes.

* Corresponding author: Dr. Hiroyasu Endo, Department of Oral Diagnosis, Nihon University School of Dentistry at Matsudo, 2-870-1 Sakaecho Nishi, Matsudo Chiba, Japan 271-8587, TEL: 81-47-360-9423, FAX: 81-47-360-9426, E-mail address: endo.hiroyasu@nihon-u.ac.jp.

Introduction

Mucous membrane pemphigoid (MMP) is a group of putative autoimmune, chronic inflammatory, subepithelial blistering diseases that predominantly affect mucous membranes [1]. MMP is characterized by linear deposition of IgG, IgA, IgM or C3 along the epithelial basement membrane zone in direct immunofluorescence testing [1, 2]. Most patients with MMP are between 60 and 80 years of age. However, on relatively rare occasions, blistering disorders such as MMP have been reported in children, adolescents or young adults [3]. It affects women at a greater ratio of at least 2:1 compared to men [1, 4, 5]. Oral lesions are observed in 85-90% cases, and the primary lesions often appear in the oral cavity [1, 4, 5]. MMP can involve any oral mucosal site: gingival, buccal or labial mucosa, hard or soft palate, alveolar ridge, or tongue, although the gingiva is affected far more often than other oral tissues. In more than half of early cases, the gingiva is the only site of lesions [4, 6, 7]. Patients with MMP often initially report only oral symptoms of pain and discomfort (Table 1) and therefore often visit the dentist before other health care workers. Desquamative gingivitis (DG) is a common manifestation of MMP, probably because the usual mouth functions such as chewing, exposure to hot foods and liquids, and oral hygiene measures traumatize the gingiva, resulting in tissue sloughing [4, 7, 8]. This chapter presents the clinical and diagnostic features of DG, as a common oral manifestation of MMP. The current literature on the diagnostic and therapeutic modalities of DG associated with MMP is reviewed.

Table 1. Reported oral symptoms in patients with MMP

gingival pain
burning sensation, particularly after eating salty or spicy foods
easy bleeding
blister formation
redness of gum
gingival desquamation

Modified from Endo et al. [4], Endo and Rees [9], Nisengard and Levine [10]

Desquamative Gingivitis

DG is a clinical manifestation that is common to several diseases or disorders [9-11]. It is characterized by localized or generalized epithelial desquamation, erythema, erosion of the gingival epithelium, and/or blister formation on the gingiva (Figure 1). Nikolsky's sign often shows a positive reaction in patients with DG (Figure 2). This sign involves the application of a shearing force on normal-appearing gingiva, producing epithelial desquamation [12]. Most cases of DG are caused by mucocutaneous diseases [9, 11, 13]. The differential diagnoses include MMP, oral lichen planus, and pemphigus vulgaris [9, 11, 13]. Contact allergic reactions to various oral hygiene products have also been reported in the differential diagnosis of DG [14, 15]. It is impossible to diagnose MMP from the clinical presence of DG lesions alone. The appropriate use of biopsies to perform histopathologic and direct immunofluorescence examination of lesional and peri-lesional tissues is required to establish the final diagnosis [9, 11]. Obtaining diagnostic gingival biopsies from MMP patients is technically challenging. The excised gingival tissue tends to be fragile because disruption of the epithelial cell-to-basement membrane adhesion components is likely to occur. This situation may often result in detachment of the gingival epithelium from the underlying connective tissue, causing a failure in biopsy diagnosis. This tissue friability, coupled with an inadequate surgical technique, surgical site selection or improper tissue handling, may easily lead to the loss of the gingival epithelium, causing a failure in histopathologic and direct immunofluorescence diagnosis. Because of this, some authors have stated that if lesions are present at several mucosal sites, including the gingiva, it is usually best not to use the gingiva for biopsies [16-18]. However, in approximately 60% of the MMP patients, the gingiva was the only site of involvement [6] and in these cases, the gingiva should be selected as the biopsy site. Recently the authors developed and validated a biopsy technique (the stab-and-roll technique) to maintain the gingival epithelium/connective tissue union in DG patients [19] (Figure 3). In this technique, the operator applies gentle pressure on the gingiva with the tip of a #15 blade until the bone surface is reached, and then the blade is rolled from the tip along the entire cutting edge. If a larger specimen is needed the tip of the blade can be repositioned and the rolling stroke extended. This stab-and-roll biopsy technique prevents the occurrence of lateral shear forces. In contrast in the conventional gingival biopsy technique, the scalpel blade is pulled across the biopsy site while the tip of the blade is against the bone surface. This potentially creates a lateral shear force potentially causing the epithelium to be displaced from the biopsy specimen. A total lack of epithelium has been reported in 40% [20] - 41.2% [21] of gingival biopsy samples using the conventional biopsy technique whereas in a series of 52 gingival biopsies only 1.9% of the samples obtained using the stab-and-roll biopsy technique resulted in epithelium-connective tissue separation [19]. Some authors are concerned that gingival biopsies may result in permanent periodontal defects [20, 21]. Indeed, since many DG lesions develop in the anterior facial area, resultant periodontal defects could be an esthetic problem. To prevent this difficulty, stab-and-roll biopsies are often taken from perilesional tissues apical to the free gingival margin. This site selection also prevents the biopsy tissue from being obscured by gingival inflammation (Figure 4).

Specific Site Consideration

Extraoral MMP lesions have been reported on skin including the external genitalia and perianal skin as well as on the mucous membranes of the eye, nose, pharynx, larynx, esophagus, and anus [1, 22]. Although scarring is rarely a feature of oral MMP, in extraoral sites scar formation may lead to an irreversible loss of function of the affected areas. Sight-threatening ocular scarring [23-25] and life-threatening upper airway obstruction [26-28] have been reported. In contrast, only one case report has described oral scarring. Sato et al. [29] reported microstomia associated with MMP exhibiting anti-laminin 332 autoantibodies. Scar contracture was ring-shaped and localized on the oral mucosa. A commissuroplasty was performed in treatment using 5-flap Z-plasty on the upper lip and 2-flap Z-plasty on the lower lip. The patient was reported to be satisfied with the postoperative esthetics and the size of the oral aperture.

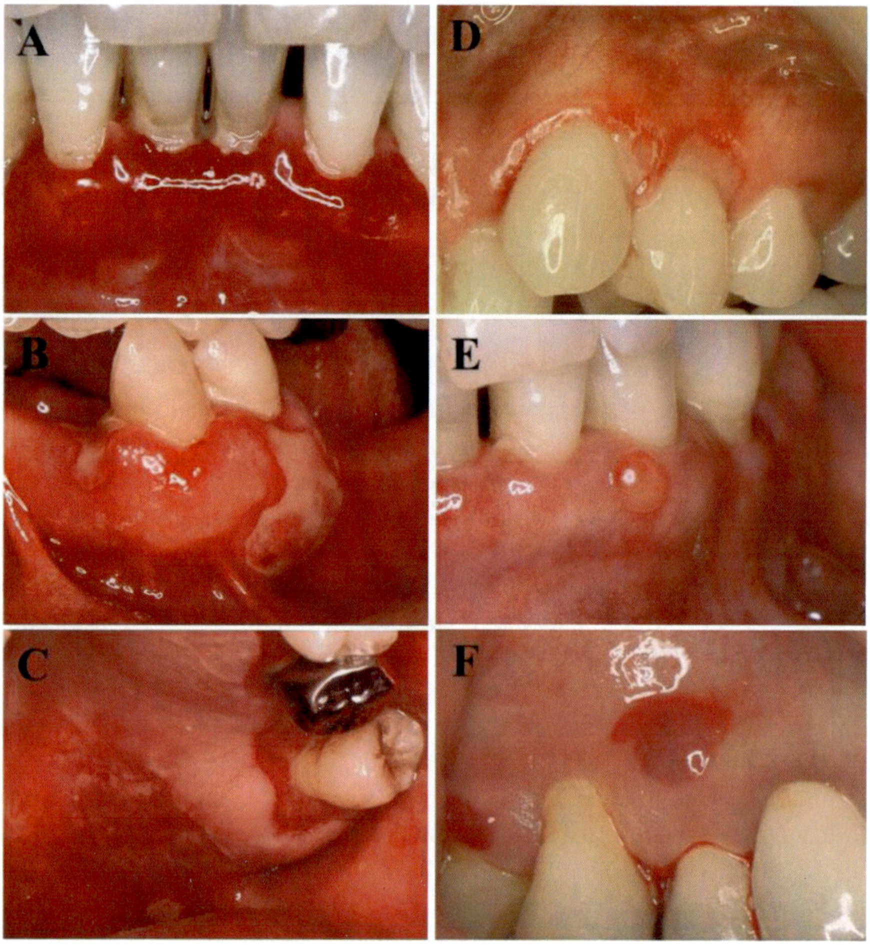

Figure 1. Clinical presentation of DG associated with MMP. (A) Erythema. (B) Pseudomembrane-covered erosion. (C) Erosion. (D) Ulceration. (E) Blister formation. (F) Localized blood-filled blister formation.

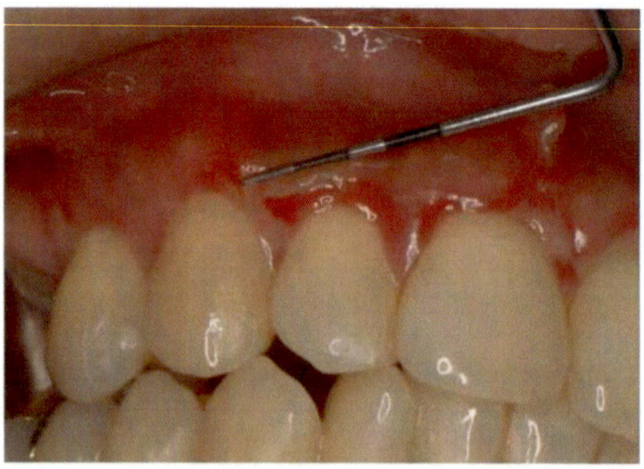

Figure 2. Positive Nikolsky's sign in a patient with MMP. Gentle palpation with the periodontal probe elicited some desquamation of the gingival surface.

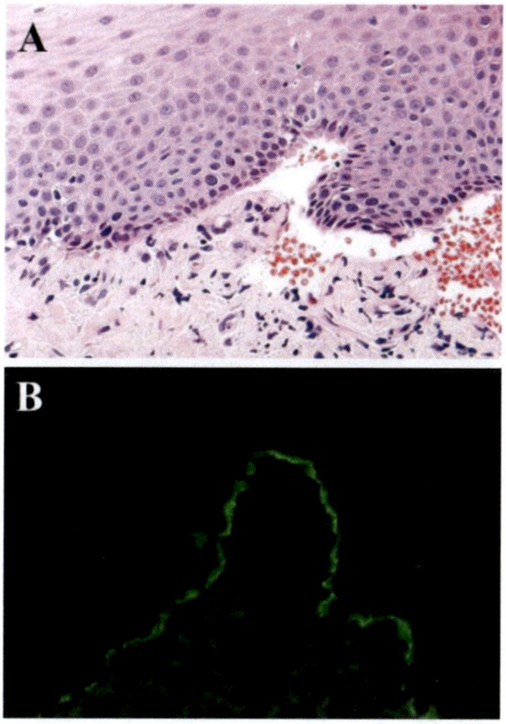

Figure 3. Histopathologic and direct immunofluorescence features of MMP. Gingival biopsies were performed using the stab-and-roll technique. (A) Hematoxylin- and eosin-stained section (Original magnification x400). Subepithelial bulla formation. (B) Direct immunofluorescence section (Original magnification x200). A linear deposition of IgG along the basement membrane zone.

In a previous study, an incidence of only 10.4% (10/96) ocular lesions was reported in MMP associated DG patients [30]. Consequently, patients with exclusively intraoral MMP were thought to have a less severe disease that might not be associated with ocular involvement [7, 31]. However, a recent study indicated 30% (9/30) of patients with oral MMP had ocular involvement at presentation to an opthalmologist [24]. Another study of 25 patients who initially had only oral involvement reported that 4 (16%) developed ocular lesions within 5 years [25]. These studies indicate that MMP patients with initial oral lesions have a risk of developing ocular involvement with a calculated incidence rate from 0.03 [24] to 0.05 [25] person per year. Some specific oral symptoms are common in individuals likely to have oral MMP (Table 1). The presence of these symptoms should increase the healthcare provider's level of suspicion of a mucocutaneous disease such as MMP. Symptoms suggestive of possible ocular involvement in patients with MMP are shown in Table 2. MMP patients with oral involvement, however, frequently have asymptomatic ocular lesions, especially in the early stages of ocular disease [24, 25]. These observations indicate that all patients diagnosed with intraoral or extraoral MMP should undergo ophthalmic examination by an ophthalmologist (Figure 5). Patients with oral MMP should have regular opthalmologic monitoring every 6 to 12 months, even if no ocular involvement is identified at initial diagnosis [24].

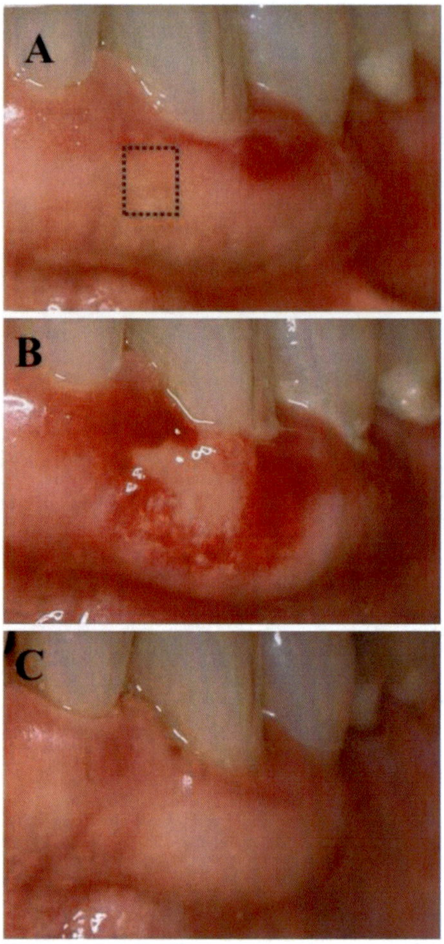

Figure 4. Periodontal conditions after gingival biopsy. The periodontal defects or recessions did not occur after the gingival biopsy using the stab-and-roll technique. (A) Before biopsy. The gingival sample was removed from the dotted-line area. (B) 1 week after biopsy. (C) 6 months after biopsy.

Table 2. Symptoms possibly related to ocular involvement in patients with MMP

burning sensation
dryness
foreign body sensation
irritation
excess tearing
mucous production
photophobia
blurry vision
decreased visual acuity

Modified from Fleming and Korman [5], Kourosh and Yancey [22]

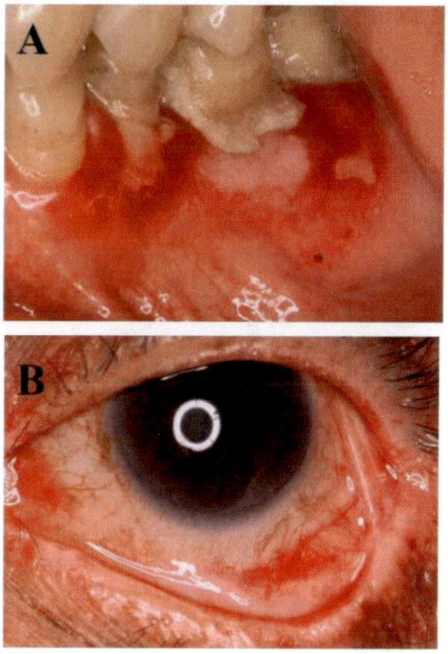

Figure 5. Ocular involvement in a DG patient with MMP. (A) Desquamative lesions featuring gingival erythema. (B) Ophthalmic examination by an opthalmologist revealed lower conjunctiva symblepharon in the same patient.

Patients with MMP restricted to the upper airway tract are rarely observed [26, 27]. More than 84% of MMP patients with upper airway involvement had oral lesions [26, 27]. Despite this, reports of the upper airway involvement in DG patients are scarce. One report described a case of MMP in a young patient presenting with DG and laryngeal manifestations that resulted in severe life-threatening sequels of events [32]. Symptoms that should raise suspicion regarding the presence of upper airway involvement in patients with MMP are shown in Table 3. When DG patients complain of these symptoms, they should be seen by an otolaryngologist for evaluation and possible endoscopic examination of the upper airway tract (Figure 6).

Table 3. Symptoms suggestive of possible upper airway involvement in patients with MMP

nasal stuffiness
nasal bleeding or blood-tinged mucous discharge
cough
hoarseness
difficult or labored breath
continuous inspiratory musical sound of variable pitch
sore throat
pain on swallowing
dysphonia

Modified from Alexandre et al. [26], Higgins et al. [27]

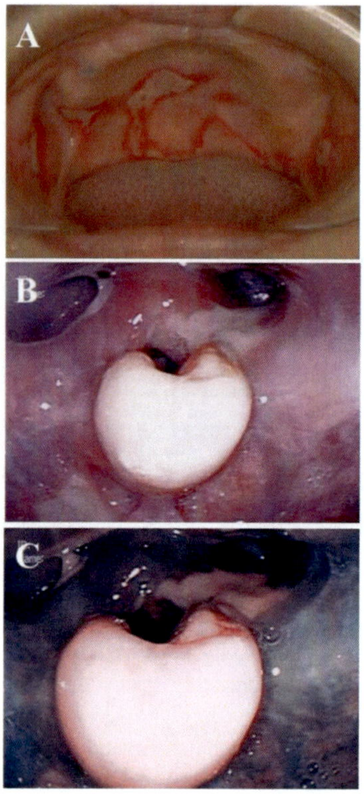

Figure 6. Laryngeal involvement in a DG patient with MMP. (A) Desquamative lesions of soft palate in addition to gingiva. The patient complained of chronic cough and sore throat. (B) Conventional endoscopic examination revealed white coat of the epiglottis and the aryepiglottic fold. The involvements are consistent with MMP early lesions. (C) Narrow band image (NBI) enhanced and defined white coat MMP.

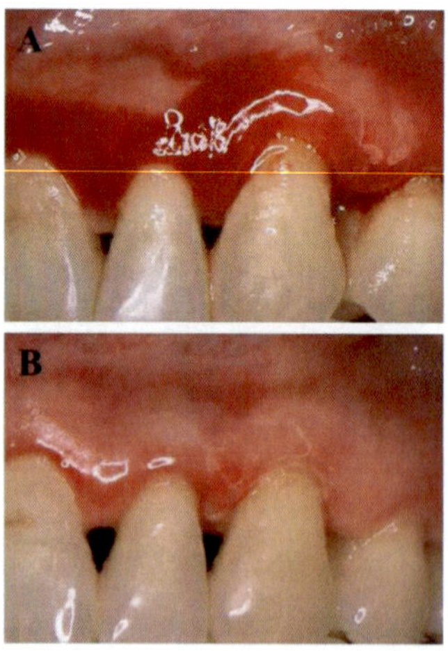

Figure 7. Topical corticosteroid therapy in a DG patient with MMP. (A) The initial examination revealed localized erythematous gingiva. (B) The gingival lesions went into remission with the topical corticosteroid therapy.

Managing Patients with Desquamative Gingivitis

The therapeutic goal for DG lesions is the remission or suppression of the clinical signs and symptoms. The severity of the DG lesions, the presence or absence of extraoral lesions, and the medical history of the patient are key factors in determining the selection of a topical or systemic treatment. In most cases, topical therapy alone is sufficient to achieve resolution of lesions when MMP is diagnosed and treated in its early stages. When MMP affects the oral cavity as the sole involvement, moderate to very high-potency topical corticosteroids are effective and widely used for treatment [6, 9] (Figure 7). The absorption of topical corticosteroids may increase in the presence of DG, since the continuity of intact epithelium may be disrupted. In 1990, Plemons et al. [33] studied the systemic uptake of high-potency topical corticosteroid gel (0.05% fluocinonide gel) applied to oral desquamative diseases three times daily for 3 weeks. They found no evidence of adrenal suppression in the study population. Occlusive steroid therapy using a plastic stent may be used to enhance the effect of topical corticosteroid therapy by maximizing the contact between the corticosteroids applied on the gingiva [34, 35] (Figure 8). In this therapy, the topical corticosteroid is in contact with the gingiva for a longer time period and the systemic absorption is probably increased thus enhancing the effect of the topical agent. To date there are no studies documenting medical complications related to the intraoral use of very high potency topical corticosteroids, but caution should be used when providing occlusive steroid therapy for patients afflicted with hypertension, gastrointestinal ulcers or diabetes mellitus, pending further study. Secondary candidosis is the most common side effect from topical corticosteroid therapy (Figure 9). Oral candidosis should be suspected in patients that continue to complain of oral symptoms despite several days or weeks of topical therapy.

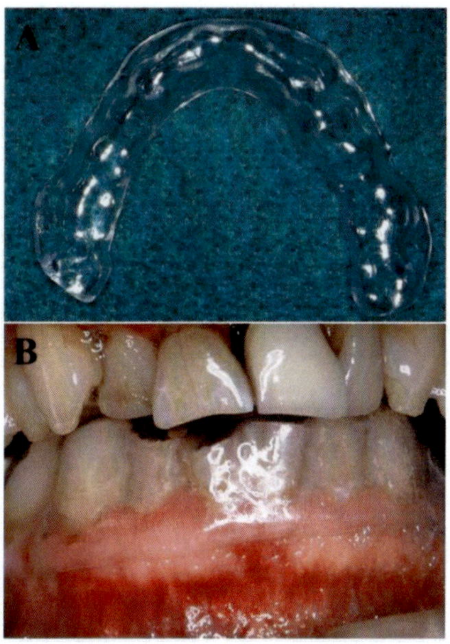

Figure 8. Occlusive steroid therapy using a plastic stent in a DG patient with MMP. (A) Plastic stent for mandibular arch. (B) Stent in place.

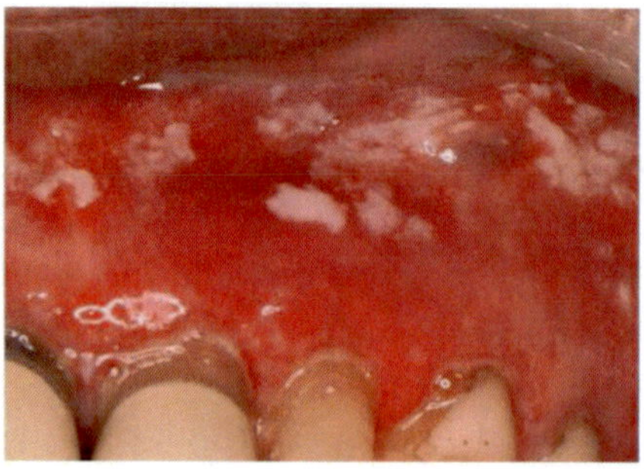

Figure 9. Secondary candidosis in a DG patient with MMP. During the topical steroid therapy period, gingival candidosis occurred. The symptoms disappeared after an antifungal medication was administered.

Patients with severe and/or multiple oral lesions, or recalcitrant lesions, may need aggressive systemic treatment [36]. The presence of extraoral lesions also may require systemic corticosteroids and/or immunosuppressive drugs for effective MMP management. Careful medical management is necessary to monitor the patient for adverse effects of systemic drugs and to manage concomitant systemic diseases. Although extraoral MMP lesions involving erythema, erosion, ulceration, or blister formation will respond well to medical immunosuppressive therapy, the treatment will be highly resistant if fibrosis and scarring has occurred [22]. The complications caused by scarring and associated loss of function often require surgical and/or medical intervention. Airway obstruction is the most serious complication and may necessitate an emergency tracheotomy [26-28]. Ocular lesions occur most often in association with DG and may induce inflammation, loss of tear film, progressive scarring and adherence of the eyelid to the eyeball (symblepharon), inward turning of the eyelashes (triachiasis), and inward turning of the eyelids (entropion) [5, 22]. Unless treated aggressively, these lesions can lead to loss of vision in one or both eyes [37]. Early diagnosis of MMP is critical and immunosuppressive treatment may prevent scar formation in mucous membrane.

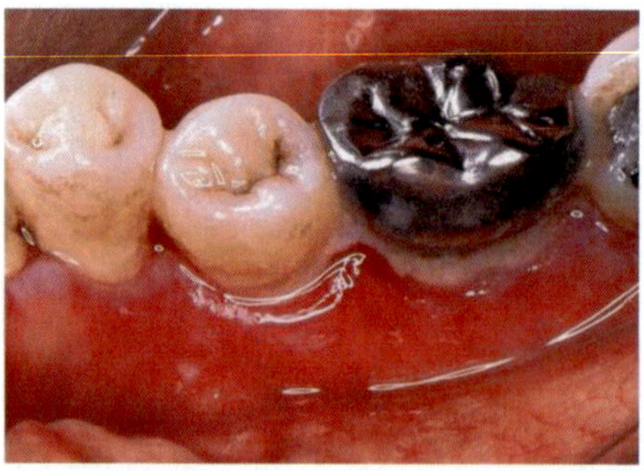

Figure 10. Poor oral hygiene status in a DG patient with MMP. Dental plaque and calculus deposits were recognized around teeth.

Periodontal Considerations

It is often very difficult for DG patients to clean their teeth due to pain and bleeding, and patients often fear to create new lesions on the gingiva. Therefore, their oral hygiene is likely to be ineffective, making it difficult to treat this condition (Figure 10). For this reason, some authorities have stated that desquamative lesion of the gingiva could lead to periodontal destruction and bone loss, necessitating tooth extractions [5, 37]. However, little information is available regarding the periodontal conditions of patients with DG associated with MMP. The relationship between the existence of MMP lesions and progression of periodontal diseases is inconclusive. Arduino et al. [38] demonstrated that periodontal status is worse in MMP patients compared with healthy controls because of substantial differences in oral hygiene. Conversely, Tricamo et al. [39] and Schellinck et al. [40] suggested that MMP patients demonstrate higher levels of gingival inflammation, but not chronic periodontitis compared to healthy age and sex matched controls even after at least a 5 year history of MMP. Plaque accumulation may be an aggravation factor to make DG worse. Plaque-related gingivitis is almost universal in patients with painful gingival lesions and an effective therapeutic protocol should include non-surgical periodontal therapy consisting of oral hygiene instruction, scaling, and root planing [41]. Orrico et al. [42] affirmed that plaque control performed by a professional and the application of 0.12% chlorhexidine digluconate resulted in 90% improvement of gingival lesions in MMP patients. Professional oral hygiene treatment and detailed oral hygiene instructions are connected with improvement of gingival status and a decrease in gingival-related pain in patients affected by MMP with DG lesions [43]. Combined treatment and long-term maintenance of MMP and periodontal disease are effective at improving and stabilizing the gingival conditions in MMP patients [44-46].

Conclusion

Early signs and symptoms of MMP develop in the oral cavity in almost all cases, and DG is a common manifestation. After MMP is diagnosed from DG or concomitant lesions, patients should undergo examination by medical specialists including an opthalmologist and an otolaryngologist, and the presence or absence of extraoral mucosal lesions should be determined. Scarring may lead to an irreversible loss of function of the affected extraoral mucous membranes in some MMP cases. Early recognition and treatment of the diseases is very important and can significantly improve the prognosis.

References

[1] Chan, LS; Ahmed, AR; Anhalt, GJ; et al. The first international consensus on mucous membrane pemphigoid: definition, diagnostic criteria, pathogenic factors, medical treatment, and prognostic indicators. *Arch Dermatol*, 2002, 138(3), 370-379.

[2] Rinaggio, J; Crossland, DM; Zeid, MY. A determination of the range of oral conditions submitted for microscopic and direct immunofluorescence analysis. *J Periodontol*, 2007, 78(10), 1904-1910.

[3] Cheng, YS; Rees, TD; Wright, JM; Plemons, JM. Childhood oral pemphigoid: a case report and review of the literature. *J Oral Pathol Med*, 2001, 30(6), 372-377.
[4] Endo, H; Rees, TD; Kuyama, K; Kono, Y; Yamamoto, H. Clinical and diagnostic features of mucous membrane pemphigoid. *Compend Contin Educ Dent*, 2006, 27(9), 512-516, quiz 517-518.
[5] Fleming TE; Korman NJ. Cicatricial pemphigoid. *J Am Acad Dermatol*, 2000, 43(4), 571-591, quiz 591-594.
[6] Lamey, PJ; Rees, TD; Binnie, WH; Rankin, KV. Mucous membrane pemphigoid. Treatment experience at two institutions. *Oral Surg Oral Med Oral Pathol*, 1992, 74(1), 50-53.
[7] Mobini, N; Nagarwalla, N; Ahmed, AR. Oral pemphigoid. Subset of cicatricial pemphigoid? *Oral Surg Oral Med Oral Pathol Oral Radiol Endod*, 1998, 85(1), 37-43.
[8] Carrozzo, M; Cozzani, E; Broccoletti, R; et al. Analysis of antigens targeted by circulating IgG and IgA antibodies in patients with mucous membrane pemphigoid predominantly affecting the oral cavity. *J Periodontol*, 2004, 75(10), 1302-1308.
[9] Endo, H; Rees, TD. Diagnosis and management of desquamative gingivitis. In: Panagakos FS, Davies RM, eds. Gingival Diseases - Their Aetiology, Prevention and Treatment. Rijeka, Croatia: InTech; 2011; 171-188. Available from: http://www.intechopen.com/articles/show/title/diagnosis-and-management-of-desquamative-gingivitis
[10] Nisengard, RJ; Levine, RA. Diagnosis and management of desquamative gingivitis. *Periodontal Insights*, 1995, 2, 4-10.
[11] Rees, TD. Desquamative gingivitis/mucocutaneous diseases commonly affecting the gingiva. In: Harpenau LA, Kao RT, Lundergan WP, Sanz M, eds. Hall's Critical Decisions in Periodontology and Dental Implantology, 5th ed. Shelton, Connecticut : People's Medical Publishing House, 2013, 68-73.
[12] Mignogna, MD; Fortuna, G; Leuci, S; Ruoppo, E; Marasca, F; Matarasso, S. Nikolsky's sign on the gingival mucosa: a clinical tool for oral health practitioners. *J Periodontol*, 2008, 79(12), 2241-2246.
[13] Endo, H; Rees, TD; Kuyama, K; Matsue, M; Yamamoto, H. Use of oral exfoliative cytology to diagnose desquamative gingivitis: a pilot study. *Quintessence Int*, 2008, 39(4), e152-161.
[14] Endo, H; Rees, TD. Clinical features of cinnamon-induced contact stomatitis. *Compend Contin Educ Dent*, 2006, 27(7), 403-409, quiz 410, 421.
[15] Endo, H; Rees, TD; Sisilia, F; et al. Atypical gingival manifestations that mimic mucocutaneous diseases in a patient with contact stomatitis caused by toothpaste. *The Journal of Implant and Advanced Clinical Dentistry*, 2010, 2(2),101-106.
[16] Casiglia, J; Woo, SB; Ahmed, AR. Oral involvement in autoimmune blistering diseases. *Clin Dermatol*, 2001, 19(6), 737-741.
[17] Daniels, TE; Quadra-White, C. Direct immunofluorescence in oral mucosal disease: a diagnostic analysis of 130 cases. *Oral Surg Oral Med Oral Pathol*, 1981, 51(1), 38-47.
[18] Siegel, MA. Intraoral biopsy technique for direct immunofluorescence studies. *Oral Surg Oral Med Oral Pathol*, 1991, 72(6), 681-684.
[19] Endo, H; Rees, TD; Allen, EP; et al. A stab-and-roll biopsy technique to maintain gingival epithelium for desquamative gingivitis. *J Periodontol*, 2014, 85(6), 802-809.

[20] Siegel, MA; Anhalt, GJ. Direct immunofluorescence of detached gingival epithelium for diagnosis of cicatricial pemphigoid. Report of five cases. *Oral Surg Oral Med Oral Pathol*, 1993, 75(3), 296-302.

[21] Sano, SM; Quarracino, MC; Aguas, SC; et al. Sensitivity of direct immunofluorescence in oral diseases. Study of 125 cases. *Med Oral Patol Oral Cir Bucal*, 2008, 113(5), e287-291.

[22] Kourosh, AS; Yancey, KB. Pathogenesis of mucous membrane pemphigoid. *Dermatol Clin*, 2011, 29(3), 479-484.

[23] Chan, LS. Ocular and oral mucous membrane pemphigoid (cicatricial pemphigoid). *Clin Dermatol*, 2012, 30(1), 34-37.

[24] Higgins, GT; Allan, RB; Hall, R; Field, EA; Kaye, SB. Development of ocular disease in patients with mucous membrane pemphigoid involving the oral mucosa. *Br J Ophthalmol*, 2006, 90(8), 964-967.

[25] Thorne, JE; Anhalt, GJ; Jabs, DA. Mucous membrane pemphigoid and pseudopemphigoid. *Ophthalmology*, 2004, 111(1), 45-52.

[26] Alexandre, M; Brette, MD; Pascal, F; et al. A prospective study of upper aerodigestive tract manifestations of mucous membrane pemphigoid. *Medicine (Baltimore)*, 2006, 85(4), 239-252.

[27] Higgins, TS; Cohen, JC; Sinacori, JT. Laryngeal mucous membrane pemphigoid: a systematic review and pooled-data analysis. *Laryngoscope*, 2010, 120(3), 529-536.

[28] Miziara, ID; Sperandio, F; Bohadana, SC; Braga, N; Romano, FR; Miniti, A. Cicatricial pemphigoid: report of five cases. *Ear Nose Throat J*, 2002, 81(7), 442-448.

[29] Sato, H; Toriyama, K; Yagi, S; et al. Surgical correction of microstomia in a patient with antilaminin 332 mucous membrane pemphigoid. *Ann Plast Surg*, 2014, 72(5), 553-555.

[30] Nisengard, RJ; Rogers, RS; 3rd. Desquamative gingivitis. In: Beutner EH, Chorzelski TP, Kumar V, eds. Immunopathology of the skin 3rd ed. New York : A Wiley medical publication; 1987, 361-369.

[31] Dayan, S; Simmons, RK; Ahmed, AR. Contemporary issues in the diagnosis of oral pemphigoid: a selective review of the literature. *Oral Surg Oral Med Oral Pathol Oral Radiol Endod*, 1999, 88(4), 424-430.

[32] Ojha, J; Bhattacharyya, I; Stewart, C; Katz, J. Cicatricial pemphigoid with severe gingival and laryngeal involvement in an 18-year-old female. *Oral Surg Oral Med Oral Pathol Oral Radiol Endod*, 2007, 104(3), 363-367.

[33] Plemons, JM; Rees, TD; Zachariah, NY. Absorption of a topical steroid and evaluation of adrenal suppression in patients with erosive lichen planus. *Oral Surg Oral Med Oral Pathol*, 1990, 69(6), 688-693.

[34] Endo, H; Rees, TD; Kuyama, K; Matsue, M; Yamamoto, H. Successful treatment using occlusive steroid therapy in patients with erosive lichen planus: a report on 2 cases. *Quintessence Int*, 2008, 39(4), e162-172.

[35] Lamey, PJ; Jones, CM. Desquamative gingivitis treated with occlusive steroid therapy: a pilot study. *Gerodontics*, 1988, 4(4),188-190.

[36] Scully, C; Lo Muzio, L. Oral mucosal diseases: mucous membrane pemphigoid. *Br J Oral Maxillofac Surg*, 2008, 46(5), 358-366.

[37] Yancey, KB. Cicatricial pemphigoid. In: Wolff K, Goldsmith LA, Katz SI, Gilchrest BA, Paller AS, Leffell DJ. eds. Fizpatrick's Dermatology in General Medicine, 7th ed. New York : McGraw Hill Inc; 2008, 481-485.
[38] Arduino, PG; Farci, V; D'Aiuto, F; et al. Periodontal status in oral mucous membrane pemphigoid: initial results of a case-control study. *Oral Dis*, 2011, 17(1), 90-94.
[39] Tricamo, MB; Rees, TD; Hallmon, WW; Wright, JM; Cueva, MA; Plemons, JM. Periodontal status in patients with gingival mucous membrane pemphigoid. *J Periodontol*, 2006, 77(3), 398-405.
[40] Schellinck, AE; Rees, TD; Plemons, JM; Kessler, HP; Rivera-Hidalgo, F; Solomon, ES. A comparison of the periodontal status in patients with mucous membrane pemphigoid: a 5-year follow-up. *J Periodontol*, 2009 80(11), 1765-1773.
[41] Rees, TD. Vesiculo-ulcerative diseases and periodontal practice. *J Periodontol*, 1995, 66(8), 747-748.
[42] Orrico, SR; Navarro, CM; Rosa, FP; Reis, FA; Salgado, DS; Onofre, MA. Periodontal treatment of benign mucous membrane pemphigoid. *Dent Today*, 2010, 29(7), 100-102; quiz 102-103.
[43] Arduino, PG; Lopetuso, E; Carcieri, P; et al. Professional oral hygiene treatment and detailed oral hygiene instructions in patients affected by mucous membrane pemphigoid with specific gingival localization: a pilot study in 12 patients. *Int J Dent Hyg*, 2012, 10(2),138-141.
[44] Damoulis, PD; Gagari, E. Combined treatment of periodontal disease and benign mucous membrane pemphigoid. Case report with 8 years maintenance. *J Periodontol*, 2000, 71(10), 1620-1629.
[45] Lilly, JP; Spivey, JD; Fotos, PG. Benign mucous membrane pemphigoid with advanced periodontal involvement: diagnosis and therapy. *J Periodontol*, 1995, 66(8), 737-741.
[46] Lorenzana, ER; Rees, TD; Hallmon, WW. Esthetic management of multiple recession defects in a patient with cicatricial pemphigoid. *J Periodontol*, 2001, 72(2), 230-237.

In: Advances in Dermatology Research
Editor: James P. Vega
ISBN: 978-1-63482-226-8

Chapter 8

Associations between Bullous Pemphigoid and Internal Malignancies: A Literature Review

Yuta Kurashige[*,1], *Norihiro Ikoma*[1], *TomotakaMabuchi*[1], *Akira Ozawa*[1] *and Kenichi Iwashita*[2]
[1]Department of Dermatology, Tokai University School of Medicine, Kanagawa, Japan
[2]Yochomachi dermatology clinic, Tokyo, Japan

Abstract

The correlation between bullous pemphigoid (BP) and internal malignancies has been argued over for more than half a century, and remains controversial. In this chapter, we review the literature in three categories. First, we examine the historical perspective of the association between BP and malignancies; the first case report was probably mentioned by Forman in 1960, and the first case series (seven cases) was described by Parsons and Savin in 1968. Second, we look at the incidence of malignancy in BP patients; among 17 previous studies, six concluded that BP carries an increased risk of internal malignancy, while nine denied such an association. The most recent cohort study found no correlation. Third, we examine the incidence of BP among cancer patients; one cohort study reported no evidence of overall correlation, but a sub-analysis in the study suggested that kidney cancer alone was linked to an elevated risk of BP. Considering the results of these studies, an overall association between BP and malignancies is not shown, while restricted associations depending on the type of cancer or ethnic background of the BP patient might be possible.

* Corresponding author: Dr. Yuta Kurashige, Department of Dermatology, Tokai University School of Medicine, 143 Shimokasuya, Isehara-shi, Kanagawa 259-1193, Japan. E-mail: kurasige@is.icc.u-tokai.ac.jp, phone: +81. 463.93.1121, fax: +81.463.93.9387.

Introduction

Bullous pemphigoid (BP), the most common form of acquired autoimmune bullous dermatosis, occurs mostly in elderly people and is characterized by autoimmune reactions to hemidesmosomal proteins BP180 and BP230, located at the dermo-epidermal junction [1]. For more than fifty years, some autoimmune bullous dermatoses such as pemphigus and pemphigoid have been considered to be associated with internal malignancies. Regarding BP, the literature has described some clinical findings as strongly suggestive of the presence of internal malignancy, including bullae on gyrate erythema [2], negative findings of indirect immunofluorescence [3], and existence of autoantibodies against BP180 [4]. A large number of case reports and clinical studies have examined associations between BP and internal malignancies, but the association remains controversial. This chapter reviews the publications that represent the historical perspective and that refer to either the incidence of malignancy in BP patients or the incidence of BP in cancer patients.

Historical Perspective

In 1953, Lever [5] first established distinct criteria for the diagnosis of BP, distinguishing this entity from other bullous diseases. To the best of our knowledge, the 1960 report by Forman [6] represents the first description of BP in association with internal malignancy; a 70-year-old man was diagnosed with rectal adenocarcinoma 1 year after the diagnosis of BP. In that patient, BP had initially been under successful control. Nevertheless, severe relapse was seen after surgery. At that time, Wilson [6] mentioned BP with carcinoma of the breast and stomach, and Hellier [6] also referred to two cases of BP with carcinoma of the breast and uterus. Hellier suggested that a search for neoplasm should be made in all BP patients. In 1968, as first case series, Parsons and Savin [7] reported seven cases in which BP and malignancies occurred at the same time: the malignancies involved the skin (two cases), cervix, bronchus, uterus, gallbladder, and anus. However, the authors denied a close relationship between BP and malignancies. In the same year, Lim et al. [8] investigated the incidence of internal malignancy among BP patients using patient data collected from dermatologists and pathologists in the eastern counties of England. As a result, malignancy was found in 12 of 103 BP patients and no correlation was apparent. Since then, as shown in Table 1, various clinical studies have aimed at revealing associations or confirming their absence.

Incidence of Internal Malignacies among BP Patients

Table 1 shows 17 representative English-language investigations concerning the incidence of internal malignancy in BP patients [3, 8-23]. Among these, six simply described the incidence of internal malignancies, while 10 conducted comparisons of the incidences of malignancy between BP patient and control groups. In addition, only one study was designed as a cohort study.

Table 1. Studies concerning the incidence of internal malignancies in bullous pemphigoid

Authors	Country	Institution	Data collection period	Incidence of malignancies (Total/ With malignancy) BP	Controls	Conclusion
Lim CC et al. (1968) [8]	UK	Multiple hospitals	1950-1965	103/ 12 (11.7%)	No controls	No association
Stone SP and Schroeter AL (1975) [9]	US	Single hospital	1960-1972	73/ 8 (11.0%)	146/ 11 (7.5%) Other skin diseases	No association
Ahmed AR et al. (1977) [10]	US	Single hospital	ND	33/ 1 (3.0%)	No controls	No association
Moss AA and Hanelin LG (1977) [11]	US	Single hospital	ND	29/ 3 (10.3%)	120/ 11 (9.2%) Diabetes mellitus	Increased risk
Person J and Rogers RS 3rd (1977) [12]	US	Single hospital	1968-1975	84/ 11 (13.1%)	No controls	No association
Chorzelski TP et al. (1978) [13]	Poland	ND	1968-1977	110/ 12 (10.9%)	Nationwide health information	Increased risk $P< 0.01$
Hodge et al. (1981) [14]	UK	Single hospital	ND	124/ 12 (9.7%)	No controls	Increased risk OR 3.63, $P< 0.05$
Venencie et al. (1984) [3]	US	Single hospital	1970-1980	93/ 9 (9.7%)	No controls	Increased risk in negative IIF patients
Lindelöf B et al. (1990) [15]	Sweden	Single national laboratory	1975-1985	497/ 61 (12.3%)	Nationwide health information	No association
Venning VA and Wojnarowska F (1990) [16]	UK	Single hospital	1975-1989	84/ 15 (17.9%)	168/ 9 (5.4%) Other skin diseases	Increased risk
Ogawa H et al. (1995) [17]	Japan	393 hospitals	1981-1986	1113/ 64 (5.8%)	Nationwide health information	Increased risk
Chang YT et al. (1996) [18]	Taiwan	Single hospital	1977-1994	86/ 13 (15.1%)	172/ 27 (15.7%) Other skin diseases	No association $P> 0.5$
Cozzani E et al. (2001) [19]	Italy	11 hospitals	1996-1997	32/ 6 (18.8%)	No controls	No association
Iwashita K et al. (2007) [20]	Japan	Single hospital	1975-2006	115/ 12 (10.4%)	Nationwide health information	Increased risk
Jedlickova H et al. [21]	Czech Republic	Single hospital	1991-2006	89/ 19 (21.3%)	89/ 14 (15.7%) Other skin diseases	No association OR 1.74, 95%CI 0.43-6.96, $p=0.33$ (Age<80)
Li J et al. (2013) [22]	China	Single hospital	1992-2012	190/ 13 (6.8%)	190/ 4 (2.1%) Other skin diseases	Increased risk AOR 4.226, 95%CI 1.176-15.180
Ong E et al. (2014) [23]	UK	Nationwide hospital admission dataset	1999-2011	4,720/ 502 (10.6%)	Nationwide hospital admission dataset	No association RR 1.00, 95%CI 0.92-1.09

RR; Relative risk, OR; Odds ratio, CI; Confidential interval, AOR; Adjusted prevalence odds ratio.

Among these, five studies were from the United States, four from the United Kingdom, two from Japan, and one each from Poland, Sweden, Taiwan, the Czech Republic, and China. The incidence of internal malignancies in BP patients varied from 3.0% to 21.3%. It should be noted that, among these studies, six concluded that BP was associated with an increased risk of internal malignancy, while nine found no such correlation. Although the majority of studies used relatively small samples, some made use of large samples or nationwide patient data. For example, the 1990 investigation by Lindelof et al. [15] reported that 61 of 497 BP patients had internal malignancies, whereas the expected number of malignancies based on nationwide information on cancer incidence in Sweden was 82.6 (relative risk [RR], 0.84; 95% confidence interval [CI], 0.65-1.06). Accordingly, the authors concluded that pemphigoid might not be associated with malignancy. On the other hand, in 1995, Ogawa et al. [17] reviewed 1113 BP patients recruited from a nationwide survey of patients with autoimmune blistering disease in Japan. The survey revealed 64 patients with internal malignancies, and this incidence rate of 5.8% was significantly higher than that of Japanese controls. These increased risks were corroborated in another Japanese study from our department [20]. Concerning the cohort study, Ong et al. [23] used nationwide hospital admission data from the United Kingdom and evaluated the risk of concurrent and subsequent malignancies. As a result, the "BP cohort" of 4,720 BP patients showed no increased risk compared with the "reference cohort" of individuals without a diagnosis of BP (RR, 1.00; 95%CI, 0.92-1.09).

Incidence of BP in Patients with Internal Malignancy

Dermatologists tend to have an interest in whether BP can provide a good predictor of latent malignancies. Accordingly, a large proportion of studies on BP from dermatologists have stressed investigation of the incidence of malignancies among BP patients. However, confirmation of an association between these entities naturally requires investigation of the incidence of BP among cancer patients. To the best of our knowledge, only one study has examined this theme; Ong et al. [23] performed another cohort study using the above-mentioned nationwide dataset. The result showed that the "cancer cohort" of 2.87 million people with a diagnosis of various types of cancer did not show any increased risk of concurrent or subsequent BP compared to the "reference cohort" of individuals without internal malignancy (RR, 0.96; 95%CI, 0.88-1.04). The authors then undertook additional analyses to investigate whether "sub-cohorts" involving specific cancers showed any increased risk of BP compared to the reference cohort. Kidney cancer alone showed an elevated risk of BP (RR, 2.23; 95%CI, 1.48-3.24; $p<0.001$).

Discussion and Summary

The argument about associations between BP and internal malignancies has been ongoing for a long time, but a definitive conclusion remains elusive. As mentioned above, previous studies have shown inconsistent outcomes between no correlation and increased risk. Factors that might contribute to this state are as follows. First, the different study designs including patient numbers, settings, and statistical methods might lead to different results. Second, the reliability of the diagnoses of BP and malignancies in early studies might be dissimilar to those of recent studies, given the advances in medical technologies. Third, because these studies were undertaken in various countries, differences in patient backgrounds in relation to lifestyle, environment or genes might have affected the results. The 17 studies are thus not directly comparable. Nonetheless, from an epidemiological perspective, the results from the recent, well-designed cohort study by Ong et al. [24] can be plausibly taken into account.

Considering the results from that study and others [8-10, 12, 15, 18, 19, 21], we suspect that the balance of evidence favors a lack of overall correlation between BP and malignancies. On the other hand, restricted associations depending on two factors are plausible: type of cancer, e.g., kidney cancer [23]; and the ethnic background of BP patients, e.g., Japanese [17, 20].

References

[1] Kasperkiewicz, M., Zillikens, D. The pathophysiology of bullous pemphigoid. *Clin. Rev. Allergy Immunol.* 2007 Oct; 33(1-2): 67-77.

[2] Gilmour, E., Bhushan, M., Griffiths, C. E. Figurate erythema with bullous pemphigoid: a true paraneoplastic phenomenon? *Clin. Exp. Dermatol.* 1999 Nov; 24: 446-448.

[3] Venencie, P. Y., Rogers, R. S. 3rd, Schroeter, A. L. Bullous pemphigoid and malignancy: relationship to indirect immunofluorescent findings. *Acta Derm. Venereol.* 1984; 64: 316-319.

[4] Muramatsu, T., Iida, T., Tada, H., Hatoko, M., Kobayashi, N., Ko, T., Shirai, T. Bullous pemphigoid associated with internal malignancies: identification of 180-kDa antigen by western immunoblotting. *Br. J. Dermatol.* 1996 Nov; 135: 782-784.

[5] Lever, W. F. Pemphigus. *Medicine* (Baltimore). 1953 Feb; 32: 1-123.

[6] Forman, L. Pemphigoid occurring with carcinoma of the rectum. *Proc. R Soc. Med.* 1960 Jul; 53: 563.

[7] Parsons, R. L., Savin, J. A. Pemphigoid and malignancy. *Br. J. Cancer.* 1968 Dec; 22: 669-672.

[8] Lim, C. C., Macdonald, R. H., Rook, A. J. Pemphigoid eruptions in the elderly. *Trans. St Johns Hosp. Dermatol. Soc.* 1968; 54: 148-151.

[9] Stone, S. P., Schroeter, A. L. Bullous pemphigoid and associated malignant neoplasms. *Arch. Dermatol.* 1975 Aug; 111: 991-994.

[10] Ahmed, A. R., Chu, T. M., Provost, T. T. Bullous pemphigoid: clinical and serologic evaluation for associated malignant neoplasms. *Arch. Dermatol.* 1977 Jul; 113: 969.

[11] Moss, A. A., Hanelin, L. G. Occult malignant tumors in dermatologic disease. The futility of radiological search. *Radiology.* 1977 Apr; 123: 69-71.

[12] Person, J. R., Rogers, R. S. 3rd. Bullous and cicatricial pemphigoid. Clinical, histopathologic, and immunopathologic correlations. *Mayo Clin. Proc.* 1977 Jan; 52: 54-66.

[13] Chorzelski, T. P., Jablonska, S., Maciejowska, E., Beutner, E. H., Wronkowski, L. Coexistence of malignancies with bullous pemphigoid. *Arch. Dermatol.* 1978 Jun; 114: 964.

[14] Hodge, L., Marsden, R. A., Black, M. M., Bhogal, B., Corbett, M. F. Bullous pemphigoid: the frequency of mucosal involvement and concurrent malignancy related to indirect immunofluorescence findings. *Br. J. Dermatol.* 1981 Jul; 105: 65-69.

[15] Lindelöf, B., Islam, N., Eklund, G., Arfors, L. Pemphigoid and cancer. *Arch. Dermatol.* 1990 Jan; 126: 66-68.

[16] Venning, V. A., Wojnarowska, F. The association of bullous pemphigoid and malignant disease: a case control study. *Br. J. Dermatol.* 1990 Oct; 123: 439-445.

[17] Ogawa, H., Sakuma, M., Morioka, S., Kitamura, K., Sasai, Y., Imamura, S., Inaba, Y. The incidence of internal malignancies in pemphigus and bullous pemphigoid in Japan. *J. Dermatol. Sci.* 1995 Mar; 9: 136-141.

[18] Chang, Y. T., Liu, H. N., Wong, C. K. Bullous pemphigoid--a report of 86 cases from Taiwan. *Clin. Exp. Dermatol.* 1996 Jan; 21: 20-22.

[19] Cozzani, E., Parodi, A., Rebora, A., Delmonte, S., Barile, M., Nigro, A., Priano, L., Troiano, G., Patri, P. L.; Gruppo Ligure di Studi in Dermatologia (GLISID). Bullous pemphigoid in Liguria: a 2-year survey. *J. Eur. Acad. Dermatol. Venereol.* 2001 Jul; 15:317-319.

[20] Iwashita, K., Matsuyama, T., Akasaka, E., Mizutani, K., Yamamoto, K., Kondoh, A., Nozawa, M., Yagi, Y., Ikoma, N., Mabuchi, T., Shinagawa, H., Tamiya, S., Nuruki, H., Ohta, Y., Umezawa, Y., Ozawa, A. The incidence of internal malignancies in autoimmune bullous diseases. *Tokai J. Exp. Clin. Med.* 2007 Mar. 20; 32: 42-47.

[21] Li, J., Zuo, Y. G., Zheng, H. Y., Qiu-Ning, S. Association between bullous pemphigoid and internal diseases. *J. Dtsch. Dermatol. Ges.* 2013 Mar; 11: 263-264.

[22] Jedlickova, H., Hlubinka, M., Pavlik, T., Semradova, V., Budinska, E., Vlasin, Z. Bullous pemphigoid and internal diseases - A case-control study. *Eur. J. Dermatol.* 2010 Jan-Feb; 20: 96-101.

[23] Ong, E., Goldacre, R., Hoang, U., Sinclair, R., Goldacre, M. Associations between bullous pemphigoid and primary malignant cancers: an English national record linkage study, 1999-2011. *Arch. Dermatol. Res.* 2014 Jan; 306: 75-80.

In: Advances in Dermatology Research
Editor: James P. Vega
ISBN: 978-1-63482-226-8

Chapter 9

Perinatal Cyanosis: Neuropsychological Functioning

Ashlee R. Loughan, MEd, PhD*[*,1],
Robert Perna, RN, PhD[2] and Hana Perkey, MS[1]
[1]NeuroBehavioral Associates, LLC., Augusta, Georgia, US
[2]TIRR Memorial Herman, Houston, TX, US

Abstract

Perinatal cyanosis is the expression of pathological low arterial blood oxygen saturation in children surrounding the time of birth. The birth process is very complicated and through many different mechanisms can lead to low oxygen levels in the fetus or newborn. The passage through the birth canal and potential placental or umbilical cord issues can interrupt CNS blood supply. Moreover, after birth the newborn must oxygenate its own blood for the first time and many newborns have lungs which are not sufficiently mature for this process. Thus, any respiratory immaturity or cardiac anomalies may quickly diminish efficient oxygenation. While acute medical issues can often be corrected with the newborn appearing fully intact, a brief period of insufficient oxygen to the brain can result in issues which are not readily apparent. Research suggests that instability of circulation or oxygenation is the leading cause of perinatal brain damage (1 – 6 out of every 1000 newborns) and can result in long-term neurological consequences, significant cognitive dysfunction, and subsequent academic challenges. Although medical practitioners often investigate the cause of a cyanotic event, parents and educators are frequently ill-informed as to the future developmental and long-term learning and social implications. This chapter will investigate perinatal cyanotic populations (i.e., cardiac, respiratory, prematurity, and hypoxic-ischemic) and their distinct neurocognitive and behavioral profiles. Specific focus will be placed on empirical literature which identifies cognitive, academic, and emotional deficits. The impact of perinatal cyanosis on all domains of cognitive functioning (i.e., intellect, language,

* Address all correspondence to: Ashlee R. Loughan, M.Ed., Ph.D. Neurobehavioral Associates, 639 13th Street, Augusta, GA, E-mail: Aspicer88@yahoo.com.

motor, memory, attention and executive functioning) will be explored. Finally, general developmental and academic recommendations will be reviewed.

Perinatal or neonatal cyanosis is an expression of pathological low arterial blood oxygen saturation in children surrounding the time of birth and may provide the earliest sign of major medical pathology. The recognized underlying causes of cyanosis can vary and include, for example, intrauterine hypoxia; asphyxia, often combined with decreased cerebral blood flow (CBF); or respiratory distress (The World Health Organization, 1993). These conditions often result from a number of medical pathologies involving the heart and lungs or other issues related to adverse events during childbirth (e.g., uterine rapture), prenatal infections (e.g., rubella), umbilical cord issues, immature lungs, congenital heart disease, and poorly controlled gestational diabetes. The nature and duration of a cyanotic episode, as well as oxygen saturation levels determine the severity of its consequences (Perna & Cooper, 2012). Though quick correction of the cyanotic episode will cause a newborn to turn a healthy shade of pink, the temporary depletion of oxygen can result in negative long-term consequences. Research suggests that instability of circulation or oxygenation is the leading cause of perinatal brain damage (1 – 6 out of every 1000 newborns) and can result in long-term neurological consequences, significant cognitive dysfunction, and academic challenges. The outcomes of cyanosis have been shown to range from mild, transient changes in behavior (e.g., irritability, inattention, poor feeding, or excessive crying) to severe acute effects, profound long-term deficits (e.g., seizures & intellectual disabilities), or even death (Triulzi, Parazzini, & Righini, 2006, 2013; van Handel, Swaab, de Vries, & Jongmans, 2007; Zhang et al., 2013). Although medical practitioners often investigate the cause of a cyanotic event, parents and educators are frequently ill-informed as to the future developmental and long-term learning and social implications.

Common Cyanotic Populations

Cardiac Etiologies

Cardiac pathology is among the most common and researched causes of perinatal cyanosis. Typical brain growth and development is dependent upon adequate volume and content of oxygenated blood supply (Limperopoulos, 2009). In order for the brain to receive ample oxygenated blood, it requires sufficient circulation from the heart, which can be negatively impacted by an abnormal cardiovascular system or event (Limperopoulos, 2009). Poor oxygen supply or cardiac procedures, such as those resulting from a congenital defect, can produce a significant impact on a child's developing cognitive abilities. Specific neurologic abnormalities have been found by multiple congenital heart defects (CHD) group and longitudinal studies (Bellinger et al., 1995, 1999, 2003; Green, 2004; Hovels-Gurich et al., 1997, 2002; Limperopoulos et al., 1999, 2000).

Approximately eight out of every 1,000 newborns have congenital heart defects, which can range from mild to severe (Green, 2004; Hoffman & Kaplan, 2002; Karsdorp, Everaerd, Kindt, & Mulder, 2006; Limperopoulos et al., 1999; Miatton, de Wolf, Francois, Thiery, & Vingerhoets, 2006). A multitude of heart defects have been known to cause some level of cyanosis (e.g., coarctation of the aorta, hypoplastic left heart syndrome, Tetralogy of Fallot, transposition of the great arteries, etc.). As a result, researchers have begun investigating the neuroanatomical structures of children with CHD and found irregularities both pre- and post-surgical intervention (Donofrio et al., 2003; Donofrio & Massaro, 2010; Johnston, 2007; Limperopoulos et al., 2010; McQuillen & Miller, 2010). This suggests that children with CHD may be exposed to numerous cyanotic risk factors including poor circulation in utero, oxygen deprivation post-delivery, surgical procedures during correction, and for some, all of the above (Donofrio et al., 2003; Donofrio & Massaro, 2010; Johnston, 2007; McQuillen & Miller, 2010). Though the cardiac issues may be fully corrected, there is the risk of persistent, yet often subtle effects on brain functioning. Compared to peers in the general population, children with CHD have an increased probability of abnormalities in the central nervous system resulting in some form of brain injury (Green, 2004; Majnemer et al., 2008). Identified reasons include "chronic hypoxemia, congestive heart failure, poor nutrition, polycythemia, right-to-left shunting with the risk of embolic events or brain abscess, episodes of arrhythmia or cardiac arrest, and other organ system abnormalities" (Bellinger et al., 1991, p.702). A common factor investigated is the insufficient circulation prior to and after surgical repair as even brief periods of hypoxia can cause adverse effects and neurologic injury (McElhinney & Wenovsky, 2001; Perna & Cooper, 2012).

Respiratory Etiologies

Respiratory distress in neonates interferes with effective intake of oxygen which often leads to cyanosis. Neonatal respiratory distress is quite frequent and, in its more severe manifestations, contributes significantly to infant mortality rates (Hermansen & Lorah, 2007; Kumar & Bhat, 1996). The most common cause of respiratory distress in newborns is from incomplete removal of fluid from the lungs following the dilation of lymphatic vessels post-delivery. The resulting transient tachypnea typically resolves in a matter of a few hours to two days. A more serious issue leading to neonatal respiration difficulties is respiratory distress syndrome (RDS). Associated with structural and functional lung immaturity, RDS is most prevalent in infants born before the 28th week of gestation. In more severe cases, RDS can develop into bronchopulmonary dysplasia and chronic oxygen dependence (Campbell, McAllister, Volpe, 1988; Hermansen & Lorah, 2007).

Meconium Aspiration Syndrome (MAS) is another common cause of infant respiratory distress (Hermansen & Lorah, 2007). Related to the release of meconium into amniotic fluid, MAS can lead to hypoxia if aspiration occurs in utero (Hermansen & Lorah, 2007; Karatekin, Kesim, & Nuhoğlu, 1999). Current research links more severe cases of MAS to other factors (e.g., prolonged fetal compromise or intrauterine infections) rather than the aspiration of meconium alone (Ghidini & Spong, 2001). Other, less frequent, conditions, such as infections, pulmonary hypertension, or pneumothorax, can also compromise respiration following delivery and increase the risk for hypoxia and cyanosis. Current literature has established a relationship between more severe cases of respiratory distress and deficits of neurological functioning (Campbell, McAllister, Volpe, 1988; Meisels, Plunkett, Roloff, Pasick, & Stiefel, 1986). Specifically, RDS and bronchopulmonary dysplasia are both linked to subsequent motor and cognitive developmental delays, and, in some cases, progressive neurological disease (Campbell, McAllister, Volpe, 1988; Meisels, Plunkett, Roloff, Pasick, & Stiefel, 1986).

Prenatal Etiologies Related to Low Birth Weight and Nenonatal Prematurity

As a group, infants who are born preterm and/or have low birth weight overlap significantly with the two previously mentioned populations—children with CHD and pulmonary disease; as both low birth weight and neonatal prematurity are associated with cardiac and pulmonary pathology. According to Cole, Hagadorn, and Kim (2002) and Fanaroff et al. (2007), the majority of neonatal complications (specifically surrounding preterm birth) include collapsed lungs or chronic lung disease, cardiac abnormalities, shallow or arrested breathing, infection or nutritional disturbances, and brain abnormalities evident in neonatal cranial ultrasounds (i.e., intraventricular hemorrhage, periventricular leukomalacia, & ventricular dilation). This cerebral pathology, especially in neonates with low birth weight, is attributed primarily to hypoxic-ischemic events which can result from many of the cardiac and respiratory issues described above (Inder & Volpe, 2000). Brain damage most often occurs in the subcortical structures and circuits connecting these structures to the frontal and parietal regions. Dysfunction in these areas has the potential to negatively impact the development of executive functions, attention, and self-regulation.

Both preterm birth and low birth weight are complex variables that may carry different risks for different individuals. Highly correlated with each other, many additional factors (e.g., previous miscarriages and preterm pregnancies, maternal age, maternal stress, other psychosocial factors, and exposure to toxins; Perna, Loughan, Perkey, & Tyson, 2014; Pitzer et al., 2001; Wadhwa, Sandman, Porto, Dunkel-Schetter, & Garite, 1993) can play a role in preterm and low birth weight delivery and thus increase the risk for cyanosis. In recent decades, advances in neonatal intensive care, including resuscitation, assisted ventilation, drug treatments, intravenous nutrition, and phototherapy for jaundice (Hack & Fanaroff, 1999) have led to increasing survival rates of children with low birth weight (2,500g) or preterm birth (<37 weeks). According to the National Center for Health Statistics, infants with low birth weight comprise 1-8% of US live births, and 2-12% of those, depending on exact classification requirements met the criteria for preterm births. Along with the decreasing mortality and morbidity, these statistics suggest that the preterm and low birth weight group constitutes a large and continually growing high risk population for cyanotic attacks and associated outcomes. For example, children with very low birth weight have been shown to be at much higher risk for brain insults and abnormalities in cognitive development, behavior, and learning compared to their normal weight peers (Aarnoudse-Moens, Weisglas-Kuperus, van Goudoever, & Oosterlaan, 2009). Additionally, although prematurity can result in a generalized cognitive impairment, many children display more subtle deficits.

Hypoxic-Ischemic Brain Injury

Many of the conditions discussed above result in cerebral insults that fall under the umbrella of hypoxic-ischemic brain injuries. This term signifies the importance of the role that both reduced levels of oxygen (i.e., hypoxia) and/or diminished cerebral blood perfusion (i.e., ischemia) play in the type and severity of the outcomes (Arciniegas, 2012; Stevens, Raz, & Sander, 1999) from these injuries. The same two factors---hypoxia and ischemia---are also prerequisite in the manifestation of cyanosis. The incidence rates for hypoxic-ischemic encephalopathy (HIE) are reported at two – five per 1000 live births in the current literature

(Graham, Ruis, Hartman, Northington, & Fox, 2008; Huang et al., 2013; Zhang et. al., 2013). Research identifies neonatal HIE as one of the most prominent causes of moderate to severe neurological deficits in children (Huang et al., 2013; de Vries & Jongmans, 2010). Furthermore, even mild cases of HIE have been associated with later cognitive impairments (Huang et al., 2013, de Vries & Jongmans, 2010). Because the long brain developmental period, these impairments may not occur for several years.

Hypoxic-ischemic brain injuries are described and investigated in both animal (Huang et al., 2013; Zhang et al., 2013) and clinical research (Kurinczuk, White-Koning, & Badawi, 2010; Triulzi et al., 2006; de Vries & Groenendaal, 2010). The current animal models identify subcortical brain, hippocampus and areas surrounding lateral ventricle as vulnerable to hypoxia-ischemia, manifesting decreased brain-derived neurotrophic factor levels, leukoaraiosis (white matter abnormalities), abnormal neural cell arrangement, neuron degeneration, and cell death (Huang et al., 2013; Zhang et al., 2013). These ischemic injuries are associated with motoric and memory impairments in later development (Huang et al., 2013; Zhang et al., 2013). Animal model researchers have also highlighted the fact that the extent and location of primary damage varies depending on the gestational phase and fetal maturity at the time of hypoxic-ischemic event (Towfighi, Mauger, Vannucci, & Vannucci, 1997).

Similarly, clinical research has identified developmental stages as an important factor in HIE outcomes (Triulzi et al., 2006). Specifically, Triulzi and colleagues (2006) found that the premature brain was more vulnerable to white matter damage, whereas full-term infants showed more grey matter involvement. Additionally, the location of insult could be further specified by the severity of the hypoxic-ischemic event (Triulzi et al., 2006). Investigators have also noted a general trend of progression from more focal and circumscribed injuries resulting from mild to moderate hypoxia-ischemia to diffuse brain damage symptom pattern in more severe cases (Triulzi et al., 2006). From a developmental perspective there is also a potential for a more diffuse presentation with increasing age. Recent research using more advanced methods of imaging (e.g., diffusion-weighted imaging, DWI, and magnetic resonance imaging, MRI) have also described distinct patterns of damage, which were related to specific deficits in later development (de Vries & Groenendaal, 2010; de Vries & Jongmans, 2010). Specifically, two main patterns emerged in the MR imaging: a basal-ganglia-thalamus pattern (BGT), which was most common in cases that included an acute sentinel event (e.g., placental abruption, uterine rapture), and the watershed predominant pattern of injury (WS), typically seen in cases of prolonged partial asphyxia (de Vries & Groenendaal, 2010; de Vries & Jongmans, 2010). The former was associated with more severe disabilities, such as dyskinetic cerebral palsy and epilepsy, as well as learning disabilities, while the latter, involving the vascular WS zones, evidenced suboptimal head growth, as well as language, and behavioral problems (de Vries & Groenendaal, 2010; deVries & Jongmans, 2010). Although the focus of investigations often seems to be on the more serious HIE and the associated severe impairments, research does suggest that even mild-to-moderate incidents of perinatal and neonatal hypoxia-ischemia of either short or prolonged duration can have adverse effects on development and later cognitive functioning (Bass et al., 2004; Perna & Cooper, 2012).

Neurocognitive Implications

A review of the literature shows that severity of neurocognitive outcomes largely corresponds with the severity of the diagnosed neonatal HIE (Pin, Eldridge, & Galea, 2009; de Vries & Jongmans, 2010). Utilizing primarily the Sarnat classification of mild, moderate, and severe (Sarnat & Sarnat, 1976), researchers have shown that the short-term outcomes (i.e., under 3 years) for infants with mild HIE do not include adverse cognitive effects. Infants with moderate HIE classification tend to experience more variable outcomes, and all infants diagnosed with severe HIE incur some adverse cognitive consequences (i.e., at least two standard deviations below their age group on a measure of cognitive functioning; Dixon et al., 2002; Pin, Eldridge, & Galea, 2009; de Vries & Jongmans, 2010). The longer-term effects of perinatal and neonatal HIE are less empirically investigated, however similar relationships between the classification of the neonatal HIE and the outcomes are evident. While school-age children that were classified with mild HIE continue to perform cognitively on par with their peers, non-disabled survivors with moderate HIE and disabled children with severe HIE show a pattern of weakness in specific cognitive domains (de Vries & Jongmans, 2010, Marlow, Rose, Rands, & Draper, 2005; Mañeru, Junqué, Botet, & Guardia, 2001).

Intelligence

With regard to overall intellectual ability, researchers have found that elementary school-age children who had a medical history of moderate HIE performed similarly to healthy peers (controls) in all domains of intellectual functioning (e.g., spatial and verbal reasoning; Marlow et al., 2005). Conversely, those with a history of severe HIE performed significantly poorer than the normal developing peers (controls) as well as the moderate HIE children in all measured domains. The only exception was a non-significant difference between moderate and severe HIE children on a subscale measuring verbal ability. Similarly to Marlow's et al. (2005) findings, Mañeru and colleagues (2001) reported significant differences from control group in perceptual reasoning for their moderate HIE group, but not for their participants with history of mild HIE.

In the low birth weight population, children showed a greater downward displacement of the IQ distribution with decreasing birth weight when Taylor et al. (2004) examined 3 groups of children born at different gestational weights (<750g; 750-1499g, & full-term). In addition, a bimodal distribution of scores was most evident in the group with < 750g birth weight. The elevated subset of more severe IQ deficits suggests that those children possibly sustained more severe brain insult; however, as previously mentioned, children with low birth weight who suffered a cyanotic episode, may also have had other issues which affected brain development.

Children with congenital heart disease (CHD) have also been investigated in terms of their overall cognitive abilities. Researchers have revealed, in general, age-expected intellectual functioning (Forbess et al., 2002; Oates, Simpson, Cartmill, & Turnbull, 1995). Interestingly, even with mean IQ scores falling in the average range, children with CHD fall below the average full scale IQ of 100, more typically floating around a full scale IQ of 90; especially in specific groups of more severe cardiac pathology (Bellinger et al., 1999, 2003;

Hovels-Gurich et al., 1997; Hovels-Gurich et al., 2002; Majnemer et al., 2008; Silbert et al., 1969; Wray & Sensky, 1999).

Language

Language appears to be an area of significant weakness for the neonatal HIE population with deficits in both expressive and receptive functioning. Marlow and colleagues (2005) found that both children with moderate and severe HIE scored significantly lower on a scale of language functioning than the controls, while they did not significantly differ from each other.

With regard specifically to the preterm population, researchers have revealed that preterm children have more limited social and communicative interactions than term-birth controls (Landry, Smith, Miller-Loncar, & Swank, 1997). However, speech and language impairments appear to be less consistently evident during the school years than was demonstrated originally in early childhood (Luoma, Herrgard, Martikainen, & Ahonen, 1998). Some of these children may have sufficient cognitive reserve to eventually fully compensate for the early life hypoxic induced brain injury.

In the CHD population, Bellinger et al. (1999, 2003), Hovels-Gurich et al. (1997, 2002), and Majnemer et al. (2008) revealed decreased language ability in comparison to healthy peers with results suggesting both expressive and receptive delays. Additionally, speech dysfunction was found to be a noted concern in this population.

Motor

Many children with history of severe HIE and some in the moderate classification develop physical disabilities that dramatically impact their motor functioning (Marlow et al., 2005; de Vries & Jongmans, 2010). For example, in Marlow's et al. study (2005) more than 20% of the participants suffered with cerebral palsy with major disabilities (i.e., quadriplegia, hemiplegia, and diplegia). Mañeru et al. (2001) investigated differences between children with mild and moderate neonatal HIE and a control group on visuo-motor task (i.e., the Purdue Pegboard test; Tiffin & Asher, 1948) and a pre-motor function assessment (Luria's hand sequencing task). Their findings supported a significant difference in performance for the moderate HIE group, but not the participants with mild HIE (Mañeru et al., 2001). Similarly, low birth weight children have demonstrated deficits in motor skills, particularly at young ages (Landry et al., 1997).

Conversely, the research literature suggests that motor functioning of children with CHD is variable Although some research has found that motor skills fall within the normal range (Forbess,Visconti, Bellinger, Howe, & Jonas, 2002a; Forbess et al., 2002b; Silbert et al., 1969), most find both fine and gross motor function delays. During school age, Majnemer et al. (2006) reported that difficulty with balance and/or coordination may limit the recreational activities that CHD children can successfully participate in, affecting social interaction with their peers. Thirty to 60 percent of classroom activities involve fine motor skills, thus a reduction in motor ability can have a large impact on learning and academic success. At a 5 year follow-up, 49.4% of their population presented with gross motor deficits and 39% had fine motor challenges (Majnemer et al., 2006).

Memory

The hippocampus is one of the brain structures identified as vulnerable to HIE damage (Huang et al., 2013; Mañeru et al., 2003; Vargha-Khadem et al., 1997; Zhang et al., 2013). For example, researchers discovered hippocampal atrophy in subjects with antecedent moderate HIE that corresponded with poorer long-term memory; however in the absence of other cognitive deficits this impairment did not affect development and academic functioning (Mañeru et al., 2003; Vargha-Khadem et al., 1997). Conversely, other investigations with participants who displayed a number of cognitive impairments discovered more substantial differences in memory functioning that likely affected academic achievement. For example, Marlow et al. (2005) noted impairment in short-term auditory memory as well as poor orientation. Similarly, Mañeru et al. (2001) found that participants with history of moderate HIE performed more poorly than controls on measures of delayed recall of a word-learning task as well as the Visual Reproduction Test (Wechsler Memory Scale-Revised, WMS-R; Wechsler, 1987). Additionally, the moderate HIE subjects achieved lower scores on a measure of working memory (Digit Span, Wechsler Intelligence Scale for Children-Revised, WISC-R; Wechsler, 1974), even though they performed significantly differently only on the forward condition and not on the backward portion of the test (Mañeru et al., 2001). Yet other investigators have reported case studies of subjects with moderate antecedent HIE who experienced a significant impairment of episodic memory (Gadian et al., 2000).

Memory, assessed over both the short and long term on psychometric measures, is a cognitive domain that appears to be relatively intact within the CHD population when compared against their peers. Forbess et al. (2002) found memory and learning to be within normal limits in a sample of 243 children who underwent repair or palliation of CHD. Bellinger et al. (2003) also examined memory at the eight year follow up and found no significant difference between the control and CHD groups.

Attention and Executive Function

Research suggests that this domain of cognitive functioning is affected most in children who had been classified as having severe HIE, while children with history of moderate HIE tend to score similarly to controls on measures of attention and executive functioning (Marlow et al., 2005). Correspondingly, Mañeru and colleagues (2001) found no differences in performance of participants with mild and moderate HIE and the control group.

Similarly, the most frequent deficits found in premature children and/or low birthweight children were impairments in working memory, attention, and executive functioning. In fact, during the "School-Age Follow-up Project," out of the four composite scores investigated (Language, Memory, Visual-Motor, and Executive Functioning), there was a significantly larger group difference in the Executive Functioning deficits than any other category (Taylor et al., 2004). Children in the <750g birthweight group were more prone to specific deficits including slower rate of learning, impulsive responses, slowed processing times, and poorly organized approaches to multistep tasks (Taylor et al., 2004). Elevated rates of inattention and hyperactivity have also been demonstrated across multiple studies. For example, Botting, Powls, and Cooke (1997) found that 23% of low birthweight children were diagnosed with ADHD compared to 6% of their matched full-term peers. These executive deficits remain evident even when IQ is controlled for (Edgin et al., 2008; Espy, Stalets, McDiarmid, Senn, Cwik, & Hamby, 2002; Vicari, Caracale, Carlesimo, Casadei, & Allemand, 2004).

Minimal research has been completed on the investigation of attention and executive functioning skills in children with CHD. Overall, few researchers have suggested attention, impulse control, and organization deficits (Bellinger et al., 2003; Bernstein & Waber, 1996; Hovels-Gurich et al., 2007; O'Dougherty, Berntson, Boysen, Wright, & Teske, 1988).

Academic

Differences in academic achievement between children with neonatal HIE and comparison peers have been supported by research findings. Marlow et al. (2005) discovered lower levels of achievement in both moderate and severe HIE groups; however, while the severe HIE group evidenced poorer performance on all indicators of attainment, the moderate HIE participants underperformed on measures of spelling and reading only (Marlow et al., 2005).

Follow-up studies indicated that children with low birthweight continued to demonstrate pervasive cognitive problems both at age of school entry (Msall, Buck, Rogers, & Catanzaro, 1992; Saigal, Szatmari, & Rosenbaum, 1992; Wolke & Meyer, 1999) and throughout their academic years (Saigal, 2000; Taylor, Minich, Klein, & Hack, 2004). Testing of reading, spelling, math, written expression, and handwriting were all demonstrated as areas of lower scores when compared to the full-term controls (Anderson et al., 2006; Feder et al., 2005; Grunau, Whitfield, & Davis, 2002; Hack et al., 1992; & Taylor et al., 2006). In fact, Saigal et al. (2000) found that 58% of their sample of extremely low birthweight children (ages 12-16) had either repeated a grade or were receiving special education services. This is compared to only 13% of their peers.

For the CHD population, although overall functioning often falls within the normal range, van der Rijken et al. (2007) proposed that problems for children with CHD most likely appear at school age when they have to "rise up" and meet specific cognitive and social demands being placed upon them. Multiple researchers have suggested that children with CHD are performing below average in academic functioning and require school services. Wright and Nolan (1994) found that surgically corrected CHD children performed significantly worse on measures of academic functioning compared to their peers who had cardiac murmurs not requiring surgery. More specifically, Hovels-Gurich et al. (2002) revealed that 23.3% of their investigated population had below average academic knowledge, with 18.3% below one standard deviation from the mean and 5% below two standard deviations. During the Boston Circulatory Arrest Trail, 37% of parents reported that their child received remediation in school and 10% had repeated a grade by age eight (Bellinger et al., 2003). These numbers are similar to the study conducted with Dutch children showing 26% of CHD children were receiving special education along with an increase in the number of children repeating a grade (van der Rijken et al., 2007).

Psychosocial Functioning

Existing literature also supports an association between neonatal moderate to severe HIE and deficits in psychosocial functioning. Marlow et al. (2005) reported a significantly higher incidence in behavioral problems, mostly manifested as increased hyperactivity, more emotional difficulties and less pro-social behavior, with higher impact on daily functioning in the severe group. Conversely, children with antecedent moderate HIE faired comparably to the control group (Marlow et al., 2005).

Similarly, behavioral consequences are also evident for children with low birthweight as early as 3 and 6 months post delivery (Wolf et al., 2002). Later behavioral sequelae have also been seen in adaptive behavior skills, social competence, hyperactivity, both internalizing and externalizing problems, and atypical behavior patterns when compared to term children (Bhutta, Cleves, Casey, Cradock, & Anand, 2002; Klebanov, Brooks-Gunn, & McCormick, 1994; Taylor, Hack, & Klein, 1998). For example, parent reports showed elevated rating of social, thought, and attention problems up to 0.5 to 1.2 standard deviations above controls (Hille et al., 2001). On personality questionnaires, Allin et al. (2006) revealed lower scores on extraversion (i.e., sociability), higher scores on neuroticism (i.e., anxiety, low mood, and low self-esteem), as well as higher scores on the "lie" scale when compared to full-term controls. Additionally, more symptoms of anxiety and depression have also been reported in low birthweight children compared to their full-term peers (Elgen, Sommerfelt, & Markestad, 2002; Indredavik et al., 2004).

Psychosocial difficulties also appear to be a common finding in those with CHD (DeMaso et al., 1990; Green, 2004). Behavioral difficulties were found in 33% of children with CHD and included increased activity level, irritability, and oppositional/defiant behavior (Limperopoulos et al., 2000), as well as internalizing behaviors, including anxiety, withdrawal, sadness, low self-esteem, and somatic complaints (Kramer, Awiszus, Sterzel, van Halteren, & Calarben, 1989; Majnemer et al., 2008; van der Rijken, Maassen, Walk, Daniels, & Hulstijn-Dirkmatt, 2007). In addition, Utens et al. (1998) examined the relationship of cardiac variables to psychosocial outcomes and found that the number of operations appeared to be a significant predictor of the intensity of internalizing, and externalizing behavior patterns; with those who had more operations showing increased externalizing patterns.

Interventions

Interventions should always be individualized, but there are many general rules which warrant mention. Children who have experienced a cyanotic episode should be screened for early developmental delays. Some research suggests that those children who have experienced cyanosis may have a higher incidence of developmental disorders. Those that have emerging developmental disorders should receive early assessment and interventions. These children may be at risk for a variety of comorbidities, and this risk likely warrants a neuropsychological assessment in their early education. Some of these children will have specific learning disorders, and many will likely be responsive to intervention. Still, others may need early speech or occupational therapy. A common long-term symptom of an early life brain injury is disruption of the attention systems of the brain and the potential for difficulty with self-regulation. While there is very strong empirical research supporting the benefits of stimulant medications for these children, many behavioral strategies can be very effective also in helping support their learning. Some of the research suggests that the behavioral strategies may actually help these children develop long-term self-regulation skills, self-esteem, and a level of self-efficacy that would not be appreciated if only medication was used.

Often appropriate academic accommodations can help the child make the necessary academic progress. A structured schedule and perhaps structured tasks or cognitive and academic exercises will serve to help the child to make age appropriate educational gains. There is often a need for an Individualized Educational Plan (IEP) for many of these children. Again, earlier implementation of treatment and accommodations, if needed, may help create the setting for academic success. The following are some academic and behavioral recommendations/accommodations which may be beneficial to those with a history of cyanotic insults:

Language

- Dysfunction in the language areas of the left hemisphere of the brain can result in a diverse range of impairments at different ages. From ages 1 to 3 language issues involve delayed speech or poor speech articulation, then potentially delayed speech fluency, problems listening, and then difficulty reading.
- Speech and language problems warrant early intervention for best outcomes.
- Acquiring well developed speech requires good role modeling and feedback.
- Difficulty with reading requires many hours of structured practice.
- Seek the services of a Speech and Language Pathologist to identify specific language deficits and practice individualized strategies. Often children attend private sessions weekly to assist with either expressive or receptive language deficits.
- Regularly practice Rapid Auditory Processing tasks and various speaking and reading drills.

Motor

- Motor delays can take very subtle forms and may start as low much tone in infants and poor head control, but later during the first year may involve a delay in crawling or walking. Later it may involve gross motor issues like clumsiness and then fine motor issues like difficulty effectively using eating utensils and then difficulty with writing skills.
- Working with an Occupational Therapist can be quite beneficial to assist with fine and gross motor skills; particularly in daily living activities.
- Assistance with motor coordination tasks (i.e., cutting, tying shoes, buttoning/zipping coat)
- Having access to a Letter Strips to refer to and graph paper to write on when needing help on letter formation. Make sure the parents have the same strip at home during homework time.

- Handwriting requirements can be limited by allowing the child to give answers orally and/or having them write every other problem.
- Taking breaks during lengthy or demanding gross motor activities to reduce motor fatigue (i.e., gym class or recess)
- Practice cutting both at school and at home. Make sure you are using child scissors (small handles and shorter blades). You can start by playing puppet games to build muscle strength and memory. When practicing cutting, begin with short straight lines, then longer lines, then finally to curvy lines before proceeding to actual shapes or pictures.
- Play Simon Says, Hokey Pokey, or Animal Walk often and incorporate gross motor skills.
- Introducing assistive technology early may assist with fine motor deficits and difficulty with handwriting. This could include a word processor or verbal recording devices when required to write lengthy assignments; especially as they advance in the grade levels.

Memory

- Make the use of Acronyms. When using Acronyms to help students remember information, it is frequently found that the more unusual the phrase, the better. If a student is non-verbal, then helping them create a visual representation of the information (i.e., cartoon) may also be a useful tool.
- Use external memory compensatory strategies including recording devices, smart phones, tablets, daily planners, and To-Do lists. This can help a student who cannot retain large amounts of information or hold information in their mind long enough to take sufficient notes. Recording the lesson and listening to it later will assist retention.
- It is important to make learning meaningful experience. Children who can relate a topic to an area of interest or to an event or a topic which is already solidified in their brain is going to be beneficial when required to store new information while learning.
- Particular placement of objects in specific locations to help the child find things and more effectively complete routines like getting ready for school. For example, placing a child's coat in front of their backpack will help ensure they see their coat, and remember to bring their coat, before grabbing their bag on the way out to the dismissal bus. Getting school supplies ready and in place the night before school and establishing a specific morning (before school) routine may also greatly help children compensate for forgetfulness.

Attention / Executive Functioning

- To-Do lists or Visual lists are very helpful for students with short working memories. Often time's children will forget their routines or which step is next in a multi-step directional activity. Teachers can post to-do lists in the classroom for students to refer to. Individual children can also have personal post-it notes on their desks with reminders or tasks to complete. Checklist can be effectively used for nearly any academic task including how to get out of the house on time each morning. Some parents say posting a checklist of the morning routine can be a sanity saver: make your bed, brush your teeth, get dressed, have breakfast, grab your lunch, get your backpack.

- A time sheet is often helpful for students to help plan their homework time and schedule. Specific time-cards can be used where each student learns to fill in timeslots with specific activities needing to be performed each night before bedtime and/or each week. Models and specific instruction are even more important for use when children enter middle and high school where independent planning is expected and required in order to juggle multiple deadlines at a time.
- Planning as a class which step should be completed and when it should, will help facilitate proper planning.
- Using scoring rubrics can also help children learn to plan what needs to be included in their assignment or projects.
- When organizing class work materials, specific systems can be taught including color coding, using separate binders to organize subjects and projects, and using assignment books.
- Breaking down the writing process explicitly with organizers (i.e., essay webs), templates, and assignment sheets would be helpful to all students, not only those with organization deficits.
- Teaching organizational note-taking strategies can also assist students during lectures and when reading textbooks independently. These strategies ensure that the students are interacting with their text instead of just skimming the material passively.

Emotional / Behavioral

- Seek out the services of a Licensed Clinical Psychologist to provide individualized coping and motivational strategies.
- Develop a positive management program for appropriate emotions and behaviors. The use of "marbles" or "tokens" can help reinforce a student's appropriate behaviors.
- Parents and teachers should utilize a ratio of five praise statements to each correction or command to assist with motivation. This 5:1 ratio has been shown in research to be highly effective at treating behavioral difficulties and reducing future emotional/ mood difficulties.
- Help the child with concrete visual strategies to understand their emotions. For example, the child might work with a professional to develop a "thermometer" or "speedometer" metaphor for measuring emotions. They should label each temperature or speed to reflect degrees of specific emotions (i.e., anger, anxiety, etc.). Each level should then be tied to a specific concrete behavior, such as counting to delay responses, terminating the conversation, seeking adult intervention, or immediately leaving the situation.
- It is important to identify triggers and observe when children are becoming overloaded and frustrated. Triggers often exacerbate the emotions and behaviors, leading to increased irritability, inattention, impulsivity, inflexibility, or aggression.

When they become overloaded, provide them with a break or down time away from other children in which they can engage in quiet pleasurable activities

Conclusion

Frequently, perinatal and postnatal cyanosis is the manifestation of low arterial blood oxygen saturation in neonates. Passage through the birth canal can induce trauma. Numerous problems can negatively affect the placenta and the umbilical cord, leading to an interruption of CNS blood supply. Moreover, upon emerging, the newborn must oxygenate its own blood for the first time. Thus, any respiratory immaturity or cardiac anomalies may quickly diminish efficient oxygenation. While acute medical issues can often be corrected with the newborn appearing fully intact, a brief period of insufficient oxygen to the brain can result in issues which are not readily apparent. As outlined in this text many medical issues can cause cyanosis and some may be sufficiently severe enough to cause a hypoxic-ischemic episode and result in brain dysfunction. The effects of these episodes can be very apparent in some cases such as when a child develops cerebral palsy. Yet, often the consequences of hypoxia-ischemia may not be fully apparent in newborns and infants. In fact, in some cases, the full impact of the injury may not be evident for many years. Documentation of the event may be important and may subsequently allow for the correct diagnosis and intervention. Physicians should be made aware of children who have experienced an episode of hypoxia-ischemia and monitor their development with follow-up assessments. Such ongoing evaluation and care may afford the timely implementation of any necessary interventions. There is certainly at least some risk that children with antecedent hypoxic-ischemic injuries may be misdiagnosed at some point during their childhood if the examining clinician is not alerted to their medical history and the hypoxic-ischemic event. Possible misdiagnoses may include ADHD or other disorders involving executive dysfunction, impulse control, or even psychiatric issues. Thus, inquiry during the clinical interview should always explore possible early life HIE, especially when there are unexplained cognitive impairments or delays.

References

Aarnoudse-Moens, C. S. H., Weisglas-Kuperus, N., van Goudoever, J. B., & Oosterlaan, J. (2009). Meta-analysis of neurobehavioral outcomes in very preterm and/or very low birth weight children. *Pediatrics, 124,* 717-728. doi:10.1542/peds.2008-2816

Allin, M., Rooney, M., Cuddy, M., Wyatt, J., Walshe, M., Rifkin, L., & Murray, R. (2006). Personality in young adults who are born preterm. *Pediatrics, 117,* 309-316.

Anderson, P., Doyle, L. W., & the Victorian Infant Collaborative Study Group (2006). Neurobehavioral outcomes of school-age children born extremely low birth weight or very preterm in the 1990's. *Journal of the American Medical Association, 289*, 3264-3272.

Arcinegas, D. B. (2012). Hypoxic-ischemic brain injury. Retrieved from http://www.internationalbrain.org/articles/hypoxicischemic-brain-injury/

Bass, J. L., Corwin, M., Gozal, D., Moore, C., Nishida, H., Parker, S., … Kinane, T. B. (2004). The effect of chronic or intermittent hypoxia on cognition in childhood: A review of the evidence. *Pediatrics, 114,* 805–816. doi:10.1542/peds.2004-0227

Bellinger, D. C., Jonas, R. A., Rappaport, L. A., Wypij, D., Wernovsky, G., Kuban, K. C. K., Barnes, P. D., Holmes, G. L., Hickey, P. R., Strand, R. D., Walsh, A. Z., Helmers, S. L., Constantinou, J. E., Carraxana, E. J., Mayer, J. E., Hanley, F. L., Castaneda, A. R., Ware, J. H., & Newburger, J. W. (1995). Developmental and neurologic status of children after heart surgery with hypothermic circulatory arrest or low-flow cardiopulmonary bypass. *The New England Journal of Medicine, 332*(9), 549-555.

Bellinger, D. C., Wernovsky, G., Rappaport, L. A., Mayer, J. E., Castaneda, A. R., Farrell, D. M., Wessel, D. L., Lang, P., Hickey, P. R., Jonas, R. A., & Newburger, J. W. (1991). Cognitive development of children following early repair of transposition of the great arteries using deep hypothermic circulatory arrest. *Pediatrics, 87*, 701-707.

Bellinger, D. C., Wypij, D., Kuban, K. C. K., Rappaport, L. A., Hickey, P. R., Wernovsky, G., Jonas, R. A., &Newburger, J. W. (1999). Developmental and neurological status of children at 4 years of age after heart surgery with hypothermic circulatory arrest or low-flow cardiopulmonary bypass. *Circulation, 100*, 526-532.

Bellinger, D. C., Wypij, D., du Plessis, A. J., Rappaport, L. A., Jonas, R. A., Wernovsky, G., & Newburger, J. W. (2003). Neurodevelopmental status at eight years in children with dextra-transposition of the great arteries: The Boston circulatory arrest trial. *The Journal of Thoracic and Cardiovascular Surgery, 126*, 1385-2003.

Bernstein, J.H., &Waber, D.P. (1996). *Developmental scoring system for the Rey-Osterrieth complex figure*. Odessa, FL: Psychological Assessment Resources.

Bhutta, A. T., Cleves, M. A., Casey, P. H., Cradock, M. M., & Anand, K. J. S. (2002). Cognitive and behavioral outcomes of school-aged children who were born preterm. *Journal of the American Medical Association, 288,* 728-737.

Botting, N., Powls, A., & Cooke, R. W. I. (1997). Attention deficit hyperactivity disorders and other psychiatric outcomes in a very low birthweight children at 12 years. *Journal of Child Psychology and Psychiatry, 8*, 931-941.

Campbell, R. L., McAllister, W., & Volpe, J. J. (1988). Neurologic aspects of bronchopulmonary dysplasia. *Clinical pediatrics, 27,* 7-13.

Cole, C., Hagadorn, J., & Kim, C. (2002). *Criteria for determining disability in infants and children: Low birth weight.* Rockville, MD: Agency for Healthcare Research and Quality.

DeMaso, D. R., Beardslee, W. R., Silbert, A. R., & Fyler, D. C. (1990). Psychological functioning in children with cyanotic heart defects. *Developmental and Behavioral Pediatrics, 11*(6), 289-294.

Dixon, G., Badawi, N., Kurinczuk, J. J., Keogh, J. M., Silburn, S. R., Zubrick, S. R., & Stanley, F. J. (2002). Early Developmental Outcomes After Newborn Encephalopathy. *Pediatrics, 109,* 26-33. doi: 10.1542/peds.109.1.26

Donofrio, M. T., Bremer, Y. A., Schieken, R. M., Gennings, C., Morton, L. D., Eidem, B. W., Cetta, F., Falkensammer, C. B., Huhta, J. C., & Kleinman, C. S. (2003). Autoregulation of cerebral blood flow in fetuses with congenital heart disease: The brain sparing effect. *Pediatric cardiology, 24,* 436-443. doi:10.1007/s00246-002-0404-0

Donofrio, M. T. & Masaro, A. N. (2010). Impact of congenital heart disease on brain development and neurodevelopmental outcome. *International journal of pediatrics, 2010,* doi:10.1155/2010/359390

Edgin, J. O., Inder, T. E., Anderson, P. J., Hood, K. M., Clark, C. A. C., & Woodward, L. J. (2008). Executive functioning in preschool children born very preterm: Relationship with early white matter pathology. *Journal of the International Neuropsychological Society, 14,* 90-101.

Elgen, I., Sommerfelt, K., & Markestad, T. (2002). Population based, controlled study of behavioural problems and psychiatric disorders in low birth weight children at 11 years of age. *Archives of Disease in Childhood: Fetal and Neonatal Edition, 87,* F128-F132.

Espy, K. A., Stalets, M. M., McDiarmid, M. M., Senn, T. E., Cwik, M. F., & Hamby, A. (2002). Executive functions in preschool children born preterm: Application of cognitive neuroscience paradigms. *Child Neuropsychology, 8,* 83-92.

Fanaroff, A. A., Stoll, B. J., Wright, L. L., Carlo, W. A., Ehrenkranz, R. A., Stark, A. R.,...Poole, K. W. (2007). Trends in neonatal morbidity and mortality for very low birthweight infants. *American Journal of Obstetrics and Gynecology, 196,* 147.e1-147.e8.

Feder, K. P., Majnemer, A., Bourbonnais, D., Platt, R., Blayney, M., & Synnes, A. (2005). Handwriting performance in preterm children compared with term peers at age 6 to 7 years. *Developmental Medicine and Child Neurology, 47,* 163-170.

Forbess, J. M., Visconti, K. J., Bellinger, D. C., Howe, R. J., & Jonas, R. A. (2002a). Neurodevelopmental outcomes after biventricular repair of congenital heart defects. *The Journal of Thorasic and Cardiovascular Surgery, 123,* 631-639.

Forbess, J. M., Visconti, K. J., Hancock-Friesen, C., Howe, R. C., Bellinger, D. C., & Jonas, R. A. (2002b). Neurodevelopmental outcomes after congenital heart surgery: Results from an institutional registry. *Circulation, 106,* 95-102. doi: 10.1161/01.cir.0000032915.33237.72

Gadian, D. G., Aicardi J., Watkins, K.E., Porter, D. A., Mishkin, M., & Vargha-Kadem, F. (2000). Developmental amnesia associated with early hypoxic-ischaemic injury. *Brain, 123,* 499-507.

Ghidini, A. & Spong, C. Y. (2001). Severe meconium aspiration syndrome is not caused by aspiration of meconium. *American journal of obstetrics and gynecology, 185,* 931-938.

Graham, E. M., Ruis, K. A., Hartman, A. L., Northington, F. J., Fox. H. E. (2008) A systematic review of the role of intrapartum hypoxia-ischemia in the causation of neonatal encephalopathy. *American journal of obstetrics and gynecology, 199,* 587–595. doi:10.1016/j.ajog.2008.06.094

Green, A. (2004). Outcomes of congenital heart disease: A review. *Pediatric Nursing, 30,* 280-284.

Grunau, R. E., Whitfield, M. F., & Davis, C. (2002). Pattern of learning disabilities in children with extremely low birth weight and broadly average intelligence. *Archives of Pediatrics and Adolescent Medicine, 156,* 615-620.

Hack, M., Breslau, N., Aram, D., Weissman, B., Klein, N., & Borawski-Clark, E. (1992). The effect of very low birthweight and social risk on neurocognitive abilities at school age. *Journal of Developmental and Behavioral Pediatrics, 13,* 412-420.

Hack, M., & Fanaroff, A. (1999). Outcomes of children of extremely low birth weight and gestational age in the 1990's. *Early Human Development, 53,* 193-218.

van Handel, M., Swaab, H., de Vries, L. S., & Jongmans, M. J. (2007). Long-term cognitive and behavioral consequences of neonatal encephalopathy following perinatal asphyxia: A review. *European journal of pediatrics, 166,* 645-654. doi: 10.1007/s00431-007-0437-8

Hermansen, C. L. & Lorah, K. N. (2007). Respiratory distress in the newborn. *American family physician, 76,*987-994.

Hille, E. T. M., den Ouden, A. L., Saigal, S., Wolke, D., Lambert, M., Whitaker, A., …Paneth, M. (2001). Behavioural problems in children who weigh 1000g at birth in four countries. *Lancet, 357*, 1641-1643.

Hoffman, J. I. E., & Kaplan, S. (2002). The incidence of congenital heart disease. *Journal of the American College of Cardiology, 39*, 1890-1900.

Hovels-Gurich, H. H., Konrad, K., Skorzenski, D., Herpertz-Dahlmann, B., Messmer, B. J., & Seyhaye, M. C. (2007). Attentional dysfunction in children after corrective cardiac surgery in infancy. *The Annuals of Thorasic Surgery, 83*, 1425-1430.

Hovels-Gurich, H. H., Seghaye, M. C., Dabritz, S., Messmer, B. J., & Bernuth, G. V. (1997). Cognitive and motor development in preschool and school-aged children after neonatal arterial switch operation. *The Journal of Thoracic and Cardiovascular Surgery, 114*, 578-585.

Hovels-Gurich, H. H., Seghaye, M. C., Schnitker, R., Wiesner, M., Huber, W., Minkenberg, R., Kotlarek, F., Messmer, B. J., & van Bernuth, G. (2002). Long-term neurodevelopmental outcomes in school-aged children after neonatal arterial switch operation. *The Journal of Thoracic and Cardiovascular Surgery, 124*, 448-458.

Huang, Y., Lai, H., Xu, H., Wu, W., Lai, X., Ho, G., …Chen, Y. (2013). Impact of perinatal systemic hypoxic–ischemic injury on the brain of male offspring rats: an improved model of neonatal hypoxic–ischemic encephalopathy in early preterm newborns. *PlosOne, 8,* e82502. doi:10.1371/journal.pone.0082502

Inder, T. E., Huppi, P. S., Warfield, S., Kikinis, R., Zientara, G. P., Barnes, P.D.,…Volpe, J. J. (1999). Periventricular white matter injury in the premature infant is followed by reduced cerebral cortical gray matter volume at term. *Annals of Neurology, 46*, 755-760.

Inder, T. E. & Volpe, J. J. (2000). Mechanisms of perinatal brain injury. *Seminars in Neonatology, 5,* 3-16.

Indredavik, M. S., Vik, T., Heyerdahl, S., Kulseng, S., Farers, P., & Brubakk, A. (2004). Psychiatric symptoms and disorders in adolescents with low birth weight. *Archives of Disease in Childhood: Fetal and Neonatal Edition, 89,* F445-F450.

Johnston, M. V. (2007). Congenital heart disease and brain injury. *The New England Journal of Medicine, 357*, 1971-1973.

Karatekin, G., Kesim (Dönmez), M., & Nuhoḡlu, A. (1999). Risk factors for meconium aspiration syndrome. *International journal of gynecology and obstetrics, 65,* 295-297.

Karsdorp, P. A., Everaerd, W., Kindt, M., & Mulder, J. M. (2006). Psychological and cognitive functioning in children and adolescents with congenital heart disease: A meta-analysis. *Journal of Pediatric Psychology, 32*, 527-541.

Klebanov, P. K., Brooke-Gunn, J., & McCormick, M. C. (1994). School achievement and failure in very low birth weight children. *Journal of Developmental and Behavioral Pediatrics, 15,* 248-256.

Kramer, H. H., Awiszus, D., Sterzel, U., van Halteren, A., & ClaBen, R. (1989).Development of personality and intelligence in children with congenital heart disease. *Journal of Child Psychology and Psychiatry, 30*(2), 299-308.

Kumar, A. & Bhat, V. (1996). Epidemiology of respiratory distress of newborns. *The Indian journal of pediatrics, 63,* 93-98.

Kurinczuk, J. J., White-Koning, M., & Badawi, N. (2010). Epidemiology of neonatal encephalopathy and hypoxic–ischaemic encephalopathy. *Early human development, 86,* 329-338. doi:10.1016/j.earlhumdev.2010.05.010

Landry, S. H., Smith, K. E., Miller-Loncar, C. L., & Swank, P. R. (1997). Predicting cognitive-language and social growth curves from early maternal behaviors in children at varying degrees of biological risk. *Developmental Psychology, 33*, 1040-1053.

Limperopoulos, C. (2009). Disorders of the fetal circulation and the fetal brain. *Clinics in perinatology, 36,* 561-577. doi:10.1016/j.clp.2009.07.005

Limperopoulos, C., Majnemer, A., Shevell, M. I., Rosenblatt, B., Rohlicek, C., &Tchervenkov, C. (1999). Neurologic status of newborns with congenital heart defects before open heart surgery. *Pediatrics, 103*, 402-408.

Limperopoulos, C., Majnemer, A., Shevell, M. I., Rosenblatt, B., Roblicek, C., &Tchervenkov, C. (2000). Neurodevelopmental status of newborns and infants with congenital heart defects before and after open heart surgery. *Journal of Pediatrics, 137*, 638-645.

Limperopoulos, C., Twiretzky, W., McElhinney, D.B., Newburger, J.W., Brown, D.W., Robertson, R.L., Guizard, N., McGrath, J.W., Geva, J., Annese, D., Dunbar-Masterson, C., Trainor, B., Laussen, P.C., & duPlessis, A.J. (2010). Brain volume and metabolism in fetuses with congenital heart disease: Evaluation with quantitative magnetic resonance imaging and spectroscopy. *Circulation, 121*, 26-33.

Lou, H. C., (1996). Etiology and pathogenesis of attention-deficit hyperactivity disorder (ADHD): Significance of prematurity and perinatal hypoxic-haemodynamic encephalopathology. *Acta Paediatrica, 85,* 1266-1271.

Luoma, L., Herrgard, E., Martikainen, A., & Ahonen, T. (1998). Speech and language development of children born at <32 weeks gestation: A 5 year prospective follow-up study. *Developmental Medicine and Child Neurology, 40*, 380-387.

Mañeru, C., Junqué, C., Botet, F., Tallada, M., & Guardia, J. (2001). Neuropsychological long-term sequelae of perinatal asphyxia. *Brain injury, 15,* 1029-1039. doi:10.1080/02699050110074178

Mañeru, C., Serra-Grabulosa, J. M., Junqué, C., Salgado-Pineda, P., Bargalló, N., Olondo, M., ... Mercader J. M. (2003). Residual hippocampal atrophy in asphyxiated term neonates. *Journal of neuroimaging, 13,* 68-74. doi:10.1177/1051228402239720

Majnemer, A., Limperopoulos, C., Shevell, M., Rohlicek, C., Rosenblatt, B., & Tchervenkov, C. (2008). Developmental and functional outcomes at school entry in children with congenital heart defects. *The journal of pediatrics, 153,* 55-60. doi:1016/j.jpeds.2007.12.019

Majnemer, A., Limperopoulos, C., Shevell, M., Rosenblatt, B., Rohlicek, C., & Tchervenkov, C. (2006). Long-term neuromotor outcome at school entry of infants with congenital heart defects requiring open-heart surgery. *Journal of Pediatrics, 148*, 72-77.

Marlow, N., Rose, A. S., Rands, C. E., & Draper, E. S. (2005). Neuropsychological and educational problems at school age associated with neonatal encephalopathy. *Archives of disease in childhood. Fetal and neonatal edition, 90,* F380-F387. doi:10.1136/adc.2004.067520

McQuillen, P. S. & Miller, S. P. (2010). Congenital heart disease and brain development. *Annals of the New York Academy of Sciences, 1184,* 68-86. doi:10.1111/j.1749-6632.2009.05116.x

McElhinney, D. G., &Wenovsky, G. (2001). Outcomes of neonates with congenital heart disease. *Current Opinion in Pediatrics, 13*, 104-110.

Meisels, S. J., Plunkett, J. W., Roloff, D. W., Pasick, P. L., & Stiefel, G. S. (1986). Growth and development of preterm infants with respiratory distress syndrome and bronchopulmonary dysplasia. *Pediatrics, 77,* 345-352.

Miatton, M., de Wolf, D., Francois, K., Thiery, E., &Vingerhoets, G. (2006). Neurocognitive consequences of surgically corrected congenital heart defects: A review. *Neuropsychology Review, 16*, 65-85.

Msall, M. E., Buck, G. M., Rogers, B. J., & Catanzaro, N. L. (1992). Kindergarten readiness after extreme prematurity. American Journal of Disease of Children, 146-1371-1378.

O'Dougherty, M., Berntson, G. G., Boysen, S. T., Wright, F. S., & Teske, D. (1988).Psychophysiological predictors of attentional dysfunction in children with congenital heart defects. *Psychophysiology, 25*, 305-315.

Oates, R. K., Simpson, J. M., Cartmill, T. B., & Turnbull, J. A. B. (1995). Intellectual function and age of repair in cyanotic congenital heart disease. *Archives of Disease in Childhood, 72*, 298-301.

Perna, R. & Cooper, D. (2012). Perinatal cyanosis: Long-term cognitive sequelae and behavioral consequences. *Applied neuropsychology: Child, 1,* 45-52. doi:10.1080/09084282.2011.643946

Perna, R., Loughan, A., Perkey, H., & Tyson, K. (2014). Terbutaline and Associated Risks for Neurodevelopmental Disorders. *Child development research, 2014,* doi:10.1155/2014/358608

Pin, T. W., Eldrgidge, B., & Galea, M. P. (2009). A review of developmental outcomes of term infants with post-asphyxia neonatal encephalopathy. *European journal of pediatric neurology, 13,* 224-234. doi:10.1016/j.ejpn.2008.05.001

Pitzer, M., Schmidt, M. H., Esser, G., & Laucht, M. (2001). Child development after maternal tocolysis with b-sympathomimetic drugs. Child Psychiatry and Human Development, 31, 165-182.

van der Rijken, R. E. A., Maassen, B. A. M., Walk, T. L. M., Daniels, O., & Hulstijn-Dirkmatt, G. M. (2007). Outcome after surgical repair of congenital cardiac malformations at school age. *Cardiology in the Young, 17*, 64-71.

Saigal, S. (2000). Follow-up of very low birth weight babies to adolescence. *Seminars in Neonatology, 5,* 107-118.

Saigal, S., Szatmari, P., & Rosenbaum, P. (1992). Can learning disabilities in children who were extremely low birth weight be identified at school entry? *Journal of Developmental and Behavioral Pediatrics, 13*, 356-362.

Sarnat, H. B. & Sarnat, M. S. (1976). Neonatal encephalopathy following fetal distress. A clinical and electroencephalographic study. *Archives of Neurology, 33*, 696–705.

Silbert, A., Wolff, P. H., Mayer, B., Rosenthal, A., & Nados, A. S. (1969).Cyanotic heart disease and psychological development. *Pediatrics, 43*(2), 192-200.

Stevens, C. P., Raz, S., & Sander, C. J. (1999). Peripartum hypoxic risk and cognitive outcome: A study of term and preterm birth children at early school age. *Neuropsychology, 13,* 598-608.

Taylor, H.G., Hack, M., & Klein, N. (1998). Attention deficits in children with <750gm birthweight. *Child Neuropsychology, 4*, 21-34.

Taylor, H.G., Klein, N., Drotar, D., Schluchter, M., & Hack, M. (2006). Consequences and risks for <1000g birth weight for neuropsychological skills, achievement, and adaptive functioning. *Journal of Developmental and Behavioral Pediatrics, 27*, 459-469.

Taylor, H.G., Minich, N., Bangert, B., Filipek, P.A., & Hack, M. (2004). Long-term neuropsychological outcomes of very low birth weight: Associations with early risks for periventricular brain insults. *Journal of the International Neuropsychological Society, 10*, 987-1004.

Taylor, H.G., Minich, N.M., Klein, N., & Hack, M. (2004). Longitudinal outcomes of very low birth weight: Neuropsychological findings. *Journal of the International Neuropsychological Society, 10*, 149-163.

Tiffin, J. & Asher, E. J. (1948). The Purdue Pegboard: norms and studies of reliability and validity. *Journal of Applied Psychology, 32*, 234-247. doi: 10.1037/h0061266

Towfighi, J., Mauger, D., Vannucci, R. C., & Vannucci, S. J. (1997). Influence of age on the cerebral lesions in an immature rat model of cerebral hypoxia–ischemia: a light microscopic study. *Developmental brain research, 100,* 149-160.

Triulzi, F., Parazzini, C., & Righini, A. (2006). Patterns of damage in the mature neonatal brain. *Pediatric radiology, 36,* 608-620. doi:10.1007/s00247-006-0203-5

Utens, E. M., Verhulst, F. C., Duivenvoorden, H. J., Meijboom, F. J., Erdman, R. A., & Hess, J. (1998). Prediction of behavioral and emotional problems in children and adolescents with operated congenital heart disease. *European Heart Journal, 19*, 801-807.

Vargha-Khadem, F., Gadian, D. G., Watkins, K. E., Connelly, A., Van Paesschen, W, * Mishkin, M. (1997). Differential effects of early hippocampal pathology on episodic and semantic memory. *Science, 277,* 376-380. doi:10.1126/science.277.5324.376

Vicari, S., Caravale, B., Carlesimo, G.A., Casadei, A.M., & Allemand, F. (2004). Spatial working memory deficits in children at ages 3-4 who were low birth weight, preterm infants. *Neuropsychology, 18*, 673-678.

de Vries, L. S. & Groenendaal, F. (2010). Patterns of neonatal hypoxic–ischaemic brain injury. *Neuroradiology,* doi: 10.1007/s00234-010-0674-9.

de Vries, L. S. & Jongmans, M. J. (2010). Long-term outcome after neonatal hypoxic-ischaemic encephalopathy. Archives of diseases in childhood. Fetal and neonatal edition, 95, F220-F224. doi:10.1136/adc.2008.148205

Wadhwa, P. D., Sandman, C. A., Porto, M., Dunkel-Schetter, C., & Garite, T. J. (1993). The association between prenatal stress and infant birth weight and gestational age at birth: A prospective investigation. *American journal of obstetrics and gynecology, 169,* 858-865. doi:10.1016/0002-9378(93)90016-C

Wechsler, D. (1974). *Manual for the Wechsler Intelligence Scale for Children-Revised.* New York: Psychological Corporation.

Wechsler, D. (1987). *Wechsler Memory Scale-Revised manual.* New York: Psychological Corporation.

Wolf, M., Koldewijn, K., Beelen, A., Smit, B., Hedlund, R., & de Groot, I.J.M. (2002). Neurobehavioral and developmental profile of very low birth weight preterm infants in early infancy. *Acta Paediatrica, 91,* 930-938.

Wolke, D., & Meyer, R. (1999). Cognitive status, language attainment, and prereading skills of 6-year-old very preterm children and their peers: The Bavarian Longitudinal Study. *Developmental Medicine and Child Neurology, 41*, 94-109.

World Health Organization. (1993). *ICD-10, the ICD-10 classification of mental and behavioural disorders: Diagnostic criteria for research.* Geneva: World Health Organization.

Wray, J., & Sensky, T. (1999). Controlled study of preschool development after surgery for congenital heart disease. *Archives of Disease in Childhood, 80*, 511-516.

Wright, M., & Nolan, T. (1994).Impact of cyanotic heart disease on school performance. *Archives of Disease in Childhood, 71,* 64-70.

Zhang, Q., Ding, Y., Yao, Y., Yu, Y., Yang, L., & Cui, H. (2013). Creating rat model for hypoxic brain damage in neonates by oxygen deprivation. *PLos ONE, 8,* e83589. doi:10.1371/journal.pone.0083589.

In: Advances in Dermatology Research
Editor: James P. Vega
ISBN: 978-1-63482-226-8

Chapter 10

Laryngomalacia: A Cause of Cyanosis in Pediatric Age

***Marco Berlucchi*[*,1], *Diego Barbieri*[2], *Daniela Tonni*[1], *Silvana Molinaro*[3], *Patrizia Bardini*[3] and *Nader Nassif*[1]**

[1]Department of Pediatric Otorhinolaryngology, Spedali Civili, Brescia, Italy
[2]Department of Otorhinolaryngology, University of Brescia, Brescia, Italy
[3]Department of Pediatric Anesthesiology, Spedali Civili, Brescia, Italy

Abstract

Laryngomalacia is the most common congenital laryngeal anomaly and the most frequent cause of stridor in pediatric age. The disorder involves 45–75% of all infants with congenital stridor. Signs and symptoms appear usually within the first 2 weeks of life and the spectrum of disease presentation, progression, and outcomes is variable. Most cases are mild and resolve spontaneously without surgical procedures. Such patients undergo only medical treatment for the gastroesophageal reflux that is generally associated with this disease. Only severe cases with intolerable symptoms such as dysphagia, failure to thrive, dyspnea, cyanosis, intermittent complete obstruction and/or cardiac failure must undergo surgery. Surgical therapy is in relation to the type and severity of laryngomalacia. The authors describe the different clinical pictures that every clinician can observe and summarize the different treatments available.

* Corresponding author: Marco Berlucchi, MD; Department of Pediatric Otorhinolaryngology, Spedali Civili, Piazza Spedali Civili 1, 25123 Brescia – Italy. Tel. +390303996226; Fax +390303996009; E-mail: marco.berlucchi@tin.it.

Introduction

Characterized by weak laryngeal tone, laryngomalacia is the most common congenital laryngeal anomaly. The pathological condition favors collapse of supraglottic structures into the airway causing inspiratory stridor and airway obstruction [1, 2] and represents the most frequent cause of stridor in pediatric age. Its symptomatology ranges from simple laryngeal stridor to severe dyspnea associated with cyanosis and difficultly in feeding. Thus, treatment of the disease is in relation to its clinical picture.

Terminology, and Incidence

The term laryngomalacia, or soft larynx in Latin, replaced the more antiquated term congenital laryngeal stridor, which had previously been used to describe the condition. First coined by Jackson and Jackson in 1942 [3], this term differentiated the disorder from other causes of stridor and more clearly depicted the flaccidity of the larynx [4].

Its incidence is unknown because it has been estimated in only cohorts of infants affected by stridor referred for specialist consultation. Holinger reported that 59.8% of congenital laryngeal anomalies in children presenting laryngeal stridor were due to laryngomalacia [5]. Furthermore, in a large series of congenital laryngeal anomalies, the incidence of laryngomalacia ranged from 50% to 75% [6, 7, 8]. Laryngomalacia affects males more than females [5, 8, 9, 10, 11, 12, 13, 14], but the importance of this is not known. Considering racial demographics, in 2007 Thompson showed that laryngomalacia is more common and more severe in Caucasian infants [2].

Pathological Mechanism

To date, the precise pathophysiologic anomaly causing laryngomalacia is still unknown. Several theories have been proposed to explain its pathogenesis. Anatomic, histological, and neurologic factors can all contribute to the development of laryngomalacia. Regarding an anatomic theory, this has been challenged. Since an anatomic theory is based on abnormal placement of flaccid tissue in the larynx [15], it does not explain why some children with typical anatomic laryngeal findings of laryngomalacia do not have the characteristic symptoms of laryngomalacia. Several classifications of laryngomalacia have been proposed [12, 16, 17, 18, 19, 20, 21, 22, 23]. Among these, Holinger's one is the most widely used and categorizes laryngomalacia into the following 5 types [16]:

Type 1: anterior prolapse of the arytenoid folds and corniculate cartilages (Figure 1). Obstruction occurs as the cuneiforms are drawn inward during inspiration;
Type 2: tubular epiglottis which curls upon itself, often associated with type 1 (Figure 2);
Type 3: anteromedial collapse of the arytenoids (Figure 3);
Type 4: posterior inspiratory displacement of the epiglottis against the posterior pharyngeal wall or vocal folds (Figure 4-5);

Type 5: short aryepiglottic folds leading an overly acute angle of the epiglottis at the laryngeal inlet (Figure 6).

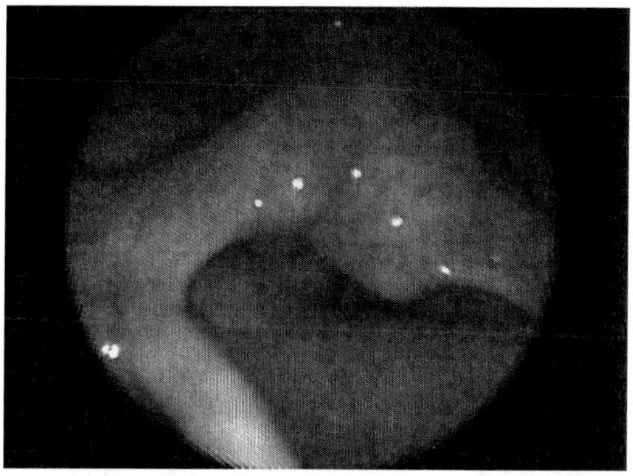

Figure 1. Anterior collapse of the arytenoids and corniculate cartilages.

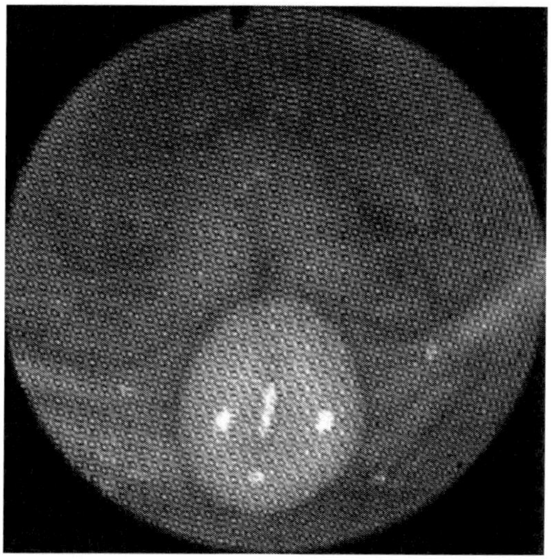

Figure 2. Tubular epiglottis curling upon itself associated with type 1.

Even if one usually dominates, two or more of these anomalies can be present simultaneously.

The histologic theory suggests that the immaturity of laryngeal cartilage may be the cause of collapse upon inspiration, but conclusive evidence of histologic abnormalities has not been found [24]. Moreover, only a few studies have documented altered histologic structure in laryngomalacia specimens without significant conclusions [24, 25]. In addition, recent studies have shown histologically normal fibroelastic arytenoid cartilage in infants with symptomatic laryngomalacia [26].

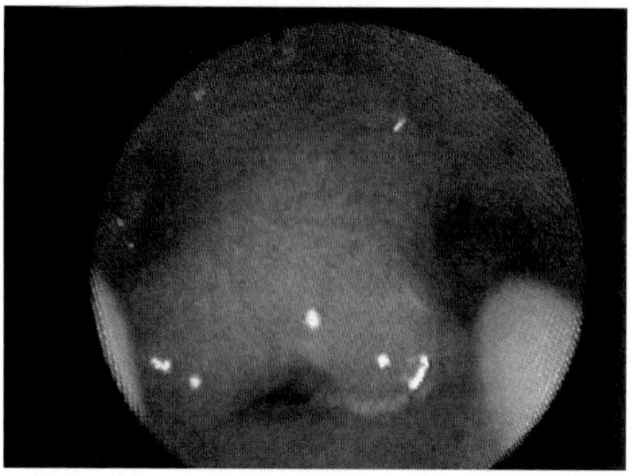

Figure 3. Anteromedial collapse of the arytenoids associated with edema retrocricoid area due to gastroesophageal reflux.

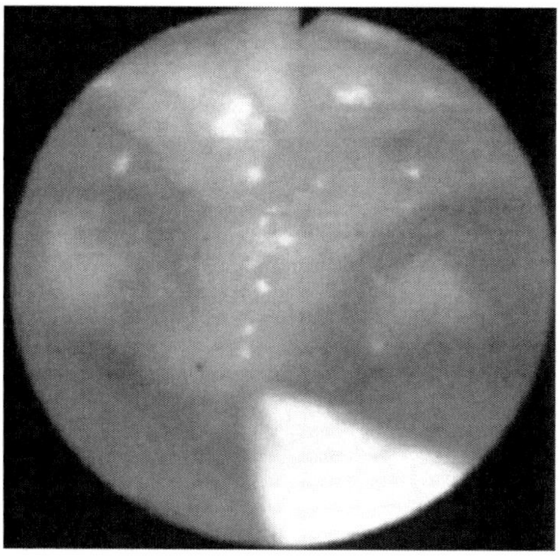

Figure 4. Posterior inspiratory displacement of the epiglottis into the laryngeal vestibule.

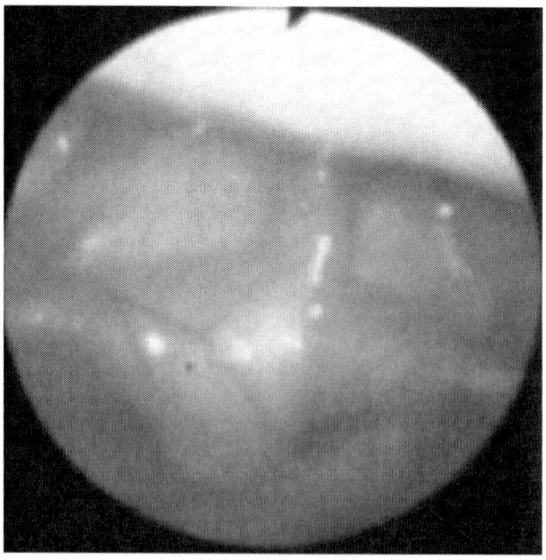

Figure 5. Close view of the posterior epiglottis displacement.

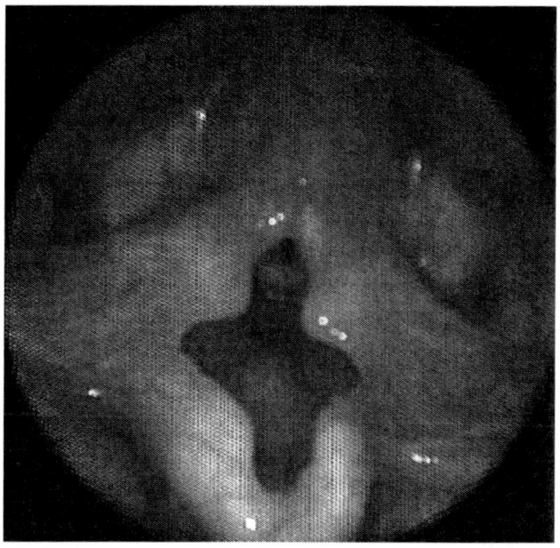

Figure 6. Short aryepiglottic folds.

At present, the neurologic theory is the best supported by the available evidence and proposes that neurosensory dysfunction leads to a lack of neuromuscular coordination of the supraglottic airway [2, 27]. Increased laryngopharyngeal sensory thresholds have been observed in patients with laryngomalacia indicating that peripheral afferent function of laryngeal sensation is altered. Such an alteration leads to changes in laryngeal motor function that appears as weak laryngeal tone in patients affected by laryngomalacia.

Symptomatology

Laryngomalacia presents with inspiratory stridor, which is the audible symptom produced by the rapid, turbulent flow of air through a narrowed segment of the respiratory tract. The symptoms usually begin at birth or within the first few weeks of life, worsen at 4–8 months, improve between 8–12 months, and generally resolves by 12–24 months [4, 28]. However, the clinical picture can sometimes persist for several years [29]. Stridor presents as a harsh, high-pitched, musical, vibrating, multiphase, inspiratory noise that typically worsens with feeding, crying, supine positioning, agitation, and flexion of the cervical spine, and improves by extension of the cervical spine, prone position, and quiet breathing. Cyanosis, supraclavicular, intercostal, and substernal retraction are signs of increasingly severe obstruction, and pectus excavatum is an example of the extreme degree of obstruction that can occur [24]. Chronic hypoxia from airway obstruction can lead to pulmonary artery hypertension if not recognized and managed [30].

However, stridor is not a specific symptom of this illness [31]. In fact, there are different causes of airway obstruction that can lead to stridor during different phases of respiration. Thus, one of the most useful ways to differentiate the causes of noisy breathing is to identify in which phase of the respiratory cycle (i.e., inspiration, expiration or both) the sound is heard. If stridor is present during inspiration, it is usually caused by partial obstruction at the level of supraglottic tissues such as in laryngomalacia. In these cases, negative pressure is created in the airway lumen causing the collapse of supraglottic structures. On the other hand, if stridor is present during expiration, it is caused by obstruction in the lower tracheal airway such as in the tracheomalacia. In this pathological situation, intrathoracic positive pressure during expiration leads a collapse of the affected portions of the trachea. Finally, if stridor is biphasic, the reason is due to fixed lesions at the level of glottic or subglottic plane that do not change dynamically with respiration. The most frequent is a viral croup, but even subglottic stenosis, subglottic cyst, subglottic hemangioma, vocal cord paralysis, laryngeal web, or respiratory papillomatosis may be present [32, 33, 34]. Moreover, stridor should be differentiated by two other noisy breathing conditions: wheezing and stertor. Wheezing is characterized by a coarse whistling sound heard on the phase of expiration and is usually due to lung disease. Stertor is a grunting or a snoring sound and is present during expiration. This sound is typically caused by adenotonsillar disease.

Other symptoms, which are related to feeding, include regurgitation, emesis, cough, choking, and slow feeding. In infants with laryngomalacia the delicate balance between the suck-swallow sequence and respiration is often disrupted [35]. The increased metabolic demand of coordinating eating and breathing against the obstruction can result in a weight loss and failure to thrive. The severity and progression of laryngomalacia are especially influenced by feeding and obstructive symptoms, APGAR score, presence of other airway lesions, or other comorbidities [2, 36].

Thompson [28] divided laryngomalacia into mild, moderate, and severe categories. Mild laryngomalacia occurs in 40% of patients and presents as inspiratory stridor with occasional feeding-related symptoms of cough and choking or regurgitation. The average resting oxygen saturation is 98−100%, and 70% of patients with mild laryngomalacia will have an uneventful course with resolution by 12 months of age. The management of these patients is based on clinical observation. The remaining 30% who present with reflux symptoms and a baseline resting SAO2 ≤96% can progress to the moderate disease category.

Moderate laryngomalacia occurs in 40% of patients. These patients complain of inspiratory stridor associated with feeding–related symptoms like cough, choking, postprandial regurgitation, and cyanosis during feeding. Their resting average SAO2 is 96%, and 72% of these patients will have resolution of symptoms by 12 months with feeding modification and acid suppression therapy. About 28% of these patients will develop severe disease requiring surgical intervention despite feeding modifications and acid suppression therapy [35].

Laryngomalacia is severe in 20% of affected infants. These patients show inspiratory stridor associated with recurrent cyanosis, apnea, feeding difficulty, aspiration, and failure to thrive. Suprasternal and subcostal retraction can lead to pectum excavatum. Their resting SAO2 is about 85%. Chronic hypoxia leads to pulmonary hypertension and cor pulmonary. These patients require surgical intervention in addition to acid suppression therapy [33].

Patient factors that do not influence severity, progression, or outcomes of the disease are: prematurity or gestational age at birth, birth weight, gender, or race [2]. On the other hand, APGAR scores, number of medical comorbidities, present of secondary air lesion [36], and baseline resting SAO2 affect evolution of the disease [28].

Synchronous Airway Lesions

Laryngomalacia may be associated with other anomalies of the airway such as laryngeal dyskinesia, vocal cord paralysis, subglottic stenosis, tracheomalacia, microretrognathism, glossoptosis, vallecular cyst, palatal anomaly, and choanal atresia [37].

The incidence of synchronous airway lesions (SALs) in children with laryngomalacia is estimated to be 19–27% [38, 39, 40], but is higher in infants with severe laryngomalacia requiring surgery. Toynton et al. [41] reported that the incidence of SALs in patients undergoing supraglottoplasty was 47%. Dickson et al. [36] reported associated lesions in 79% of cases of severe laryngomalacia and in 28.8% of cases of laryngomalacia with few signs of severity. Shroeder et al. found similar results in a cohort of 60 patients [37]: 58% of these children had SALs of whom 77% had subglottic stenosis, while 47% had tracheomalacia, bronchomalacia, or both.

SALs have an accumulative effect on airway block, leading to greater airway obstruction. Infants with mild or moderate disease that have a SAL is 4.8 times more likely to require surgical intervention [36]. Diagnosis of SAL may lead to earlier intervention and ultimately affect progression.

Comorbidities

The most common associated medical comorbidity is gastroesophageal reflux disease (GERD), which is present in 23–100% of patients with laryngomalacia [12, 16, 31, 42, 43, 44, 45]. GERD is common in neonates and infants and is characterized by emesis, dysphagia, chocking, gagging, and failure to thrive. The pathophysiology of GERD in laryngomalacia is caused by negative intrathoracic pressure that potentiates gastroesophageal and laryngopharyngeal reflux (LPR). Frequent LPR events result in inflammation and edema of laryngeal tissues, potentially leading to airway compromise [44, 46].

Neurologic diseases including hypotonia, developmental delay, cerebral palsy, mental retardation, microcephaly, and quadriparesis are the second most commonly reported medical comorbidities, with an incidence of 8–50% [9, 11, 12, 13, 18, 31, 42, 47, 48]. Moreover, congenital anomalies and genetic disorders occur in infants with laryngomalacia with an estimated incidence of 8–20% [12, 49]. Down syndrome appears to be the most commonly reported associated genetic disorder. Other syndromes associated with laryngomalacia include CHARGE association, Pierre Robin Sequence characterized by micrognathia [9, 12, 49, 50, 51, 52], George syndrome [51, 53], Larsen syndrome [54, 55, 56, 57], and arthrogryposis [49, 58].

Diagnosis

Diagnosis of laryngomalacia is suggested by its typical history, but it is confirmed by direct examination of the larynx. Awake flexible laryngoscopy is the gold standard examination (Figure 7). During execution of laryngeal endoscopy using a flexible fiberoptic nasopharyngolaryngoscope, a topical anesthetic such as lidocaine can worsen symptoms. For this reason, the use of a topical anesthetic is not indicated during this procedure [22]. Endoscopic evaluation of the upper airway in the office setting includes assessment of nasal fossae, choanae, nasopharynx, tongue base and posterior pharyngeal wall, hypopharynx, and larynx. Laryngeal dynamics is studied for supraglottic collapse and vocal fold motion. The checklist includes assessment of respiratory epithelium and the presence of edema. Routine use of rigid bronchoscopy is not usually necessary. However, in patients with severe laryngomalacia, who require surgical intervention, complete airway evaluation, including direct laryngoscopy and rigid broncoscopy, is required in order to assess the possible presence of SALs. In the operating room, endoscopic examination starts with flexible laryngoscopy without anesthesia for evaluation of vocal fold function. Following this, a careful examination of the pharynx, larynx, trachea, and bronchi is carried out under general anesthesia.

Other diagnostic procedures may be considered. Whenever aspiration events are present, modified barium swallow or functional endoscopic evaluation of swallowing can be carried out.

Furthermore, impedance pH for laryngopharyngeal reflux is reserved for patients who have failed medical treatment or who have refractory symptoms after supraglottoplasty and/or supraglottoplasty failure. Finally, the diagnostic work-up of laryngomalacia may be completed by cardiological, ophthalmological, and genetic assessment.

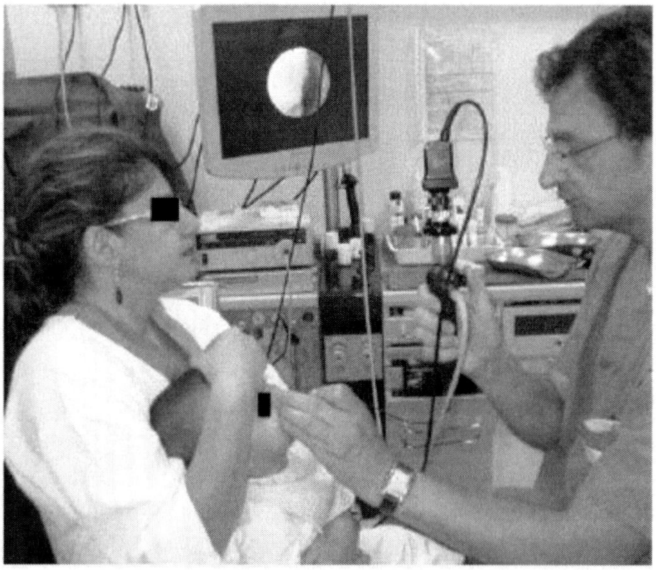

Figure 7. Execution of a flexible laryngoscopy in an infant held in the arms of a nurse in the office.

Treatment

The treatment of laryngomalacia depends on its severity, and comprises non-pharmacological, pharmacological and/or surgical procedures. Non-pharmacological treatment is reserved for children affected by mild laryngomalacia. These patients are managed with lifestyle, dietary measures, and regular monitoring of the disease with flexible laryngeal endoscopy. Lifestyle changes includes maintenance of posture after eating, no bottles of water before lying down, raising the head of the bed or mattress and weekly weight checks, whereas feeding procedures consist in the use of high-calorie formulas with smaller volumes.

Since the association between laryngomalacia and GERD has been well documented [59], pharmacological therapy of laryngomalacia involves the use of anti-reflux drugs. The treatment should be administered in patients with a confirmed diagnosis of GERD and/or in those with feeding difficulties and symptoms related to GERD. No studies have determined the optimal dose and duration H2 histamine antagonist or proton pump inhibitor (PPI) therapy or the preferred agent. Ranitidine can be used at a dose of 3 mg/kg TID and PPI can be used at the dose of 1 to 2 mg/kg/day [2]. A proton pump inhibitor is used for both refractory and breakthrough symptoms. At present, a combination of daytime PPI therapy and nighttime histamine type-2 receptor antagonist therapy is used [28]. Most infants are kept on acid suppression therapy for an average of 9 months [28].

Although laryngomalacia is a benign and self-limiting disorder, 10–20% of patients affected by severe laryngomalacia require surgical intervention [18, 41]. The presence of dyspnea with permanent and severe intercostal and/or xyphoid retraction, difficulty in feeding, failure to thrive, sleep apnea or obstructive hypoventilation, bradycardia, cyanosis, cor pulmonale, and uncontrollable reflux disease are considered indications for surgical treatment [13, 18, 60].

In the past, tracheotomy was considered the gold standard for severe laryngomalacia, although in recent years more conservative managements have been proposed. In 1898, Variot performed first the resection of excess mucosal tissue from the aryepiglotic folds based on the post-mortem findings in a neonate. In 1922, Iglauer first proposed partial epiglottectomy. After 6 years, Hasslinger performed successful endoscopic division of the aryepiglottic folds by forceps in three patients [61]. In the 1970s, Fearon and Ellis [62] described the suture of the epiglottis to the base of the tongue. In France, in the same years, hyomandibulopexy was reported with satisfactory initial results [8], but was subsequently abandoned. In 1981, Templer et al. carried out a resection of the epiglottis, ventricular folds, and aryepiglottic folds via lateral pharyngotomy in an 18-year-old patient with satisfactory results [63]. In 1984, Lane et al. reported the endoscopic resection of the excess supra-arytenoid and epiglottic mucosa using micro instruments [24]. In 1985, Seid et al. divided the short aryepiglottic folds by CO2 laser in 3 patients [64]. Following this, several authors used endoscopic treatment to resolve severe laryngomalacia. At present, this technique, called supraglottoplasty, is considered the standard surgical treatment [16, 48, 65]. The mean timing of supraglottoplasty is approximately 3 months [2], but can range from 1−12 months of age [66].

Different methods can be used for anesthesia: 1) mechanically controlled ventilation via a small caliber endotracheal tube is rarely used, as it may interfere with the surgical procedure; 2) spontaneous breathing anesthesia is generally the technique of choice; 3) the intermittent apnea technique provides only a limited time to the surgeon to perform the surgical procedure before re-intubation; and 4) jet ventilation [67, 68].

Although jet ventilation, spontaneous breathing anesthesia, and apnea techniques have the advantage of providing optimal view, maximum space, and operating time, the airway is not protected by tracheal intubation. Thus, particulate debris, smoke, gastric contents and/or blood may contaminate the patient's lungs.

After inhalation induction of anesthesia and intravenous access are established, the mobility of the true vocal folds should be assessed using a flexible fiberoptic nasopharyngoscope with the patient spontaneously breathing. This procedure also allows observation of the dynamic collapse of structures of the supraglottis into the airway. After this, anesthesia is deepened and the patient is placed supine, with a shoulder roll, head drape, and eye protection in place. The larynx is exposed with a Parson's laryngoscope, and the laryngeal inlet and supraglottic structures are sprayed with lidocaine (maximum 4 mg/kg) to blunt sympathetic stimulation [67]. Next, the larynx is exposed by inserting a Parson's or Benjamin-Lindholm laryngoscope. At this point, endoscopic procedures in the supraglottic area may be carried out using different surgical techniques.

Surgical techniques such as division of short aryepiglottic folds, resection of excess supra-aryetenoid mucosal tissue, sectioning of the median glossoepiglottic ligament with suspension of the epiglottis to the base of the tongue, partial epiglottectomy [69] and/or a combination of these procedures are in relation to the laryngeal structures involved [70]. Supraglottoplasty is usually bilateral, but some authors have also proposed a unilateral technique highlighting the lower risk of supraglottic stenosis after unilateral treatment [13]. In 1995, Kelly and Gray first analyzed the results of unilateral supraglottoplasty, reporting a success rate of 94% in a cohort of 18 patients. Only 3 children required a bilateral approach [71].

Several instrumented can be used for resection of excess tissue, and the use of cold microinstruments, microdebriders [70], or CO_2, thulium [72], and diode laser all provide similar results [73]. However, some authors believe that management of laryngomalacia by CO_2 laser and a microdebrider can reduce the risk of intraoperative bleeding and postoperative edema. Laser and microdebriders are more expensive than traditional laryngeal microsurgery instruments. Furthermore, laser techniques require special precautions to avoid the risk of fire during surgery. For this reason, a special orotracheal tube must be utilized.

Complications of supraglottoplasty are rare and are divided into major and minor groups [67]. Major complications include intraoperative and postoperative complications. The former comprise airway fire, whereas the latter include supraglottic and glottic stenosis. Damage to teeth or gums from pressure caused by the laryngoscope, airway edema, hoarseness, aspiration, bleeding, infection, granuloma, and granulation tissue represent the minor complications. Moreover, pneumonia can be present in 7−10% of cases [47, 73, 74].

Finally, revision supraglottoplasty and/or tracheotomy is required in 19−45% of infants and is influenced by the number and type of medical comorbidities [75]. In particular, tracheotomy is performed in patients who continue to have life-threatening airway obstruction and who fail to improve after supraglottoplasty.

Non-invasive Ventilation

Although there are no guidelines, several authors have proposed the use of non-invasive ventilation (NIV) for children affected by severe laryngomalacia [~~76, 68~~ 68, 76]. The aim of NIV for these patients is to decrease the exertion of breathing, which is increased due to collapse of sopraglottic structures during inspiration. In particular, positive-end-expiratory-pressure (PEEP) keeps the airway patent and increases the residual functional capacity of the patient [77, 78].

This therapeutic procedure can be utilized when a patient is waiting for surgical treatment, there are severe comorbid diseases, and/or whenever surgery has been unsuccessful [68].

PEEP can be performed by the following NIV-techniques: 1) continuous positive airway pressure (CPAP) and 2) bilevel positive airway pressure (BiPAP). The use of CPAP provides positive pressure throughout the respiratory cycle, while inspiration is not supported [79]. On the other hand, BiPAP involves the use of a ventilator that provides two different levels of pressure in view of the diverse patient efforts during the respiratory cycle. During inspiration, ventilatory support is greater, whereas it is less during the expiratory phase [80].

The choice of the devices with which to perform NIV is fundamental. Facial devices must ensure minimal air leak and at the same time be well tolerated. Nasal devices are often preferred in younger patients and are better tolerated than total-face masks and/or oro-nasal methods. Moreover, it is important to keep in mind that children are growing, and thus facial deformities that could be favored by pressure exerted by the mask on the facial structures must be avoided [81, 82].

NIV can be used in case of sudden progression and/or long-lasting disease. In this latter situation, NIV is generally carried out during sleep [80]. Finally, it is sometimes necessary to use NIV at the home. In this case, training of caregivers and compliance of parents is mandatory [83].

Conclusion

Laryngomalacia is the most frequent laryngeal congenital disease. Clinical picture ranges from simple laryngeal stridor to severe dyspnea associated with cyanosis. Its treatment, which includes non-pharmacological, pharmacological and/or surgical managements, is in relation to symptomatology. Every children affected by this disorder must be carefully assessed to decide his/her more adequate therapy.

References

[1] Daniel, SJ. The upper airway: congenital malformations. *Paediatr. Respir. Rev.* 2006; 7, S260-263.

[2] Thompson, DM. Abnormal sensorimotor integrative function of the larynx in congenital laryngomalacia: a new theory of etiology. *Laryngoscope* 2007; 117 (6Pt 2 Suppl 114), 1-31.

[3] Jackson, C; Jackson, CS. Diseases and inijuries of the larynx. New York: The Mac-Millan Company 1942; p.xi.

[4] Richter, GT; Thompson, DM. The surgical management of laryngomalacia. *Otolaryngol. Clin. North Am.* 2008; 41, 837-864.

[5] Holinger, LD. Etiology of stridor in the neonate, infant and child. *Ann. Otol. Rhinol. Laryngol.* 1980; 89, 397-400.
[6] Holinger, PH; Johnson, KC; Shiller, F. Congenital anomalies of the larynx. *Ann. Otol. Rhinol. Laryngol.* 1954; 63, 581-606.
[7] Ferguson; CF. Pediatric Otolaryngology. Vol.2 Saunders, Philadelphia. 1972; p.1168.
[8] Narcy, P; Bobin, S; Contencin, P; Le Pajolec, C; Manac'h, Y. Laryngeal anomalies in newborn infants. Apropos of 687 cases. *Ann. Otolaryngol. Chir. Cervicofac.* 1984; 101, 363-373.
[9] Apley, J. The infant with stridor; a follow-up survey of 80 cases. *Arch. Dis. Child.* 1953; 28, 423-435.
[10] Polonovski, JM; Contencin, P; Francois, M; Viala, P; Narcy, P. Aryepiglottic fold excision for the treatment of severe laryngomalacia. *Ann. Otol. Rhinol. Laryngol.* 1990; 99, 625-627.
[11] Prescott, CA. The current status of corrective surgery for laryngomalacia. *Am. J. Otolaryngol.* 1991; 12, 230-235.
[12] Olney, DR; Greinwald, JH Jr; Smith, RJ; Bauman, NM. Laryngomalacia and its treatment. *Laryngoscope* 1999; 109, 1770-1775.
[13] Reddy, DK; Matt, BH. Unilateral vs. bilateral supraglottoplasty for severe laryngomalacia in children. *Arch. Otolaryngol. Head Neck Surg.* 2001; 127, 694-699.
[14] Toynton, SC; Saunders, MW; Bailey, CM. Aryepiglottoplasty for laryngomalacia: 100 consecutive cases. *J. Laryngol. Otol.* 2001; 115, 35-38.
[15] Manning, SC; Inglis, AF; Mouzakes, J; Carron, J; Perkins, JA. Laryngeal anatomic differences in pediatric patients with severe laryngomalcia. *Arch. Otolaryngol. Head Neck Surg.* 2005; 131, 340-343.
[16] Holinger, LD; Konior, RJ. Surgical management of severe laryngomalacia. *Laryngoscope* 1989; 99, 136-142.
[17] Nussbaum, E; Maggi, JC. Laryngomalacia in children. *Chest* 1990; 98, 942-944.
[18] Roger, G; Denoyelle, F; Triglia, JM; Garabedian, EN. Severe laryngomalacia: surgical indications and results in 115 patients. *Laryngoscope* 1995; 105, 1111-1117.
[19] Lee, KS; Chen, HL; Yang, CC. Surgical management of severe laryngomalacia. *J. Taiwan Otolaryngol. Soc.* 1997; 32, 235-240.
[20] Shah, UK; Wetmore, RF. Laryngomalacia: a proposed classification form. *Int. J. Pediatr. Otorhinolaryngol.* 1998; 46, 21-26.
[21] Liu, HC; Lee, KS, Hsu, CH; Hung, HY. Neonatal vallecular cyst: report of eleven cases. *Changgeng Yi Xue Zsa Zhi* 1999; 22, 615-620.
[22] Nielson, DW; Ku, PL; Egger, M. Topical lidocaine exaggerates laryngomalacia during flexible broncoscopy: *Am. J. Respir. Crit. Care Med.* 2000; 161, 147-151.
[23] Kay, DJ; Goldsmith, MD. Laryngomalacia: a classification system and surgical treatment strategy. *Ear Nose Throat J.* 2006; 85, 328-331.
[24] Lane, RW; Weider, DJ; Steinem, C; Marin-Padilla, M. Laryngomalacia: a review and case report of surgical treatment with resolution of pectus escavatum. *Arch. Otolaryngol.* 1984; 110, 546-551.
[25] Shulman, JB; Hollister, DW; Thibeault, DW; Krugman, ME. Familial laryngomalacia: a case report. *Laryngoscope* 1976; 86, 84-91.
[26] Chandra, RK; Gerber, ME; Holinger, LD. Histological insight into the pathogenesis of severe laryngomalacia. *Int. J. Pediatr. Otorhinolaryngol.* 2001; 61, 31-38.

[27] Munson, PD; Saad, AG; El-Jamal, SM; Dai, Y; Bower, CM; Richter, GT. Submucosal nerve hypertropy in congenital laryngomalacia. *Laryngoscope* 2011; 121, 627-629.
[28] Thompson, DM. Laryngomalacia: factors that influence disease severity and outcomes of management. *Curr. Opin. Otolaryngol. Head Neck Surg.* 2010; 18, 564-570.
[29] Smith, GJ; Cooper, DM. Laryngomalacia and inspiratory obstruction in later childhood. *Arch. Dis. Child.* 1981; 56, 345-349.
[30] Jacobs, IN; Teague, WG; Bland, JW Jr. Pulmonary vascular complications of chronic airway obstruction in children. *Arch. Otolaryngol. Head Neck Surg.* 1997; 123, 700-704.
[31] Belmont, JR; Grundfast, K. Congenital laryngeal stridor (laryngomalacia): etiologic factors and associated disorders. *Ann. Otol. Rhinol. Laryngol.* 1984; 93, 430-437.
[32] Zoumalan, R; Maddalozzo, J; Holinger, LD. Etiology of stridor in infants. *Ann. Otol. Rhinol. Laryngol.* 2007; 116, 329-334.
[33] Landry, AM; Thompson, DM. Laryngomalcia: disease presentation, spectrum, and management. *Int. J. Pediatr.* 2012; 2012, article ID 753526.
[34] Dobbie, AM; White, DR. Laryngomalacia. *Pediatr. Clin. North Am.* 2013; 60, 893-902.
[35] Richter, GT; Wootten, CT; Rutter, MJ; Thompson, DM. Impact of supraglottoplasty on aspiration in severe laryngomalacia. *Ann. Otol. Rhinol. Laryngol.* 2009; 118, 259-266.
[36] Dickson, JM; Richter, GT; Meinzen-Derr, J; Rutter, MJ; Thompson, DM. Secondary airway lesions in infants with laryngomalacia. *Ann. Otol. Rhinol. Laryngol.* 2009; 118, 37-43.
[37] Schroeder, JW Jr; Bhandarkan, ND; Holinger, LD. Synchronous airway lesions and outcomes in infants with severe laryngomalcia requiring supraglottoplasty. *Arch. Otolaryngol. Head Neck Surg.* 2009; 135, 647-651.
[38] Gonzalez, C; Reilly, JS; Bluestone, CD. Synchronous airway lesions in infancy. *Ann. Otol. Rhinol. Laryngol.* 1987; 96, 77-80.
[39] Mancuso, RF; Choi, SS; Zalzal, GH; Grundfast, KM. Laryngomalacia: the search for the second lesion. *Arch. Otolaryngol. Head Neck Surg.* 1996; 122, 302-306.
[40] Yuen, HW; Tan, HK; Balakrishnan, A. Synchronous airway lesions and associated anomalies in children with laryngomalacia evaluated with rigid endoscopy. *Int. J. Pediatr. Otorhinolaryngol.* 2006; 70, 1779-1784.
[41] Toynton, SC; Saunders, MW; Bailey, CM. Aryepiglottoplasty for laryngomalacia: 100 consecutive cases. *J. Laryngol. Otol.* 2011; 115, 35-38.
[42] McClurg, FL; Evans, DA. Laser laryngoplasty for laryngomalacia. *Laringoscope* 1994; 104, 247-252.
[43] Giannoni, C; Sulek, M; Friedman, EM; Duncan, NO 3rd. Gastroesophageal reflux association with laryngomalacia: a prospective study. *Int. J. Pediatr. Otorhinolaryngol.* 1998 ;43, 11-20.
[44] Matthews, BL; Little, JP; McGuirt, WF Jr; Koufman, JA. Reflux in infants with laryngomalacia: results of 24-hour double-probe pH monitoring. *Otolaryngol. Head Neck Surg.* 1999; 120, 860-864.
[45] Yellon, RF; Coticchia, J; Dixit, S. Esophageal biopsy for the diagnosis of gastroesophageal reflux-associated otolaryngologic problems in children. *Am. J. Med.* 2000; 108 Suppl 4a, 131S-138S.

[46] Koufman, JA; Aviv, JE; Casiano, RR; Shaw, GY. Laryngopharyngeal reflux: position statement of the committee on speech, voice, and swallowing disorders of the American Academy of Otolaryngology-Head and Neck Surgery. *Otolaryngol. Head Neck Surg.* 2002; 127, 32-35.

[47] Denoyelle, F; Mondain, M; Gresillon, N; Roger, G; Chaudre, F; Garabedian, EN. Failures and complications of supraglottoplasty in children. *Arch. Otolaryngol. Head Neck Surg.* 2003; 129, 1077-1080.

[48] Solomon, NB; Prescott, CA. Laryngomalacia. A review and the surgical management for severe cases. *Int. J. Pediatr. Otorhinolaryngol.* 1987; 13, 31-39.

[49] Master, IB; Chang, AB; Patterson, L; Wainwright, C; Buntain, H; Dean, BW et al. Series of laryngomalacia, tracheomalacia, and bronchomalacia disorders and their associations with other conditions in children. *Pediatr. Pulmonol.* 2002; 34, 189-195.

[50] Schwartz, L. Congenital laryngeal stridor (inspiratory laryngeal collapse): A new theory as to its underlying cause and the desirability of a change in terminology. *Arch. Otolaryngol.* 1944; 39, 403-412.

[51] Markert, ML; Majure, M; Harville, TO; Uhulka, G; OldHam, K. Severe laryngomalacia and bronchomalacia in DiGeorge syndrome and CHARGE association. *Pediatr. Pulmonol.* 1997; 24, 364-369.

[52] Werner, JA; Lippert, BM; Dünne, AA; Ankermann, T; Folz, BJ; Seyberth; H. Epiglottopexy for the treatment of severe laryngomalacia. *Eur. Arch. Otorhinolaryngol.* 2002; 259, 459-464.

[53] Huang, RY; Shapiro, NL. Structural airway anomalies in patients with DiGeorge syndrome: a current review. *Am. J. Otolaryngol.* 2000; 21,326-330.

[54] Crowe, AV; Kearns, DB; Mitchell, DB. Tracheal stenosis in Larsen's syndrome. *Arch. Otolaryngol. Head Neck Surg.* 1989; 115, 626.

[55] Grundfast, KM; Mumtaz, A; Kanter; R; Pollack, M. Tracheomalacia in an infant with multiplex congenita (Larsen's) syndrome. *Ann. Otol. Rhinol. Laryngol.* 1981; 90, 303-306.

[56] Rock, MJ; Green, CG; Pauli, RM; Peters, ME. Tracheomalacia and bronchomalacia associated with Larsen syndrome. *Pediatr. Pulmonol.* 1988; 5, 55-59.

[57] Karakas, K; Percin, EF; Percin, S. Surgical risk factors in Larsen's syndrome. *Acta Orthop. Belg.* 2000; 66, 495-498.

[58] Cohen, SR; Isaacs, H Jr. Otolaryngological manifestations of arthrogryposis multiplex congenita. *Ann. Otol. Rhinol. Laryngol.* 1976; 85, 484-490.

[59] Apps, JR; Flint, JD; Wacogne, I. Towards evidence based medicine for paediatricians. Question 1. Does anti-reflux therapy improve symptoms in infants w ith laryngomalacia? *Arch. Dis. Child.* 2012; 97, 385-387.

[60] Kavanagh, RT; Babin, RW. Endoscopic surgical management for laryngomalacia. Case report and review of the literature. *Ann. Otol. Rhinol. Laryngol.* 1987; 96, 650-653.

[61] Senders, CW; Navarette, EG. Laser supraglottoplasty for laryngomalacia: are specific anatomical defects more influential than associated anomalies on outcome? *Int. J. Pediatr. Otorhinolaryngol.* 2001; 57, 235-244.

[62] Fearon, B; Ellis, D. The management of long-term airway problems in infants and children. *Ann. Otol. Rhinol. Laryngol.* 1971; 80, 669-677.

[63] Templer, J; Hast, M; Thomas, JR. Congenital Laryngeal stridor secondary to flaccid epiglottis, anomalous accessory cartilages and redundant aryepiglottic folds. *Laryngoscope.* 1981; 91, 394-397.

[64] Seid, AB; Park, SM; Kearns, MJ; Gugenheim, S. Laser division of the aryepiglottic folds for severe laryngomalacia. *Int. J. Pediatr. Otorhinolaryngol.* 1985; 10, 153-158.

[65] Zalzal, GH; Anon, JB; Cotton, RT. Epiglottoplasty for the treatment of laryngomalacia. *Ann. Otol. Rhinol. Laryngol.* 1987; 96, 72-76.

[66] Pinto, JA; Wambier, H; Mizoguchi, EI; Gomes, LM; Kohler, R; Ribeiro, RC. Surgical treatment of severe laryngomalacia: a retrospective study of 11 cases. *Braz. J. Otorhinolaryngol.* 2013; 79, 564-568.

[67] Rawlings, BA; Derkay, CS; Chu, MW; John, J. Surgical treatment of laryngomalacia. *Op. Tech. Otolaryngol. Head Neck Surg.* 2009; 20, 222-228.

[68] Ayari, S; Aubertin, G; Girschig, H; Van Den Abbeele, T; Denoyelle, F; Couloignier, V et al. Management of laryngomalacia. *Eur. Ann. Otorhinolarygol., Head Neck Dis.* 2013; 130, 15-21.

[69] Golz, A; Goldenberg, D; Westerman, ST; Catalfumo, FJ; Netzer, A; Westerman, LM et al. Laser parzial epiglottidectomy as a treatment for obstructive sleep apnea and laryngomalacia. *Ann. Otol. Rhinol. Laryngol.* 2000; 109, 1140-1145.

[70] Zalzal, GH; Collins, WO. Microdebrider-assisted supraglottoplasty. *Int. J. Pediatr. Otorhinolaryngol.* 2005; 69, 305-309.

[71] Kelly, SM; Gray, SD. Unilateral endoscopic supraglottoplasty for severe laryngomalacia. *Arch. Otolaryngol. Head Neck Surg.* 1995; 121, 1351-1354.

[72] Ayari-Khalfallah, S; Fuchsmann, C; Froehlich, P. Thulium laser in airway diseases in children. *Curr Opin Otolaryngol. Head Neck Surg.* 2008; 16, 55-59.

[73] O'Donnell, S; Murphy, J; Bew, S; Knight, LC. Aryepiglottoplasty for laryngomalacia: results and recommendations following a case series of 84. *Int. J. Pediatr. Otorhinolaryngol.* 2007; 71, 1271-1275.

[74] Whymark, AD; Clement, WA; Kubba, H; Geddes, NK. Laser epiglottopexy for laryngomalacia: 10 years' experience in the west of Scotland. *Arch. Otolaryngol. Head Neck Surg.* 2006; 132, 978-982.

[75] Day, KE; Discolo, CM; Meier, JD; Wolf, BJ; Halstead, LA; White, DR. Risk factors for supraglottoplasty failure. *Otolaryngol. Head Neck Surg.* 2012; 146, 298-301.

[76] Fauroux, B; Pigeot, J; Polkey, MI; Roger, G; Boulé, M; Clément, A et al. Chronic stridor caused by laryngomalacia in children: work of breathing and effects of noninvasive ventilatory assistance. *Am. J. Respir. Crit. Care Med.* 2001; 164, 1874-1878.

[77] Sullivan, CE; Issa, FG; Berthon-Jones, M; Eves, L. Reversal of obstructive sleep apnoea by continuous positive airway pressure applied through the nares. *Lancet* 1981; 1, 862-865.

[78] Strohl, KP; redline, S. Nasal CPAP therapy, upper airway muscle activation, and obstructive sleep apnea. *Am. Rev. Respir. Dis.* 1986; 134, 555-558.

[79] Boldrini, R; Fasano, L; Nava, S. Noninvasive mechanical ventilation. *Curr. Opin. Crit. Care* 2012; 18, 48-53.

[80] Pavone, M; Verrillo, E; Caldarelli, V; Ullmann, N; Cutrera, R. Non-invasive positive pressure ventilation in children. *Early Hum. Dev.* 2013; 89 Suppl 3, S25-31.

[81] Li, KK; Riley, RW; Guilleminault, C. An unreported risk in the use of home nasal continuous positive airway pressure and home nasal ventilation in children: mid-face hypoplasia. *Chest* 2000; 117, 916-918.
[82] Villa, MP; Pagani, J, Ambrosio, R; Ronchetti, R; Bernkopf, E. Mid-face hypoplasia after long-term nasal ventilation. *Am. J. Respir. Crit. Care Med.* 2002; 166, 1142-1143.
[83] Norregaard, O. Noninvasive ventilation in children. *Eur. Respir. J.* 2002; 20, 1332-1342.

In: Advances in Dermatology Research
Editor: James P. Vega

ISBN: 978-1-63482-226-8

Chapter 11

THE VISUAL RECOGNITION OF CYANOSIS AND THE INFLUENCE OF LIGHTING AND COLOR VISION

Stephen J. Dain*
School of Optometry and Vision Science,
University of New South Wales, Sydney, NSW, Australia

Abstract

The use of pulse oximeters has minimized the need for the visual recognition of cyanosis. However, there are times when this is still valuable. Lighting is important for this visual task and it is also a difficult task for some people with color vision deficiencies. There were fluorescent tubes that permitted the accurate recognition of cyanosis but they used less efficient halophosphate technology. In the 1990s the change in fluorescent tube technology to give greater energy efficiency introduced tri-phosphor technology. This created some problems most notably for anesthetists. A standard for lighting to permit the accurate identification of cyanosis was written (Australian/New Zealand Standard 1680.2.5:1997) based on measurements of isolated blood that were later confirmed by measurements of lips, nail beds and palm creases. Using these data, the basis of the problem for people with color vision deficiencies was also illustrated. The standard introduced the concept of the Cyanosis Observation Index (COI), its calculation and compliance values. Since then, there have been many attempts to produce complying sources for hospital lighting using fluorescent tube technology. The solutions tended to be energy inefficient (using halophosphate technology) or expensive. As a consequence, there was no successful solution to the problem using fluorescent lamps (straight tube or compact fluorescent). The other, less demanding, visual tasks in clinical observation (like observation of rashes etc.) were satisfied using modified tri-phosphor technology. The future of lighting is now firmly with light emitting diode (LED) technology. LEDs are more efficient than fluorescent sources and have advantages of compactness and no warm-up time. There are a number of white LED products available that have a COI that

* Phone: + 61 2 93854622. Fax + 61 2 9313 8602. E-mail: s.dain@unsw.edu.au.

easily complies with AS/NZS 1680.2.5. As a consequence, there has been a renewed interest in the COI as an appropriate and achievable measure in hospital lighting.

In this chapter the basis of the COI will be reviewed. The issues with color vision deficiencies will be discussed. The reasons why tri-phosphor technology fails to deliver a good solution will be outlined and the results of suitable LED sources will be provided.

Introduction

Technology has largely reduced the need for visual observation of patients and the unfortunate events like the demise of Mrs. Arnott-Smith [1] are, hopefully, now largely a thing of the past. However, visual observation of the color of lips, skin, nail beds and palm creases is still needed. [2, 3]

In the measurement of color, there are a number of influences;

1. spectral reflection characteristics of the object viewed,
2. spectral characteristics of the lighting and
3. spectral characteristics of the observer.

For the perception of color, we need to add;

4. size of the object,
5. state of visual adaptation of the observer and
6. color of the background.

1. The Spectral Reflection Characteristics of the Object Viewed

This is the primary feature and the direct relation of blood oxygen concentration. The measurements of spectral reflectance characteristics of such small and heterogeneous objects as lips, nail beds and palm creases on a subject that is not totally motionless is a challenging exercise for a color metrologist. In the past such an exercise took a few minutes per subject and the need for that subject to hold still and for the blood oxygen concentration to be maintained constant made the task very difficult, if not impossible. As a proxy for *in vivo* color, the author's early work on lighting for cyanosis observation used the spectral reflectance of blood. [4, 5] It seemed safe to assume that the overlying dermis and epidermis (or nail) constituted a constant so that any color change would be directly related and proportional to the color change of the blood. It was actually suggested, albeit a long time ago, that visual examination of drawn blood is a better measure than visual examination of the lips etc. [6] The ability to measure spectral reflectances in the visible range for oxygen saturations from 0.7 to 99.4% provided the basis to an averaged set of data in 10% oxygen saturation. The upper and lower limits of this scale are shown in Figure 1 along with the difference between the two, to highlight that the vast majority of the change in reflectance is in the red part of the spectrum, 600-700 nm.

From this, the change in color of the blood with oxygenation can be calculated. This is shown in Figures 2 and 3 (redrawn from [4]). In Figure 2, CIE L^* is the measure of lightness and is related to the total amount of light reflected. It is a perceptually linear scale. This shows that L^* reduces, almost linearly, with decreasing oxygen saturation. This is a quantification of the visual observation that blood (and lips etc.) gets darker with decreasing oxygen saturation. In Figure 3, a^* is redness (+ve) - greenness (-ve) and b^* is yellowness (+ve)-blueness (-ve). Again the scale is perceptually approximately linear and quantitatively the same as Figure 2. That is, a change of a given magnitude looks the same whether it is in L^*, a^* or b^* or a combination of them. The origin has been included in Figure 2. This represents greys. It may be seen that the overall change in color is a move towards the origin, so the change in blood color is that it becomes less colorful, loses redness and yellowness, rather than is changed in hue, becoming bluer. Color metrologists use the term "saturation" [7] for this metric, but in the present context, that would be confusing. That is, it does not turn blue despite the popular term. The total change in lightness (Figure 2) is about 10 units and the total change in chromaticity (Figure 3) is about 37 units, so the change in chromaticity is a much more visible clue than the change in lightness. This difference may also be seen ophthalmoscopically. In the eyes, veins look a darker red rather than blue. The apparent visual blueness in cyanosis arises, therefore, because of the structures overlying the blood supply and also the colors that surround the structure observed.

The measurements on isolated blood were made and used because the problems in measuring the color of lips, nail beds and palm creases were considerable. As the technology for making spectral reflectance measurements improved, the viability of making *in vivo* measurements has improved. The measurement now takes about 5 seconds [8] rather than the 3-4 minutes previously. [4, 5] Spectral reflectance measurements *in vivo* have been reported for chronically cyanosed patients before and after exercise. [8] In general, they confirm the direction of color shifts, but the measurements still show a high degree of variability.

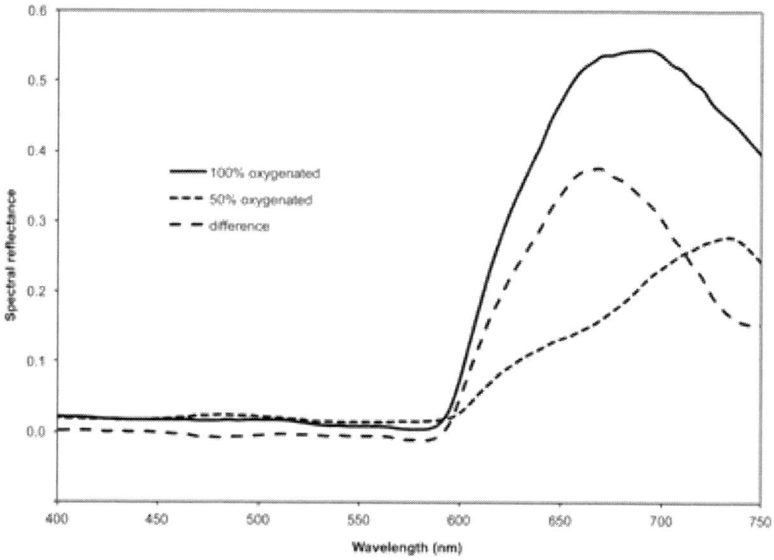

Figure 1. Spectral reflectance of blood in the visible region for two oxygen levels and showing the difference in reflectance (which is primarily in the region around 650 nm.

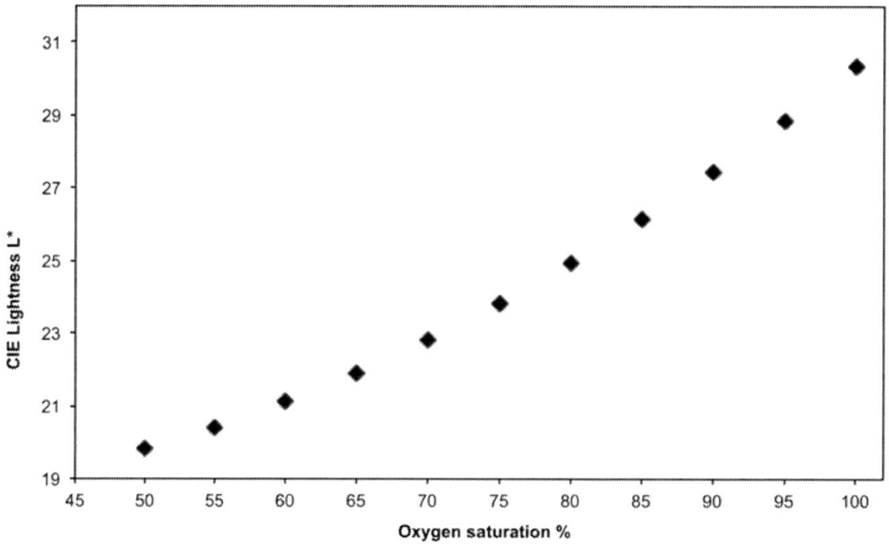

Figure 2. Change of CIE Lightness L* as a function of oxygen saturation. The reduction is about 10 units and in a monotonic fashion.

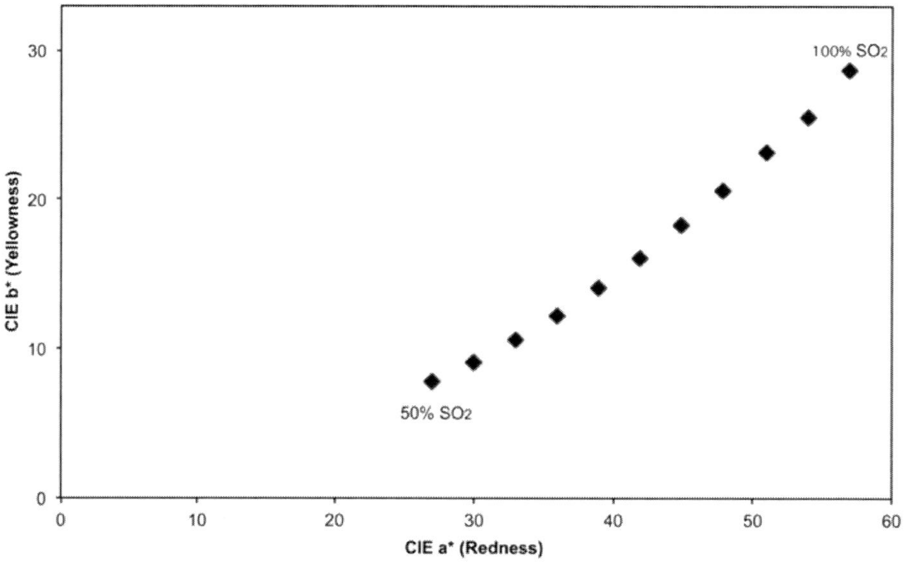

Figure 3. Change of CIE a* and b* as a function of oxygen saturation. The reduction is about 37 units and in a monotonic fashion. Extrapolated it passes close to the origin which is the location of grey.

2. The Spectral Characteristics of the Lighting

This is normally characterized by the correlated color temperature (CCT, T_c) expressed in Kelvin and the CIE color rendering index (R_a). The CCT is the temperature of the ideal source or of a reference daylight most closely resembling the source under test. It is a convenient way of characterizing the color of a nominally white source in one number. Typical examples are set out in Table 1. A CCT of about 4000 K has become the benchmark for clinical observation (see later).

Sources with identical CCTs are not necessarily spectrally the same. In an extreme case, a mixture of monochromatic blue and yellow-green could form a white source and this will perform differently from a white source that has approximately equal energy at all visible wavelengths. This phenomenon is known as "metamerism". The measure of the fidelity with which a source renders colors is the CIE Color Rendering Index, R_a. This is calculated from the change in color of 8 reference samples under the test source and reference source. [9] There are a further 6 reference samples that are not included in the general color rendering index but may be used for specific situations. The reference sample 9 is a red and R_9 is traditionally accepted as a good indication of the quality of a source for assessing skin tones. Color rendering is a scale running from 100 for a perfectly color rendering source to 0 or even negative. For many applications $R_a \geq 80$ is considered adequate and for the more critical applications $R_a \geq 90$ is often specified. The model numbers of modern fluorescent sources now often incorporate these numbers so that the first digit is the more significant digit in the color rendering and the second and third digits are the two most significant digits in the correlated color temperature. Thus a fluorescent tube designated 840 has a color rendering index in the range 80 to 89 and a correlated color temperature of 3500 K to 4500 K.

In 1965, a Medical Research Council study recommended an optimal light source for clinical purposes. The study was based on the observations of dermatology and pathology specimens and a few cyanosed patients. The recommended light source had a CCT of around 4000 K. The Crawford method of specifying color rendering was used at first to indicate acceptable color rendering limits of the light source. [10-12] The Crawford method has since been superseded by the Internationally accepted Commission Internationale de l'Éclairage (CIE) Color Rendering Index (CRI) [9] and the recommended sources were defined in the new system as a function of CCT and CRI. The form of this specification, in this case in an Australian Standard) may be seen in Figure 4. [13] Consistent with the advice of the time, hospitals were often uniformly lit using the same fluorescent tube type. [14]

Table 1. Examples of the correlated color temperature of common light sources

Correlated color temperature	Typical description	Example sources
About 2850 K		Tungsten filament lamps
2900-3300 K	Warm white	Quartz halogen tungsten filament lamps Fluorescent tubes Compact fluorescent lamps Light emitting diodes
Around 4000 K	White	Fluorescent tubes
Around 5000 K	Cool white	Compact fluorescent lamps
5500 to 7500 K	Daylight	Light emitting diodes

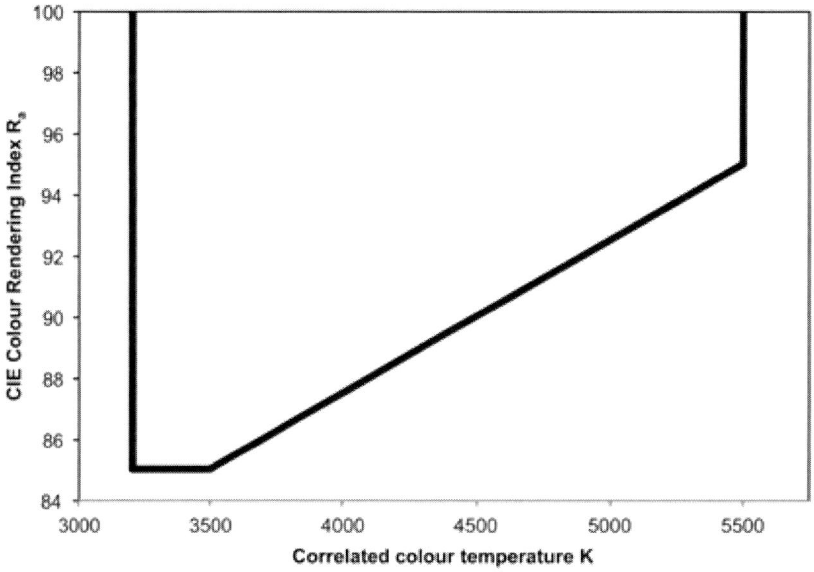

Figure 4. The limits of Correlated Color Temperature and CIE Color Rendering Index for clinical observation. [13]

The technology in fluorescent tubes at the time was halophosphates. The spectral emittance was a combination of the mercury discharge lines and the broad-band emission of the phosphors coating the tube. See Figure 5. It was relatively easy to design fluorescent lighting with high values of color rendering and a wide range of CCTs. Their broadband emission was not dissimilar to the reference 4000 K source (see Figure 5). However, these sources were relatively inefficient. They have been superseded by the triphosphor technology that is cheaper to produce and more energy efficient. This technology includes a red phosphor that has a "spikey" spectral emittance that is also relatively deficient in the 650-700 nm region of the spectrum, Figure 5, which is where the reflectance change of blood occurs. There are some modified triphosphor lamps that have higher general color rendering but low energy levels in this wavelength region are still relatively low and R_9 is low. Dissatisfaction with these tubes led to the studies reported above. [4, 5] From the measurements on blood and the conventional wisdom on which tubes were successful, a measure called the "Cyanosis Observation Index" (COI) was developed and incorporated into a new standard. [15] Elsewhere, studies in hospital lighting reported difficulty making measurements relating to cyanosis (probably because the light sources in use had little energy in the significant spectral region) and the recommendations were made on the basis of the needs of dermatological observation rather than cyanosis. [16-18] For surgical luminaires, the limits are set as 3000 K $\leq T_c \leq$ 6700 K and 85 $\leq R_a \leq$ 100. [19] Cyanosis observation is more likely to be carried out under general lighting.

In the author's experience, there have been no triphosphor tubes that comply with the COI requirements, so the measure did not achieve much recognition. What has changed the prospect is the coming of light emitting diode (LED) sources. Where the fluorescent tubes use a mercury arc to "pump" the phosphor, white LEDs contain a blue (around 470 nm) or, more recently, a violet (around 445 nm) LED as the pumping source and a yellow phosphor or mixture of phosphors. These have a broadband emission more in the style of the halophosphate. There are a number of different ways of obtaining the required CCT, CRI > 90 and a COI < 3.3 to comply with AS/NZS 1680.2.5. They also embody all the other advantages of LEDs including higher efficiency, no warm up time, long life, stability and robustness. Figure 5 includes such a white LED source. Table 2 contains the CCT and CRI values for these sources and also a modified triphosphor with a good CRI. Measurements were made with a Topcon SR-3 telespectroradiometer having a wavelength accuracy ± 0.9 nm (mercury and neon spectral lines), spectral half band width of 1.1 (mercury line at 546.1 nm) and calibrated using sources calibrated at the National Measurement Laboratory of Australia. The COI superiority of the halophosphate and LED sources is evident in Table 2.

Table 2. Characteristics of some white sources. See also Figure 5

Measure	Halophosphate	Triphosphor		LED
		840	940	
Correlated color temperature K	3986	3691	3970	3982
General color rendering index R_a	87.7	83.0	90.5	94.5
R_9	88.4	10.6	55.8	78.7
Cyanosis observation index	0.9	6.4	3.9	1.6
AS/NZS 1680.2.5	Pass	Fail	Fail	Pass

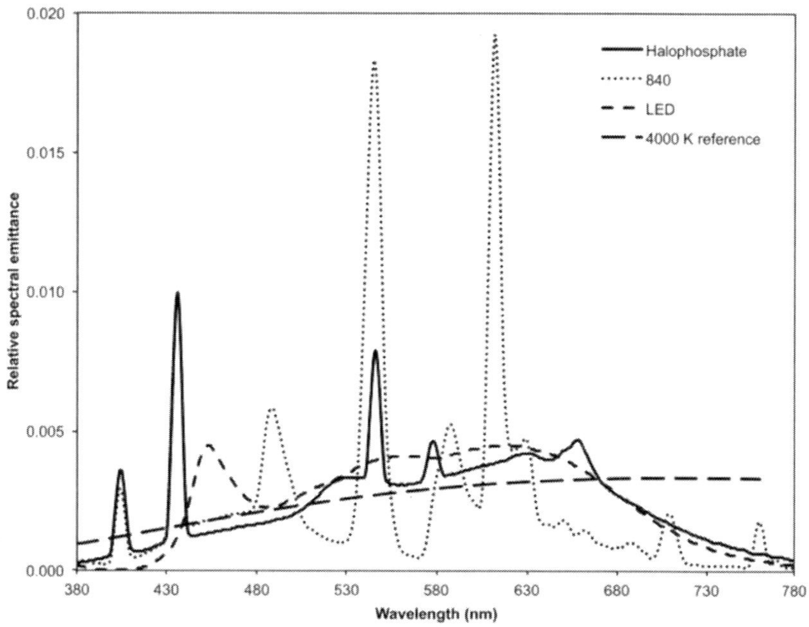

Figure 5. Spectral emittance of some representative sources for clinical observation. The halophosphate is an old technology inefficient source that is compliance with AS/NZS 1680.2.5 [15]. Color 840 is a source with moderate colour rendering and considered suitable for dermatological observation but which is deficient in the region of 650 nm and not compliant. The LED source is a source that is compliant. See also Table 2.

This illustrates that, in addition to their superior characteristics in efficiency and longevity, LEDs can also meet the correct color for hospital lighting.

3. The Spectral Characteristics of the Observer

Just as sources vary and may be described as being metameric, observers are also described as having metamerism because they also vary. For a visual task such as identification of cyanosis, the inter-observer variation in normal color vision does not result in significant differences. However, the greater variations exhibited in congenital color vision deficiencies have the potential to affect detection and recognition of cyanosis significantly.

The common congenital color vision deficiencies are in two distinct types termed protan and deutan. They are both "red-green deficiencies". In protans, the "red" receptor that is modified (anomalous trichromats) or missing (dichromats) and in deutans it is the "green" receptor that is modified or missing. They are called protanomalous, deuteranomalous, protanopic and deuteranopic, respectively. Both types of anomalous trichromat come in a range of severities from those in which the alteration of the cone is minor, with a mild color vision deficiency, through to those who lack the red or green cone entirely and for whom the world is actually in shades of blueness, yellowness and neutrals (although they may use other clues, e.g., a yellow always reflects or emits more light in total and is seen as brighter than a red or green). The problems for color vision deficient practitioners in the detection and recognition of cyanosis have been identified by Spalding, himself a deuteranope. [20-24]

A theoretical analysis was undertaken to assess the propensity for error by comparing the direction of color change of blood with oxygenation using the same blood data. [25] The change of lightness (L^*) is little changed for deuteranopes but is about 40% reduced for protanopes. The color difference for protanopes is only about 9% that for normal observers and deuteranopes are reduced to about 23% of that for the normal observer. From this it might be concluded that deutans are the more disadvantaged than protans. However, the anecdotal reports are always about deutans. [22] The study went on to assess the possibility of enhancing the color differences to aid the color vision deficient by changing the light source. The rate of change of L^* is increased only when a warm incandescent source is used. For color vision normals, such a source is too red, tending to make even the cyanosed look healthy. In addition, the warmer sources tend to reduce the chromaticity changes for color vision normals. The reduction in color difference is less dramatic for deuteranopes and is more affected by changing the source. The bluer the source, the greater the chromaticity difference for deutans. However, the bluer the source, the less the rate of change of L^*. It is not clear which is the more powerful clue for the deutan. However, extremes of yellowness and blueness in the source disqualify its use for color vision normals.

A practical experiment using digitally altered photographs [26] confirmed that some color vision deficient subjects are less accurate at identifying cyanosis. It also showed that new ambulance officer recruits perform less well than experienced ambulance officers, so the identification of cyanosis is a learned skill unlike, for instance, signal color naming. [27]

Influences on Perception

The effects of size, adaptation and surround have received little attention. While the colorimetric system provides for stimuli with 2° or 10° subtense [28], the calculated effects of increasing size are seen, almost entirely, in blue-yellow discrimination not red-green.

At low lighting levels, color vision is impeded, however, the levels that are typically recommended for hospital lighting [15] are well within the region of optimal color vision performance.

The effects of the color of the surround, such as operating theatre drapes, have been commented upon but not systematically investigated. [3]

Conclusion

The color changes that provide visible clues to the possibility of cyanosis in a patient are relatively subtle and subject to many influences. The variable of illumination color may be taken into account by the use of limitations on the CCT and CRI of the source or by applying the requirement of the COI. While COI has effectively excluded fluorescent tube sources as a validated lighting option, the availability of LED sources (as fluorescent tube replacements and spotlight replacements and the like) means that simple, effective, energy efficient and colorimetrically accurate options are now available. Many (if not most) practitioners with a color vision deficiency are able to recognize cyanosis as accurately as those with normal color vision. However, those with the more extensive color vision deficiencies need, at least, to be aware of their potential limitations to be able to be more guarded in their dependence on visual color.

References

[1] *Transcript of Inquest before coroner and jury upon request of relatives.* Deceased: Margaret Arnott-Smith. 1979: City Coroner's Court, Glebe. Coroner: Margaret Mary Sleeman.

[2] O'Donnell, C. P. F., et al., *Clinical assessment of infant colour at delivery.* Arch Dis Child Fetal Neonatal Ed., 2007. 92: p. F465-467.

[3] Changizi, M. and Rio K., Harnessing color vision for visual oximetry in central cyanosis. *Med Hypotheses,* 2009. 74: p. 87-91.

[4] Dain, S. J., et al., A Method for Evaluating the Acceptability of Light Sources for Clinical Visual Evaluation of Cyanosis. *Color Res Appl,* 1998. 23: p. 4-17.

[5] Dain, S. J. and Hood J. W., *Lighting for cyanosis identification Lighting,* 1998. 65: p. 18-24.

[6] Morgan-Hughes, J. O. and Bartlett M. C., The colour of blood in syringes as a guide to hypoxaemia. *Brit J Anaesth,* 1968. 40(5): p. 310-314.

[7] Commission Internationale de l'Éclairage., *ILV: International Lighting Vocabulary.* 2011, Commission Internationale de l'Éclairage.: Vienna.

[8] McNamara, R., et al., Colour change in cyanosis and the confusions of congenital colour vision deficient observers. *Ophthal Physiol* Opt, 2010. 30(5): p. 699-704.

[9] Commission Internationale de l'Éclairage., *Method of measuring and specifying colour rendering properties of light sources.* 1995, Commission Internationale de l'Éclairage. Vienna.

[10] Crawford, B. H., Measurement of Color Rendering Tolerances. *J Opt Soc Am,* 1959. 49(12): p. 1147-1156.
[11] Crawford, B. H. and Palmer D. A., Further Investigations of Colour Rendering, and the Classification of Light Sources. *Stud Conserv,* 1961. 6(2-3): p. 71-82.
[12] Crawford, B. H., The colour rendering properties of illuminants: the application of psychophysical measurements to their evaluation. *Brit J Appl Phys,* 1963. 14: p. 319-328.
[13] AS, 1765, *Artificial lighting for clinical observation.* 1965, Standards Australia: Sydney.
[14] Kelman, G. R. and Nunn J. F., Clinical recognition of hypoxaemia under fluorescent lamps. *Lancet,* 1966. 287(7452): p. 1400-1403.
[15] AS/NZS, Interior lighting Part 2.5. *Hospital and medical tasks.* 1997, Standards Australia/Standards New Zealand: Sydney.
[16] Lovett, P. A., et al., The effect on clinical judgements of new types of fluorescent lamps: I. Experimental arrangements and clinical results. *Lighting Res Tech,* 1991. 25: p. 35-51.
[17] Lovett, P. A., Halstead M. B., and Hill A. R., The effect on clinical judgements of new types of fluorescent lamps: II. Colour measurements and statistical analysis. *Lighting Res Tech,* 1991. 23: p. 53-67.
[18] Lovett, P. A., Hill A. R., and Halstead M. B., The effect on clinical judgements of new types of fluorescent lamps: III. Further statistical measurements leading to a new specification for lamps. *Lighting Res Tech,* 1991. 23: p. 69-80.
[19] IEC, 60601-2-41, Medical electrical equipment Part 2-41. *Particular requirements for the basic safety and essential performance of surgical luminaires and luminaires for diagnosis.* 2013, International Electrotechnical Commission: Geneva.
[20] Spalding, J. A., The doctor with an inherited defect of colour vision: effect on clinical skills. *Brit J Gen Pract,* 1993. 43(366): p. 32-33.
[21] Spalding, J. A., Colour vision deficiency in the medical profession. *Brit J Gen Pract,* 1999. 49: p. 469-475.
[22] Spalding, J. A., Confessions of a colour blind physician. *Clin Exp Optom,* 2004. 87(4-5): p. 344-349.
[23] Spalding, J. A., Medical students and congenital colour vision deficiency: Unnoticed problems and the case for screening. *Occup Med* (Lond), 1999. 49(4): p. 247-252.
[24] Spalding, J. A., Cole B. L., and Mir F. A., Advice for medical students and practitioners with colour vision deficiency: a website resource. *Clin Exp Optom,* 2010. 93(1): p. 39-41.
[25] Dain, S. J., Color changes in cyanosis and the significance of congenital dichromasy and lighting. *Color Research and Application,* 2007. 32(6): p. 428-432.
[26] Dain, S. J., Recognition of simulated cyanosis by color-vision-normal and color-vision-deficient subjects. *J Opt Soc Am A,* 2014. 31(4): p. A303-306.
[27] Dain, S. J., et al., Color Vision and the Railways, 1. *The Railway LED Lantern Test.* Optometry Vision Sci, 2015. in press.
[28] ISO, Colorimetry Part 1, *CIE standard colorimetric observers.* 2008, International Standardization Organisation: Geneva.

In: Advances in Dermatology Research
Editor: James P. Vega
ISBN: 978-1-63482-226-8

Chapter 12

Cyanosis: Causes, Symptoms and Treatment

K. R. Ramanathan*
National University of Singapore, Department of Cardiac Thoracic and Vascular Surgery, National University Heart Centre, National University Hospital, Singapore

Abstract

Cyanosis refers to the bluish discoloration of the skin, nails or mucus membrane due to an increased amount of reduced hemoglobin [> 5 g %] in capillary blood. Cyanosis is broadly classified as being central, peripheral or differential but can also be caused by abnormal pigments circulating in the blood. Central causes of cyanosis are mainly cardiac or pulmonary while peripheral causes arise from local vasoconstriction or lack of peripheral blood supply. Differential cyanosis happens in specific cardiac conditions. Cyanosis is usually a sign of an underlying condition rather than being a disease in itself.

Patients with cyanosis may have other features like breathlessness, shortness of breath, bluish or purple discoloration of the oral mucous membranes, rapid and shallow breathing etc.

There is general tiredness or weakness in patients who suffer from long term cyanosis. There may be episodes of headaches as well.

Treatment of cyanosis focuses on the underlying disease rather than the symptom alone. Initial stabilization requires oxygenation. Treatment of central cyanosis due to congenital heart defects may often involve surgery. Peripheral cyanosis brought about by exposure to cold may be treated symptomatically using gentle warming of the fingers and toes.

Antibiotics are prescribed for treatment of pneumonia and other infections. The chapter analyses the various causes of cyanosis and the possible treatment options for patients when they are cyanosed.

* Dr. Ramanathan K.R.: Consultant CTICU, A/Prof – National University of Singapore, Department of Cardiac Thoracic and Vascular Surgery, National University Heart Centre, National University Hospital, 1E Kent Ridge Road, NUHS Tower Block, Level 9, Singapore 119228.

Introduction

Cyanosis refers to the bluish discoloration of the skin or mucus membrane due to an increased concentration of deoxygenated hemoglobin in the capillary bed [1]. Cyanosis can be caused either by reduced oxygenation of the arterial blood or by sluggish peripheral circulation with increased oxygen extraction. The normal adult has a hemoglobin concentration of 15 gm% of which 95% is saturated with oxygen in the arterial blood.

The capillaries contain 2-3 gm% of reduced or deoxygenated hemoglobin. When the level of reduced hemoglobin exceeds 5 gm% in the capillaries the blood appears dark giving the tissues a bluish hue.

This discoloration is seen earliest in warm areas with increased capillary circulation e.g., palate, tongue, inner side of lips or conjunctiva and is referred to as central cyanosis. Peripheral cyanosis occurs due to the slowing of blood which allows more time for removal of oxygen, so cyanosis is more visible on the tip of the nose, ear lobule, tip of the finger and nail bed.

Causes of Cyanosis

Cyanosis is broadly classified as central, peripheral or differential, but also can be caused by abnormal pigments in the blood.

Central Cyanosis

a. Cardiac: Circulatory conditions may cause cyanosis by mixing oxygenated and deoxygenated blood

1 Congenital cyanotic heart disease
2 Acute pulmonary edema
3 Congestive heart failure

b. Pulmonary

1 Hypoxia due to reduced fraction of inspired oxygen
2 Obstruction of airways as in Chronic Obstructive Pulmonary Disease
3 Intrinsic Lung disease as in fibrosis of lung or bronchogenic carcinoma
4 Impaired lung expansion as in tension pneumothorax.
5 Pulmonary vascular abnormalities as in primary pulmonary hypertension.
6 Hypercoagulable states like pulmonary embolism

c. High Altitude

Peripheral Cyanosis

a. Cold
b. Shock
c. Raynaud's disease
d. Polycythemia

Mixed Cyanosis

Mixed Cyanosis: Refers to a mix of central and peripheral cyanosis.

1 Acute Left Ventricular Failure
2 Mitral Stenosis [right heart failure with peripheral vasoconstriction]

Differential Cyanosis

Differential Cyanosis: Refers to cyanosis of upper or lower limbs.

a. Of lower limbs: Patent Ductus Arteriosus [PDA] with reversal of shunt
b. Of upper limbs: PDA with reversal of shunt in transposition of great arteries.

Cyanosis Due to Abnormal Pigmentation

1 Methemoglobinemia
2 Sulhemoglobinemia

Approach to a Patient with Cyanosis

History — Several historical features help determine the cause of cyanosis.

- Age – Cyanotic congenital heart disease and polycythemia are much more common etiologies for life-threatening central cyanosis in neonates. Acrocyanosis and cold exposure are common causes of peripheral cyanosis.
- Trauma – Chest wall or upper airway trauma may cause central cyanosis due to lung injury or upper airway obstruction.
- Exposures – Smoke inhalation or exposure to other low oxygen environments suggests central cyanosis from decreased inspired oxygen.
- Medications – Blue skin color may occur in patients undergoing treatment with amiodarone.

- Prior lung disease – Exacerbation of pre-existing lung disease (e.g., asthma, bronchopulmonary dysplasia) is a common cause of respiratory distress and central cyanosis.
- Congenital heart disease – Cyanotic congenital heart disease may explain profound central cyanosis in some patients.

Physical examination — Cyanosis is always a concerning finding and is often less apparent in the skin of patients with darker pigmentation. For this reason, examination should

Management of Patient with Cyanosis

An approach to diagnosis of the etiology in patients with cyanosis is outlined in Figures 1 and 2.

Treatment of cyanosis focuses on the underlying disease rather than the symptom alone. Initial stabilization requires oxygenation.

Treatment of central cyanosis due to congenital heart defects may often involve surgery. Peripheral cyanosis brought about by exposure to cold may be treated symptomatically using gentle warming of the fingers and toes.

Antibiotics are prescribed for treatment of pneumonia and other infections.

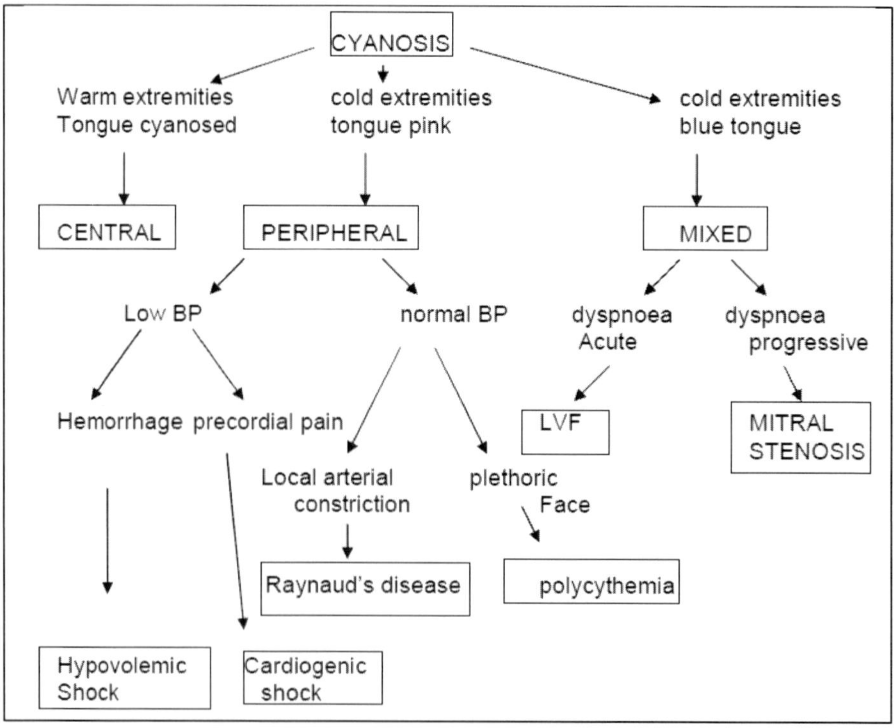

Figure 2. (Continued).

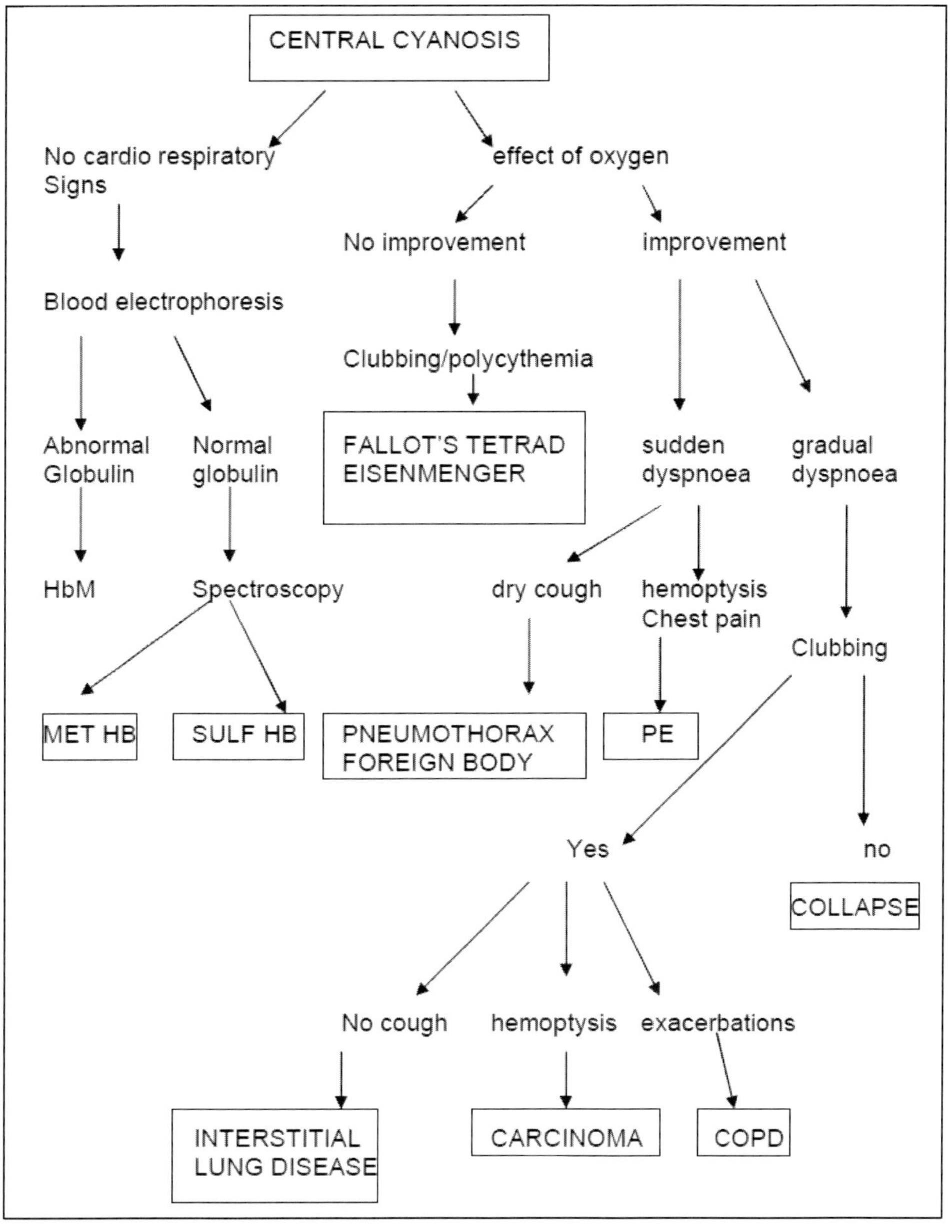

Figure 2. Differential Diagnosis for central cyanosis.

References

[1] Driscoll, D. J. Evaluation of the cyanotic newborn. *Pediatr. Clin. North Am.* 1990;37(1):1.

[2] Dahshan, A., Donovan, G. K. Severe methemoglobinemia complicating topical benzocaine use during endoscopy in a toddler: a case report and review of the literature. *Pediatrics*, 2006;117(4):e806.

In: Advances in Dermatology Research
Editor: James P. Vega
ISBN: 978-1-63482-226-8

Chapter 13

New Therapeutic Advances in the Management of Acne

Vincenzo Bettoli, Stefania Zauli [*]
and Annarosa Virgili
Department of Medical Sciences, Section of Dermatology,
University of Ferrara, Arcispedale S. Anna, Ferrara, Italy

Abstract

The treatment of acne continues to be a challenge to practicing clinicians and dermatologists.

Among the available treatment oral isotretinoin remains the more effective acne medication and oral antibiotics the more prescribed treatments. Given the restrictions placed on the use of isotretinoin and the increase in antibiotic resistant strains of *P. acnes*, there is a high clinical need for new treatment.

Acne pathogenesis is a complex mechanism in which different factors play a role. In the recent years the increased knowledge of the acne pathogenesis lead to the development of new and targeted drugs such as drugs blocking the activation of Toll-like receptor, PPAR antagonist, inhibitors of IL-1α and leukocyte chemotaxis, the antagonist of pro-inflammatory cytokines, the inhibitors of the production of reactive oxygen species and so on. A number of molecules named with abbreviations are studied and registered in the official sites.

Another problem is the tolerability of the currently available topical. In order to increase tolerability of these topical and of consequence to improve the patients' compliance, new vehicles have been tested.

Finally, also a vaccination killed *P. acnes* may lead to an innovative approach of acne management.

This indicates that the research in the field of acne is very active and so it is probably that in the next years several new drugs will hit the market.

The authors propose a review of the emerging treatments in acne field.

---

[*] Tel.: +39 0532 688129; Fax.: +39 0532 206791; E-mail: stefania.zauli@libero.it.

Introduction

Acne is a common chronic inflammatory dermatosis that affects more than 85% of adolescents and approximately 95% of the population [1].

The increased knowledge about the mechanisms of action regulating the development of acne lesions have stimulated further research in the hope of finding new active drugs [2].

A number of inducing factors, acting on a genetic predisposition, pave the way to the development of the following pathogenic events which lead to formation of acne lesions:

1) hypercornification of the infrainfundibulum and sebaceous duct,
2) hyperactivity of sebaceous glands and hyperseborrea,
3) hyperactivity of *P. acnes*,
4) inflammation and immunological host reaction.

Anatomically, the pilosebaceous unit is the cutaneous entity where the above mentioned events occur.

Hypercornification of the infrainfundibulum has been considered for a long time as the first of the sequence of events ending in the formation of inflammatory acne. More recent data have demonstrated the presence of inflammatory cells around the follicle before the appearance of the microcomedone [3]. As factors inducing hypercornification like androgens, growth factors, *P. acnes* and IL-1α may also directly induce inflammation, probably hypercornification and inflammation concur simultaneously at the start of the process leading to acne.

Clinically acne lesions are mainly localized on face, back and chest.

During active phase acne vulgaris is characterized by a mixture of different types of non inflammatory and inflammatory lesions which are concurrently present giving the dermatosis a polymorphic aspect. Non inflammatory lesions, also called comedones, include open comedones (blackheads) and closed comedones (whiteheads) depending on the presence or not of an evident opening to the surface of the skin. Inflammatory acne lesions may be superficial and relatively small like papules and pustules or deep and larger like nodules.

After the resolution of the acute inflammatory phase erythematous macules, post-inflammatory hyperpigmentations and post-acne scars can persist. Post-acne scars occur in up to 90% of the acne patients and they are socially and estetically relevant in 22% of the sufferers [4].

On the basis of acne severity, current guidelines for acne treatment suggested to use a combination of topicals (retinoid plus antimicrobial agents) in patients affected with mild-to-moderate papulopustolar acne and a systemic antibiotic, usually tetracyclines, associated with topicals in patients with severe papulopustolar/moderate-to-severe nodular acne. Oral isotretinoin can be used in patients not responsive or relapsed after the use of previous systemic treatments [5].

Given that many current treatments have potential side effects as teratogenicity of oral isotretinoin and experience-reduced responsiveness as the increase of antibiotic resistance, there is a need to develop safer and effective options to treat this common disorder. Moreover some of the treatments commonly used are contraindicated in certain groups as pregnant women.

The Centers for Disease Control defined a chronic disease as a disease "that in general terms, has a prolonged course, that does not resolve spontaneously, and for which a complete cure is rarely achieved" [6]. As acne vulgaris is characterized by prolonged course, pattern of recurrences or relapse, manifestation as acute outbreaks or slow onset, psychological and social impact, according to the aforementioned definition, it can be considered a chronic disease.

Based on that, it is reasonable to use all the available "tools" to prevent the recurrences of acne. Maintenance therapy represents an adequate strategy to maintain the achieved therapeutical results and to minimize the risk of relapse [6].

The management of acne is a problem also in term of costs. In fact there is a tremendous number of visits made to both generalists and dermatologists for the treatment of acne. The direct cost of acne treatment is estimated to be more than $1 billion per year and approximately $100 millions are spent on over-the-counter acne medication [1]. To follow the authors propose a review of some emerging treatments is acne field.

Oxidative Stress

The results of a recent study suggest that also oxidative damage may play a role in the pathogenesis of acne. In fact the serum levels of malondialdehyde and xanthine oxidase activity in patients with acne vulgaris resulted significantly higher than those of the healthy controls. A significantly lower superoxide dismutase and catalase activity has been found in the acne group than in the control group. It shows that in acne patients is present an alterations in the antioxidant defence system [7].

Fullerene

Fullerene is a spherical carbon molecule with strong radical sponge activity that penetrates deep into the epidermis. Oxidative stress plays a role in acne formation, suggesting that oxygen radical scavengers are potential therapeutic agents. In a vitro study, fullerene significantly decreases sebum production by 27.4%, suggesting another possible pathway of fullerene's effect on acne [8]. On the other hand, fullerene seems not to have antibacterial activity against *P. acnes*.

In an open trial including 11 patients with mild to moderate acne, fullerene 1% gel was given twice a day for 8 weeks [8]. At the end of the treatment comedos' number decreased only in 3 patients and this reductions was not statistically significant. Inflammatory lesions decreased in a statistically significant way in 9 patients. Also pustules decreased to 87.6% indicating that fullerene strongly suppresses neutrophil infiltration, possibly through its potential antioxidant effect on skin cells.

No apparent side effects were experienced by all patients.

The authors concluded that fullerene has a mild effect on acne and it could be used as a skin care product for acne patients.

Recently, fullerenol, a novel polyhydroxylated fullerene, with many hydroxyl groups capable of potent radical-scavenging activity has been developed. Vitro results suggest that fullerenol could be a beneficial skin care reagent for controlling acne vulgaris by suppressing sebum in the inflammatory response and by reducing *P. acnes* lipase activity [9].

Taurine Bromamine

Taurine bromamine (TauBr) is a haloamine generated by eosinophil and neutrophils at the site of inflammation, that has anti-inflammatory and anti-oxidant properties [10]. In fact TauBr reacts and inactivates H_2O_2, induces the synthesis of heme oxygenase-1 (a stress inducible enzyme with anti-inflammatory and anti-oxidant capacity), suppresses the productions of cytokines and chemokines, and inhibits the activation of NF-kB. Moreover TauBr has strong microbicidal activity and, at non-cytotoxic concentrations, is able to kill *P. acnes*. In a double blind trials 3.5 mM TauBr cream was evaluated versus 1% clindamycin gel [11]. Both were applied twice-a-day for 6 weeks. Forty patients affected by mild to moderate inflammatory facial acne were enrolled. After 6 weeks of treatment, comparable reductions of acne lesions, 65% and 68%, were observed respectively in the TauBr and clindamycin groups. No adverse events were observed. The authors support the concept that TauBr can be used in the treatment of acne, especially in patients who are already developed antibiotic resistance.

Anti-Microbial Molecules

P. acnes, a gram-positive anaerobic bacterium, attaches to pilosebaceous gland wall and secretes an extracellular polysaccharide substance, the biofilm. This biofilm acts as a barrier between the cell populations underlying and the exterior environment. *P. acnes* is the major contributor of the inflammation as it releases chemotactic factors, pro-inflammatory cytochines and corticotrophin releasing hormone (CRH), increases the expression and activation of Toll-like receptors, produces lipases and Reactive Oxygen Substances (ROS), stimulates lipogenesis, lipid peroxidation and comedogenesis, drives to production of enzymes such as metalloproteases.

Moreover membrane fractions of *P. acnes* could act as superantigens, amplifying the inflammatory reaction [12-16].

Due to the important role of *P. acnes* in the pathogenesis of acne, antibiotics have frequently used in the treatment of acne.

Among topicals clindamycin and erythromycin are the most popular. Other types of topical antibiotics are available in different countries according to the local national licences, such as nadifloxacin, tetracyclines, clarithromycin and azithromycin. Among systemic antibiotics cyclines and macrolides are the most used. Recently a decrease in term of efficacy of these antibiotics, erythromycin in particular, have been detected due to the development of antibiotic-resistant propionibacteria [17].

The management of antibiotic-resistant, and of consequence how to used antibiotics in acne treatment, is a delight question. Anyway the presence of propionibacteria resistant to the common used antibiotics has led to the development of new molecules with antimicrobial properties.

Picolinic Acid

Picolinic acid is an intermediate metabolite of the amino acid tryptophan that plays a role in zinc transport [18]. It chelates transition metal ions and is involved in the absorption and transport of transition metal ions. This molecule seems to work by perturbing zinc binding in zinc finger proteins and therefore leads to an alteration in chemokine expression. It has antibacterial properties and also modifies the immune response. In a open-label study picolinic acid 10% gel was applied twice daily on the face of 15 acne patients over a 12 week time [18]. A reduction of 58.2% ($P < 0.001$) in mean total lesion count, 55.5% ($P < 0.001$) in mean inflammatory lesion count and 59.7% ($P < 0.005$) in non-inflammatory lesion count was seen in this population. No serious adverse events or clinically significant changes in laboratory values were noted. The anti-inflammatory and antibacterial properties of lauric acid are already known, whereas recently also the anti-inflammatory and antibacterial properties of capric acid were investigated. Although to a lesser extent than lauric acid, also capric acid has bactericidal and anti-inflammatory activities against *P. acnes* probably through the inhibition of NF-κB activation and the phosphorylation of MAP kinases [19].

Calcipotriene

Calcipotriene is a vitamin D topical cream that seems to have antimicrobial properties and comedolytic activity. A study evaluating the effects of calcipotriene on the face and on the bacteria that cause acne is currently in phase of recruiting participants. In this study calcipotriene is compared with a placebo cream in a double blind way [20, 21].

Vaccines

Acne vaccine, obtained by inactivated *P. acnes*, targets a cell wall-anchored sialidase of *P. acnes*. Sialidases are thought to be used by *P. acnes* in order to catabolise sialoglycoconjugates to obtain sialic acids that ultimately act as substrates for energy production. It is also probable that sialidase may facilitate the adhesion of *P. acnes* to sebocytes [22].

Nakatsuji et al. demonstrated that intranasal immunization of mice with this vaccine generated in vivo protective immunity against *P. acnes*. The antibodies elicited attenuated IL-8 production in human sebocytes but without effect on *P. acnes* growth. So, the authors suggested that these antibodies exhibit anti-inflammatory properties sufficient for clinical improvement but without an antimicrobial effect [23].

The question is whether the results obtained in mice can be translated to the human model and if these antibodies have the potential to cross-react with other human cells.

Beside these killed pathogen-based vaccines various immunization-based approaches have been developed over the last decades, including monoclonal antibodies to the Christie, Atkins, Munch-Peterson factor of *P. acnes* and anti-Toll-like receptors vaccines.

The role of *P. acnes* in acne confers legitimacy on the possible benefits of immunization-based approaches, which may represent a solution for limiting the development of antibiotic-resistant *P. acnes* [24].

Thiazolidinedione Derivatives

Propionibacterium acnes infections are difficult to treat due to the presence of biofilms at the infection site and the associated resistance towards conventional antimicrobials.

A recent study has clearly demonstrated the effect of two thiazolidinedione derivatives on Propionibacterium acnes biofilm formation in vitro. The compounds were shown to have a moderate to strong anti-biofilm activity when used in sub-inhibitory concentrations. These compounds do not affect *P. acnes* attachment but lead to increased dispersal of biofilm cells. This dispersal results in an increased killing of the *P. acnes* biofilm cells by conventional antimicrobials [25].

Antimicrobial Peptides

Natural antimicrobial peptides could be considered as a new type of antimicrobial reagents for several reasons including their relative selectivity towards targets (microbial membranes), their rapid mechanism of action and, above all, the low frequency in selecting resistant strains.

Cathelicidines are a family of antimicrobial peptides acting as multifunctional effector molecules in innate immunity [26]. Cathelicidin-BF has been purified from snake venoms of *Bungarus fasciatus*. It is synthesized by GL Biochem (Shanghai) Ltd. In vitro cathelicidin-BF exerts a rapid antimicrobial activity against *P. acnes*. Its MIC against two *P. acnes* strains is 4.7 μg/ml, which is comparable to the anti-*P. acnes* potential antibiotics of clindamycin (2.3 μg/ml).

Cathelicidin-BF was found to inhibit O_2^- production induced by *P. acnes*. As a consequence it has anti-inflammatory properties because reduce the production of cytokines (such as IL-8, TNF-alpha, IL-1β and MCP-1) induced by O_2^-. In vivo anti-inflammatory effect of cathelicidin-BF was confirmed by relieving *P. acnes*-induced ear swelling and granulomatous inflammation in mice [26].

A designed peptide named LZ1, with 15 amino acid residues, contains strong antimicrobial activity against Propionibacterium acnes. The minimal inhibitory concentration against three strains of *P. acnes* was only 0.6 μg/ml, which is 4 times lower than that of clindamycin. In experimental mice skin colonization model, LZ1 significantly reduced the number of *P. acnes* colonized on the ear, *P. acnes*-induced ear swelling, and inflammatory cell infiltration. It ameliorated inflammation induced by *P. acnes* by inhibiting the secretion of inflammatory factors including tumor necrosis factor-α (TNF-α) and interleukin (IL)-1β. Combined with its potential bactericidal and anti-inflammatory properties, simple structure and high stability, LZ1 might be an ideal candidate for the treatment of acne [27].

ProOxy

ProOxy facial spray is a topical 15% Oxygen solution. A phase I open label pilot clinical trial evaluating the efficacy and safety of ProOxy spray in the treatment of moderate facial acne has been recently completed. In this study the spray were used twice daily for 3 months [28].

Povidone-Iodine

A mainstay in the pathogenesis of acne involves the overgrowth and proliferation of skin micro-organisms, primarily Proprionibacterium Acnes. Long term antibiotic therapy is usually prescribed for a period of 3 to 6 months or more. Povidone Iodine with its antiseptic property represents a promising avenue for the elimination of Proprionibacterium Acnes without the associated problems of long term antibiotic use, and the development of antibiotic-resistance. It is cosmetically acceptable, affordable, and easy to use. A phase II study with the aim to evaluate efficacy and safety of 3% Povidone-Iodine cream (Repigel-Mundipharma Pte Ltd.) versus placebo applied twice a day during 8 weeks has been registered in official site. Actually this study is not yet open for participant recruitment [28].

Anti-Inflammatory

Zileuton

Zileuton (Zyflo™) directly inhibits lipogenesis in human sebocytes and blocks the activity of 5-lipoxygenase, an enzyme involved in the biosynthesis of the pro-inflammatory lipids leukotriene B_4 (LTB_4) and prostaglandin-E_2 by arachidonic acid. LTB_4 is considered to be a major player in the development of tissue inflammation, and it is also a natural ligand for PPAR-alpha [29].

In the first pilot clinical study with 10 patients with papulo-pustular acne Zileuton 4 x 600 mg/day per os for 3 months decreased the acne severity index in a time-dependent manner being 41% of the initial score at week 12 ($P < 0.05$). This was mostly due to a decrease of the number of inflammatory lesions, corresponding to 29% ($P < 0.01$). In addition total sebum lipids significantly decreased (35%, $P < 0.05$) [30].

These data were in agreement with a phase II multicentric clinical study including 101 patients with moderate-to-severe inflammatory facial acne, which showed an average reduction on the total number of lesions of 25.3% in the Zileuton group and 16.4% in the placebo group [28]. In all studies Zileuton was found to be safe and well tolerate.

Afamelanotide

Afamelanotide is a super potent α-melanocyte-stimulating hormone (α-MSH) analogue [31]. α-MSH is a melanocortin peptide that increases skin pigmentation during ultraviolet light-mediated tanning. However, many experimental in vitro and in vivo studies have demonstrated that α-MSH have also anti-inflammatory and antioxidative properties [32].

It is further reported as α-MSH have anti-bacterial effects against gram-positive bacteria, but it is unknown if it has antimicrobial effect also against *P. acnes* [33]. On the other hand, α-MSH increased lipid synthesis by human sebocytes in vitro [34]. In a phase II open-label pilot study, afamelanotide 16 mg was given subcutaneously to 3 patients with mild to moderate facial acne [31]. Two patients received 3 injections at 3-week intervals, one patient 2 injections at 4-week interval. The total lesion number, as well as the number of inflammatory acne lesions, declined in all patients 56 days after the first injection. Total lesions decreased from 68 to 30 and inflammatory lesions from 46 to 23.7. The number of non-inflammatory lesions declined dramatically in 2 patients, while in the third patient only a transient improvement was seen. No adverse events, except mild and short-term fatigue in one patient, were observed. Important abnormalities in laboratory data were not detected. A placebo-controlled trial on a much larger number of acne patients will be needed to confirm the preliminary data and to determinate the optimal dose of afamelanotide capable to suppressing skin inflammation.

Apremilast

Apremilast is an oral PDE4-inhibitor agent that has been shown to inhibit the production of TNF-α, IL-8 and neutrophil infiltration. It is usually use to treat different kind of arthritis. A phase II, open-label, single-arm pilot study evaluating the efficacy and safety of apremilast in the treatment of moderate to severe acne has been recently completed [28]. In this study 20 mg of apremilast was assumed twice a day for 12 weeks.

Gevokizumab

XOMA 052 (gevokizumab) is a recombinant humanised anti-interleukin 1β antibody that seem efficacy to treat different kind of disease such as diabetes, arthritis and Behcet's disease. It is a sterile solution administered subcutaneously on day 0, 28 and 56.

A phase II, randomized, double-blind, placebo controlled study to evaluate the efficacy and safety of gevokizumab in subjects with moderate to severe acne is registered and currently in phase of recruiting participants [28].

Ectopeptidase Inhibitors

Inhibitiors of dipeptidylpeptidase IV and APN stimulate the expression of IL-1 receptor antagonist, thus they could be expected to reduce primarily comedogenesis and, secondarily, inflammation [35]. In vitro these inhibitors suppressed proliferation, enhanced terminal differentiation and slightly decreased total neutral lipid production, and suppressed proliferation and IL-2 production of *P. acnes*-stimulated T cells. Moreover the level of IL-1 receptor antagonist results significantly up-regulated.

Other

Talarozole

Talarozole (R115866-Rambazole™) is an inhibitor of cytochrome P450-mediated catabolism of endogenous all-trans retinoic acid in the skin. So it enhances intracellularly the endogenous levels of all-trans-retinoic acid. By virtue of this property, and the proven positive effects of retinoids in the treatment of acne, talarozole could potentially be an useful drug for acne [28].

It was developed by Barrier Therapeutics Inc initially under license from Johnson and Johnson and after acquired by Stiefel Laboratories Inc (GlaxoSmithKline) [36].

A phase II clinical trial of an oral formulation of talarozole in patients with psoriasis and acne, and a phase I clinical trial of a topical formulation have been completed [37].

Oral talarozole 1 mg once daily for 12 weeks was assumed by 17 males affected by moderate to severe acne in a phase II trial. At the end of the treatment a mean reduction in inflammatory lesion count of 77.4% ($P < 0.001$), in non-inflammatory lesion count of 58.3% ($P < 0.001$) and in total lesion count of 76.0% ($P < 0.001$) was observed. Nine patients complained of side effects, mainly eczema and stomach discomfort, but they were mild in most of the cases. The authors concluded that talarozole is efficacious in acne treatment and well tolerate [38].

As far as topical formulation is concerned, gels containing talarozole (0.35% and 0.07%) were applied once daily for 9 days on the buttock of 16 healthy patients in a phase I, double-blind vehicle-controlled study [39].

Talarozole treatment increased the mRNA expression of cellular retinoic acid binding protein 2 (CRABP29), cytokeratins (KRT4), CYP26A1 and CYP26B1 dose dependently, and decreased the expression of KRT2 and IL-1alpha compared with vehicle-treated skin. Both the two examined dosages showed a low irritancy [39].

An European placebo-controlled Phase II trial evaluating a topical containing talarozole 0.35% administered once-daily for 12 weeks in 80 acne patients has been conducted.

Twenty-five% of patients in talarozole group and 8% in placebo group resulted to be clear or almost clear [28].

Cortexolone 17α-Propionate

Cortexolone 17α-propionate (cortodoxone) is a new and the first topical anti-androgen that competes at the human androgen-receptor level. It seems to have also mild anti-inflammatory properties.

A randomized, double-blind, parallel-group, comparative trial, with placebo and tretinoin 0.05% cream, has been performed to evaluate the safety and efficacy of 8 weeks treatment with cortexolone 17α-propionate 1% cream applied once a day in acne patients [40].

Seventy-seven patients with mild to moderate facial acne were enrolled in the study. Cortexolone 17α-propionate 1% cream decreased the total lesion count and inflammatory lesion count; the improvement was significantly better than placebo. In comparison with tretinoin, cortexolone 17α-propionate 1% cream was always clinically more effective without reaching a statistically significant level.

The time to reach 50% improvement showed significant differences among the groups with a median time of 42.5 days for cortexolone 17α-propionate 1%, 44.0 days for tretinoin and 57.0 days for placebo.

A total of 8 subjects (11%) experienced 14 adverse events which were distributed as follows: 5 in placebo group, 6 in tretinoin group and 3 in cortexolone 17α-propionate group. None was judged serious to required treatment discontinuation.

A double-blind, placebo-controlled, dose-escalating Phase II trial in 360 patients with mild-to-moderate facial acne is ongoing to evaluating the safety and efficacy of cortexolone 17α-propionate for 12 weeks [28].

Epigallocatechin-3-Gallate

Epigallocatechin-3-Gallate (EGCG) is the major polyphenolic constituent of green tea know as a potent anti-carcinogenic, anti-inflammatory, anti-proliferative and anti-microbial activities. Also anti-androgenic properties have been reported.

In SEB-1 sebocytes EGCG reduces sebum production by modulating AMPK-SREBP-1 signalling pathway and reduces inflammation by suppressing the NK-kB and AP-1 pathway. Moreover EGCG decreases the viability of *P. acnes*, thus targeting almost all the pathogenic feature of acne.

In a 8-week randomized, split-face, clinical trial EGCG improved acne and it is well tolerated [41]. Tea tree oil gel is also under study in the treatment of mild to moderate facial acne. In a phase II open label study the gel is applied twice daily for 12 weeks.

Oligonucleotides

Inhibition of the expression of androgen receptor by antisense oligonucleotides reduces in vitro the enhanced proliferation of sebocytes challenged by testosterone and DHT [42]. They could be consider a novel strategy for the blockage of the androgen receptor and could be represent a specific therapeutic approach in androgen-associated acne.

Natural Products - Homoeopatic Medicine

A long list of natural product have been tested in the treatment of acne and in general in the treatment of cutaneous disease, including green tea, essential oil, various plant extracts, etc.

Studies on cell lines revealed that flavonoid, alkaloid, essential oil, phenol and phenolic compound, tannin, xanthone and xanthone derivative, and the bisnaphthquione derivative are effective in treatment of acne. Animal studies showed that diterpene acid, phenylpropanoid glycosides, acteoside and flavonoids have anti-inflammatory activity. Eleven human studies revealed that Camellia sinensis has 5α-reductase inhibitory and anti-inflammatory activities. Also anti-bacterial effect has been shown by oleoresin of Commiphora mukul [43].

Below we have listed only some of these studies just to underline how the research of new anti-acne molecules derived from nature is active.

Resveratrol

Resveratrol is a natural phytoalexin produced by some spermatophytes, such as grapes and other plants. It exhibits activity against *P. acnes* as well as anti-inflammatory properties [44]. In a pilot single-blind study including 20 patients with facial acne resveratrol incorporated in a carboxymethylcellulose-based gel was applied daily on the right side of the face for 60 days.

As control the hydrogel vehicle was applied to the left side [44]. Clinical evaluation showed a reduction in the acne score of 53.47% on the resveratrol-treated sides and of 6.10% on the vehicle-treated sides. No adverse events were registered. The authors concluded that resveratrol could be a valid alternative in acne treatment. This effectiveness should be tested at different concentration and formulation, and in a larger group of patients.

Curcumin

Curcumin in the vehicles significantly inhibited the growth of *P. acnes* in the skin when evaluated by the bioluminescence assay [45].

Ethanolic Rosemary Extract

Ethanolic rosemary extract (ERE) has been showed to significantly suppress the secretion and mRNA expression of pro-inflammatory cytokines, including interleukin (IL)-8, IL-1β, and tumor necrosis factor-α in *P. acnes*-stimulated monocyte THP-1 cells.

In vivo mouse model intradermal injection of ERE attenuated the *P. acnes*-induced ear swelling and granulomatous inflammation. Further studies are needed to explore the role of bioactive compounds of rosemary in mitigation of *P. acnes*-induced inflammation [46].

Essential Oil and Aromatherapy

A randomized controlled trial involving 192 participants divided in 3 groups (treatment with essential oil-aromatherapy-wait list control) has been provided high-quality evidence of the effectiveness of essential oil and aromatherapy in the treatment of acne [47].

Marine-Derived Ingredients

Potential benefits may be offered also by natural, marine-derived ingredients such as those derived from brown seaweed (Laminaria digitata) and a novel seaweed oligosaccharide-zinc complex (SOZC) [48].

Homoeopatic Medicine

The efficacy of some lesser known homoeopatic medicines in acne treatment has been recent assessed in open label phase I studies. Zingiber officinalis are pills to assumed 4 times a day for 7 days. The same is for azadurachta indica and lappa arctium [28].

Instrumental Treatment

Headheld Heat Device

A phase 4 open label study comparing a popular handheld heat devised and a topical treatment with BPO 4% in the treatment of individual acne lesions is currently registered under the sponsoritation of the University of British Columbia [28].

Acleara Needle Insert

A open-label study assessing the efficacy of Acleare Needle Insert in acne vulgaris has been completed. Fifteen subjects were enrolled. Each subject could have up to 5 lesions treated with this system and received up to 3 follow up visits [28].

Clear Device

Clear device is a light based devise. A clinical research, involving 50 patients, assessed the efficacy of this device to treat mild to moderate inflammatory acne and determined if the patients are able to use the device properly.

Two sessions a week for 4 weeks, for a total of 8 sessions, and 2 follow-up visits were performed. The patients treated themselves with the clear device.

The average improvement of acne lesions was 56.7% after one month and 57.7% after three months [28].

KLOX Biophotonic System

An opel label split face phase III study evaluating KLOX Biophotonic System versus no treatment in moderate to severe acne is ongoing. This system provides the application of KLOX KLGA0105-01 photo-convert gel and after the use of KLOX THERA lamp.

This procedure is performed twice a week for 6 weeks followed by a 6 week follow up period [28].

PhotoPneumatic System

The PhotoPneumatic System includes the use of intense pulsed light in combination with vacuum technology. This system has been used to treat mild to moderate acne in 20 adult patients in a prospective observational spilt-face study.

A significant reduction in the number of acne lesions were observed on the treated side of the faces. Most patients experienced global clinical improvement.

No severe side effects occurred during the study, with only a few patients experiencing transient erythema, purpura and/or exacerbation of pre-existing acne [49].

Photodimanic Therapy

Recently PDT with a photosensitizer, 5-aminolevulanic acid (ALA) or methyl aminolevulinate (MAL), has been proven useful in the management of inflammatory acne [50].

Twenty-four subjects with acne on both sides of the face were included in a study with the aim to evaluate the clinical efficacy and safety of chlorophyll-a photodynamic therapy. Eight treatment sessions were performed over a 4-week duration. Half of the face was irradiated using a blue and red light-emitting diode after topical application of chlorophyll-lipoid complex. The other half underwent only light-emitting diode phototherapy. On the chlorophyll-a photodynamic therapy-treated side a significant reduction in acne lesion counts, acne severity grades, and sebum levels were observed in comparison with the side treated with light-emitting diode phototherapy alone. The side effects were tolerable in all the cases [51].

Two studies using as photosensitizier respectively lemuteporfin topical solution 15 and topical visonac have been registered.

More over a study comparing PDT with a conventional acne treatment with topical adapalene gel 0.1% for 12 weeks plus doxycycline 100 mg/day for three months is ongoing [28].

Botulin

A phase II and a phase III double-blind randomized studies evaluating the efficacy and safety of the botulinum neurotoxin type A injections in subjects with acne has been terminated.

This approach already known in the treatment of post-acne scars is so currently proposed also in the treatment of active acne lesions [28].

Ultrasound Device

Currently two pilot open label studies assessing, in a small group of subjects, the efficacy of an ultrasound device in acne treatment have been registered. One has been already completed whereas the other one is in phase of recruiting of participants.

The experimental ultrasound device uses sound waves to heat the acute acne lesion and the surrounding sebaceous gland without affecting the surface of the skin. The authors hope that heating the sebaceous glands will reduce their size and the symptoms of inflamed acne [28].

Plasma Treatment System

A single center pilot study evaluating the efficacy and safety of the antimicrobial plasma treatment system to treat back acne is ongoing. Plasma is applied to back for up to 20 minutes twice/week for 4 weeks [28].

Silk'n Blue Device

The Silk'n Blue device has an array of 24 LEDs emitting a spectrum of light in the blue-violet range of light (405-460 nm). This light based technology seems safe and efficacious as home device for the treatment of mild to moderate inflammatory acne vulgaris.

The data were obtained by a study involving 70 subjects that have been received eight treatments with the Silk'n Blue device over a 4-week period. There was a statistically significant decrease in mean acne counts from baseline through the follow-up visits ($p = 0.002$).

The 36.4% of the patients have also obtained a complete clearance with the studied device [52].

Low-Level Laser Therapy (Erchonia EML)

Recent evidence indicates that low-level laser therapy (LLLT) is able to significantly diminish the expression of COX-2, resulting in the reduction of inflammation.

The ability to modulate the COX-2 pathway via LLLT is believed to inhibit the production of pro-inflammatory cytokines (i.e., TNF-α and IL- α) present in acne-prone skin.

The Erchonia® EML Laser is a dual-diode 7 mW laser of 635 nm and 405 nm wavelength. The light emitting diode is manufactured by Coherent and classified by the Center for Devices and Radiological Health (CDRH) as a Class IIIb laser diode.

A pilot study assessing the efficacy of this system to reduce the number of inflammatory and non-inflammatory acne lesions has been completed [28].

Conclusion

The treatment of acne continues to be a challenge to practicing clinicians and dermatologists. Among the available treatments oral isotretinoin remains the more effective acne medication and oral antibiotics the more prescribed treatments. Given the restrictions placed on the use of isotretinoin and the increase in antibiotic resistant strains of *P. acnes*, there is a high clinical need for new treatments. Acne pathogenesis is a complex mechanism in which different factors play a role. In the recent years the increased knowledge of the acne pathogenesis have led to the development of new and targeted drugs overall with anti-microbial and anti-inflammatory properties. In order to reduce the development of antibiotic resistant *P. acnes* also acne vaccine, obtained by inactivated *P. acnes*, may represent an innovative approach of acne management in the future. A number of molecules named with abbreviations, therefore unidentifiable, are studied and registered in the official sites. So, it is probably, that in the next years several new drugs will hit the market. Finally, various instrumental approaches have been tested in the treatment of acne range from the use of different kind of lights to mechanical insults such as ultrasound or needle insert.

All this indicates that the research in the field of acne is very active.

In the future it is likely that other new treatments will continue to appear as our knowledge of the pathogenic mechanism of acne are in continuous improvement providing an always wider array of therapeutic targets. Prospective new acne treatment may be represent by drugs blocking the activation of Toll-like receptor, PPAR antagonist, inhibitors of IL-1α and leukocyte chemotaxis, antagonist of pro-inflammatory cytokines, inhibitors of the production of reactive oxygen species, etc. Nanotechnology may facilitate follicular targeting of such treatments.

Some studies investigating dietary interventions are also registered. So, it is also probably that in the next years beside to a pharmacological prescription, a modification of patients' lifestyle could be required.

References

[1] Patel P., Lin H. C., Feldman S. R.,et al. Medication choice and associated health care outcomes and costs for patients with acne and acne-related conditions in the United States. *J. Drugs Dermatol.*, 2011; 10: 766-71.

[2] Kurokawa I., Danby F. W., Ju Q., et al. New developments in our understanding of acne pathogenesis and treatment. *Experimental Dermatology,* 2009; 18: 821-32.

[3] Jeremy A. H., Holland D. B., Roberts S. G. et al. Inflammatory events are involved in acne lesion initiation. *J. Invest. Dermatol.,* 2003; 121: 20-7.

[4] Layton A. M., Henderson C. A., Cunliffe W. J. A clinical evaluation of acne scarring and its incidence. *Clin. Exp. Dermatol.,* 1994; 19: 303.

[5] Nast A., Dréno B., Bettoli V., et al. European evidence-based (S3) guidelines for the treatment of acne. *J. Eur. Acad. Dermatol. Venereol.,* 2012; 26: 1-29.

[6] Gollnick H. P., Finlay A. Y., Shear N.; Global Alliance to Improve Outcomes in Acne. Can we define acne as a chronic disease? If so, how and when? *Am. J. Clin. Dermatol.*, 2008; 9: 279-84.

[7] Sarici G., Cinar S., Armutcu F., et al. Oxidative stress in acne vulgaris. *J. Eur. Acad. Dermatol. Venereol.,* 2010; 24: 763-7.

[8] Inui S., Aoshima H., Nishiyama A., et al. Improvement of acne vulgaris by topical fullerene application: unique impact on skin care. *Nanomedicine*, 2011; 7: 238-41.

[9] Inui S., Aoshima H., Ito M., et al. Inhibition of sebum production and Propionibacterium acnes lipase activity by fullerenol, a novel polyhydroxylated fullerene: potential as a therapeutic reagent for acne. *J. Cosmet. Sci.*, 2012; 63: 259-65.
[10] Marcinkiewicz J. Taurine bromamine (TauBr)-its role in immunity and new perspectives for clinical use. *J. Biomed. Sci.,* 2010; 17 Suppl. 1: S3.
[11] Marcinkiewicz J., Wojas-Pelc A., Walczewska M., et al. Topical taurine bromamine, a new candidate in the treatment of moderate inflammatory acne vulgaris: a pilot study. *Eur. J. Dermatol.*, 2008; 18: 433-9.
[12] Pivarcsi A., Bodai L., Rethi B., et al. Expression and function of Toll-like receptors 2 and 4 in human keratinocytes. *Int. Immunology*, 2003; 15: 721.
[13] Jappe U., Ingham E., Henwood J., et al. Propionibacterium acnes and inflammation in acne: P.acnes has T-cell mitogenic activity. *Br. J. Dermatol.,* 2002; 146: 202-9.
[14] Iinuma K., Sato T., Akimoto N., et al. *J. Invest. Dermatol.*, 2009; 129: 2113-9.
[15] Isard O., Knol A., Castex-Rizzi N., et al. Cutaneous induction of corticotrophin releasing hormone by propionibacterium acnes extracts. *Dermato-Endocrinology*, 2009; 1: 96-99.
[16] Kim J., Ochoa M. T., Krutzik S. R., et al. Activation of toll-like receptor 2 in acne triggers inflammatory cytokine response. *J. Immuno.,* 2002; 169: 1535-41.
[17] Simonart T., Dramaix M. Treatment of acne with topical antibiotics: lessons from clinical studies. *Br. J. Dermatol.*, 2005; 153: 395-403.
[18] Heffernan M. P., Nelson M. M., Anadkat M. J. A pilot study of the safety and efficacy of picolinic acid gel in the treatment of acne vulgaris. *Br. J. Dermatol.*, 2007; 156: 548-52.
[19] Huang W. C., Tsai T. H., Chuang L. T., et al. Anti-bacterial and anti-inflammatory properties of capric acid against Propionibacterium acnes: a comparative study with lauric acid. *J. Dermatol. Sci.*, 2014; 73: 232-40.
[20] Youssef D. A., Miller C. W., E-Abbassi A. M., et al. Antimicrobial implications of vitamin D. *Dermatoendocrinol.*, 2011; 3: 220-9.
[21] Nieves N. J., Ahrens J. M., Plum L. A., et al. Identification of a unique subset of 2-methylene-19-nor analogs of vitamin D with comedolytic activity in the rhino mouse. *J. Invest. Dermatol.*, 2010; 130: 2359-67.
[22] Nakatsuji T., Liu Y. T., Huang C. P., et al. .Vaccination targeting a surface sialidase of P. acnes: implication for new treatment of acne vulgaris. *PLoS One*, 2008; 3: 1551.
[23] Nakatsuji T., Liu Y. T., Huang C. P., et al. Antibodies elicited by inactivated propionibacterium acnes-based vaccines exert protective immunity and attenuate the IL-8 production in human sebocytes: relevance to therapy for acne vulgaris. *J. Invest. Dermatol.*, 2008; 128: 2451-7.
[24] Simonart T. Immunotherapy for acne vulgaris: current status and future directions. *Am. J. Clin. Dermatol.*, 2013; 14: 429-35.
[25] Brackman G., Forier K., Al Quntar A. A., et al. Thiazolidinedione derivatives as novel agents against Propionibacterium acnes biofilms. *J. Appl. Microbiol.*, 2013; doi: 10.1111/jam.12378.
[26] Wang Y., Zhang Z., Chen L., et al. Cathelicidin-BF, a snake cathelicidin-derived antimicrobial peptide, could be an excellent therapeutic agent for acne vulgaris. *PLoS One*, 2011; 6: 22120.

[27] Zhang Z., Mu L., Tang J., et al. A small peptide with therapeutic potential for inflammatory acne vulgaris. *PLoS One*, 2013; 8: e72923.
[28] clinicaltrials.gov.
[29] Zouboulis C. C. Zileuton, a new efficient and safe systemic anti-acne drug. *Dermatoendocrinol.*, 2009; 1: 188-92.
[30] Zouboulis C. C., Nestoris S., Adler Y. D., et al. A new concept for acne therapy: a pilot study with zileuton, an oral 5-lipoxygenase inhibitor. *Arch. Dermatol.,* 2003; 139: 668-70.
[31] Böhm M., Ehrchen J., Luger T. A. Beneficial effects of the melanocortin analogue Nle4-D-Phe7-α-MSH in acne vulgaris. *J. Eur. Acad. Dermatol. Venereol.,* 2014; 28: 108-11.
[32] Brzoska T., Luger T. A., Maaser C., et al. Alpha-melanocyte-stimulating hormone and related tripeptides: biochemistry, antiinflammatory and protective effects in vitro and in vivo, and future perspectives for the treatment of immune-mediated inflammatory diseases. *Endocr. Rev.,* 2008; 29: 581-602.
[33] Cutuli M., Cristiani S., Lipton J. M., et al. .Antimicrobial effects of alpha-MSH peptides. *J. Leukoc. Biol.,* 2000; 67: 233-9.
[34] Zhang L., Anthonavage M., Huang Q., et al. Proopiomelanocortin peptides and sebogenesis. *Ann. N Y Acad. Sci.,* 2003; 994: 154-61.
[35] Thielitz A., Reinhold D., Vetter R., et al. Inhibitors of dipeptidyl peptidase IV and aminopeptidase N target major pathogenetic steps in acne initiation. *J. Invest. Dermatol.*, 2007; 127: 1042-51.
[36] Geria A. N., Scheinfeld N. S. Talarozole, a selective inhibitor of P450-mediated all-trans retinoic acid for the treatment of psoriasis and acne. *Curr. Opin. Investig. Drugs*, 2008; 9: 1228-37.
[37] Geria A. N., Scheinfeld N. S. Talarozole, a selective inhibitor of P450-mediated all-trans retinoic acid for the treatment of psoriasis and acne. *Curr. Opin. Investig. Drugs*, 2008; 9: 1228-37.
[38] Verfaille C. J., Thissen C. A., Bovenschen H. J., et al. Oral R115866 in the treatment of moderate to severe plaque-type psoriasis. *J. Eur. Acad. Dermatol. Venereol.*, 2007; 21: 1038-46.
[39] Pavez Loriè E., Cools M., Borgers M. et al. Topical treatment with CYP26 inhibitor talarozole (R115866) dose dependently alters the expression of retinoid-regulated genes in normal human epidermis. *Br. J. Dermatol.,* 2009; 160: 26-36.
[40] Trifu V., Tiplica G. S., Naumescu E., et al. Cortexolone 17α-propionate 1% cream, a new potent antiandrogen for topical treatment of acne vulgaris. A pilot randomized, double-blind comparative study vs. placebo and tretinoin 0.05% cream. *Br. J. Dermatol.*, 2011; 165: 177-83.
[41] Yoon J. Y., Kwon H. H., Min S. U., et al. Epigallocatechin-3-Gallate Improves Acne in Humans by Modulating Intracellular Molecular Targets and Inhibiting P. acnes. *J. Invest. Dermatol.*, 2013; 133: 429-40.
[42] Fimmel S., Saborowski A., Térouanne B., et al. Inhibition of the androgen receptor by antisense oligonucleotides regulates the biological activity of androgens in SZ95 sebocytes. *Horm. Metab. Res.*, 2007; 39: 149-56.

[43] Azimi H., Fallah-Tafti M., Khakshur A. A., et al. A review of phytotherapy of acne vulgaris: perspective of new pharmacological treatments. *Fitoterapia,* 2012; 83: 1306-17.
[44] Fabbrocini G., Staibano S., De Rosa G., et al. Resveratrol-containing gel for the treatment of acne vulgaris: a single-blind, vehicle-controlled, pilot study. *Am. J. Clin. Dermatol.*, 2011; 12: 133-41.
[45] Liu C. H., Huang H. Y. In vitro anti-propionibacterium activity by curcumin containing vesicle system. *Chem. Pharm. Bull.*, 2013; 61: 419-25.
[46] Tsai T. H., Chuang L. T., Lien T. J., et al. Rosmarinus officinalis extract suppresses Propionibacterium acnes-induced inflammatory responses. *J. Med. Food,* 2013; 16: 324-33.
[47] Agnew T., Leach M., Segal L. The clinical impact and cost-effectiveness of essential oils and aromatherapy for the treatment of acne vulgaris: a protocol for a randomized controlled trial. *J. Altern. Complement Med.,* 2014; 20: 399-405.
[48] Ruxton C. H., Jenkins G. A novel topical ingredient derived from seaweed significantly reduces symptoms of acne vulgaris: a general literature review. *J. Cosmet. Sci.,* 2013; 64: 219-26.
[49] Lee E. J., Lim H. K., Shin M. K., et al. An open-label, split-face trial evaluating efficacy and safty of photopneumatic therapy for the treatment of acne. *Ann. Dermatol.*, 2012; 24: 280-6.
[50] Zheng W., Wu Y., Xu X., et al. Evidence-based review of photodynamic therapy in the treatment of acne. *Eur. J. Dermatol.*, 2014; 24: 444-56.
[51] Song B. H., Lee D. H., Kim B. C., et al. Photodynamic therapy using chlorophyll-a in the treatment of acne vulgaris: A randomized, single-blind, split-face study. *J. Am. Acad. Dermatol.*, 2014; doi: 10.1016/ j.jaad.2014.05.047.
[52] Gold M. H., Biron J. A., Sensing W. Clinical and usability study to determine the safety and efficacy of the Silk'n Blue Device for the treatment of mild to moderate inflammatory acne vulgaris. *J. Cosmet. Laser Ther.*, 2014; 16: 108-13.

In: Advances in Dermatology Research
Editor: James P. Vega
ISBN: 978-1-63482-226-8

Chapter 14

A Large-Scale European Observational Study to Describe the Management of Acne in Clinical Practice

***S. Seité*[*,1] *and B. Dreno*[2]**
[1]La Roche-Posay Pharmaceutical Laboratories, Asnières, France.
[2]Hôtel Dieu, Nantes, France

Abstract

Background: Acne is one of the major reasons that patients consult a dermatologist. Current recommendations for the treatment of juvenile facial acne suggest treating mild acne with topical treatments and moderate acne with a combination of topical treatments with systemic antibiotics. The aim of this investigational survey was to evaluate how European dermatologists in private practice currently manage acne.

Method: Dermatologists practicing in 12 European countries were asked how they manage patients with acne (except those undergoing isotretinoin treatment). Each dermatologist completed a written questionnaire, about patient characteristics, acne severity and the therapy they prescribed at baseline and after 2 months of treatment.

Results: In total, 5809 acneic patients were questioned. In 40% of cases (independent of severity), dermatologists prescribed up to 3 local treatments combined with up to 2 systemic therapies, and a cosmetic product. In 44% of cases, dermatologists prescribed only a dermocosmetic product for very mild acne; in 44% of cases of mild acne they prescribed one treatment, mostly topical one and in 48 and 58% of cases two treatments (mainly a combination of local and systemic therapy) to patients with moderate or severe acne respectively.

Conclusion: This observational study illustrates that dermatologists employ complex treatment regimens to manage acne. Seeing as complex regimens are harder for patients to comply with, this notably raises the question of adherence, which is a key factor in successful treatment.

* Correspondence: S. Seite, Ph.D., La Roche-Posay Pharmaceutical Laboratories, 110 Avenue Henri Barbusse, 92602 Asnières Cedex, France. Phone: + (33) 1.46.88.65.44; Fax: + (33) 1.46.88.29.22; E-mail: sophie.seite@loreal.com.

Keywords: acne, management, severity of acne, tolerance, adherence

Background

Acne is one of the most frequent reasons patients consult in dermatology (20% of consultations) and affects approximately 80% of adolescents. Acne interferes with quality of life, and requires both therapeutic and psychological support [1, 2]. Therapeutic management must balance efficacy and tolerance, otherwise defined as benefit/risk. The treatment period can be long as acne is a chronic inflammatory disease and the majority of treatments have a latent effect. Patient compliance/adherence is imperative to obtain a therapeutic success [3, 4]. Published guidelines and recommendations, review scientific and medical advances and guide practitioners on the appropriate use of different pharmaceutical products. The recommendations of the Global Alliance in 2003, updated in 2009 [5, 6] led to an algorithm for the management of acne [7] and more recently the French group published recommendations for juvenile acne [8]. These algorithms were based upon the published literature, National Health Authority recommendations, expert experience in the field, and also regulatory changes concerning the different treatments. They provide therapeutic markers for the daily use of anti-acne medication. These guidelines therefore evolve regularly over time [9, 10] to keep in line with current research. These recommendations have led to changes in prescribing habits that reflect scientific research in areas such as bacterial resistance or side effects [11]. Additionally, although not included in the treatment algorithms, dermocosmetic products are often prescribed as part of acne treatment regimens [12].

Questions Addressed

In this context, it seemed interesting to perform a survey to assess the implementation of these algorithms in daily practice of European dermatologists for patients with acne. For each level of acne severity, we set out to evaluate the number and type of medical treatments prescribed in addition to a dermocosmetic product.

Experimental Design

This observational study was conducted with dermatologists in private practice in 12 European countries including France, Spain and Portugal (Western countries), Poland, Slovakia, Hungary, Romania and Croatia (Eastern countries) and Germany, Switzerland, Italy and Slovenia. Patients, with acne, of both sexes, aged seven years or older were invited to participate. Patients undergoing isotretinoin treatment were excluded. At baseline, dermatologists were asked to complete a questionnaire to obtain information concerning the patient profile (age, sex, skin type, age of acne), and clinical severity, using the Global Evaluation Acne scale (GEA) [13]. Lastly, the prescribed treatment regimen was noted, and dermatologists were asked to prescribe the dermocosmetic (Effaclar Duo® (La Roche-

Posay)). During the second visit, planned 2 months later, dermatologists re-evaluated the acne severity, and the overall tolerance and efficacy of treatment prescribed. During these 2 visits, seborrhea was evaluated with a 10 cm visual analogic scale (VAS).

Data analysis was performed on all patients included for whom both inclusion and final questionnaires were completed by dermatologists. Some analysis was also done for GEA grade sub-groups. Variables were expressed by number of subjects (N), percentage (%), quantitative data by mean ± SD (min - max) and median.

Results

The baseline characteristics of the 5809 patients, with grade 1 to grade 4 acne, questioned during this survey are shown in Table 1. Most of the patients were female (66%) and 34% were male, with a mean age of 21 ± 7 years (7-97 years), the average length of time since their acne was diagnosed was 25 ± 31 months (0.5 to 384 months) and 82% had skin type II or III. The presence of lesions on the trunk was noted in 30% of the total population.

Table 1. Patient characteristics and degree of acne severity (GEA scale) [14]

GEA grade (n=5763)	**Gender**		**Age**		**lesions on the trunk**	
	F	**M**	**<20**	**≥20**	**Yes**	**No**
Grade 1 (n=663/11.5%)	71%	29%	56%	44%	6%	94%
Grade 2 (n=2494/43.3%)	71%	29%	56%	44%	19%	81%
Grade 3 (n=2332/40.5%)	61%	39%	59%	41%	43%	57%
Grade 4 (n=274/4.8%)	50%	50%	65%	35%	66%	34%

Prescription Therapy

Dermatologists prescribed the dermocosmetic product alone, without supplementary medical treatments for 15% of the total population. Otherwise, prescribing habits were complex, particularly for young patients (sometimes up to 6 different treatments prescribed). No correlation was noticed between the number of treatments prescribed and patient age.

In 35% of cases, dermatologists prescribed up to 3 topical treatments. In 9% of cases, up to 2 systemic treatments and in 40% of cases, they prescribed up to 3 local treatments associated with one or 2 systemic therapies.

Prescriptions made in western countries differed from those in Eastern countries (Table 2).

Table 2. Percentage of patients according to the different treatment regimens

Prescription (n=5809)	%	n	**Western countries (n=3609)**	**Eastern countries (n=1779)**
Systemic only	9%	513	9%	7%
Local only	35%	2036	**27%**	**52%**
Local + systemic	41%	2364	**52%**	**23%**
No treatment (dermocosmetic only)	15%	896	12%	18%

Eastern dermatologists prescribed twice the amount of local therapies alone than western dermatologists. Conversely, western dermatologists preferred combining topical and systemic treatments.

Therapeutic regimens prescribed in accordance with the GEA grade are presented in figures 1 to 4.

For patients with virtually no lesions or grade 1 acne, according to the GEA scale (Figure 1), 44% of prescriptions contained only the dermocosmetic product, with no additional medical treatment. If they prescribed a drug treatment, a topical one was preferred (42%). The top 3 topical treatments prescribed were: a topical antibiotic, a topical retinoid or benzoyl peroxide (BPO).

For patients with mild or grade 2 acne (Figure 2), the dermocosmetic product alone was prescribed for 18% of prescriptions. However, in most cases (44%), dermatologists prescribed one drug treatment, either a local antibiotic, a topical retinoid, or BPO. In 31% of cases, they prescribed two treatments; mostly a combination of a topical with a systemic treatment, most frequently a retinoid with a cycline. However combination therapy was mix of various products (a cycline associated with BPO or with BPO plus a retinoid). And for 6% an association of three treatments was prescribed, essentially the association of two topical with one systemic treatment.

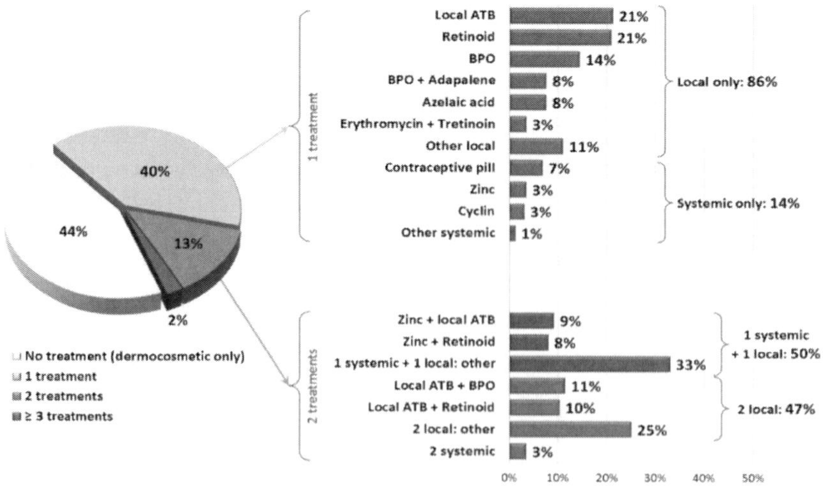

Figure 1. Regimen prescribed for Grade 1 patients (n=658).

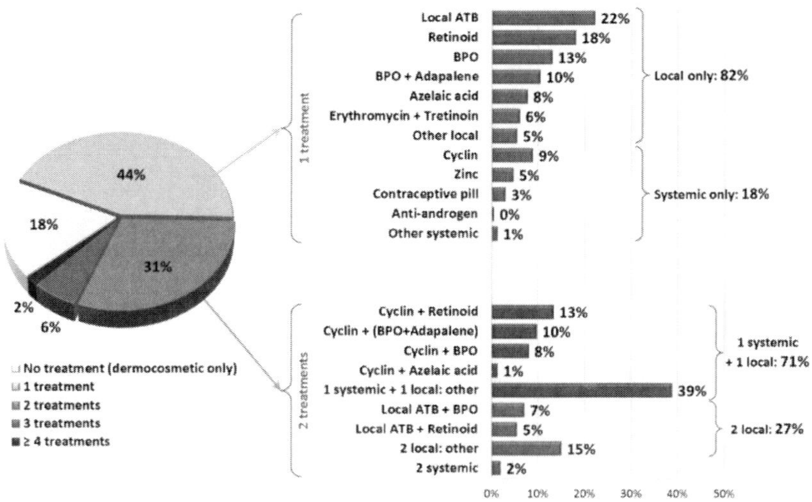

Figure 2. Regimen prescribed for Grade 2 patients (n=2486).

For patients with moderate or grade 3 acne (Figure 3), 6% of dermatologists prescribed the dermocosmetic product alone. Two-thirds (68%) of the patients were treated with combined therapy (2 to 6 associated treatments). Cyclines with retinoids or BPO were the preferred two associated prescriptions for these patients. A quarter of grade 3 patients received only one treatment, which was often a topical antibiotic (17%) or a cycline (27%).

For patients with severe or grade 4 acne (Figure 4), only 2% of prescriptions contained a dermocosmetic prescription alone. More than half of the patients were treated with combination therapy, most often consisting of a topical and a systemic drug treatment. As for grade 3, cyclines were associated with either retinoid or BPO alone or associated with Adapalene.

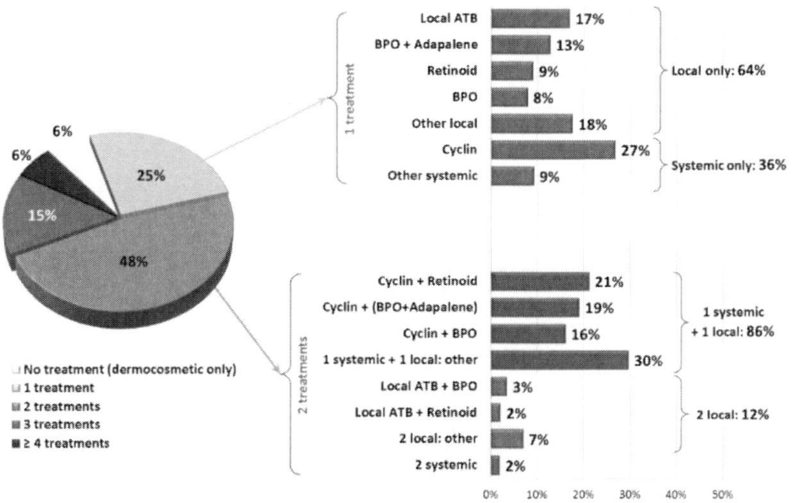

Figure 3. Regimen prescribed for Grade 3 patients (n=2324).

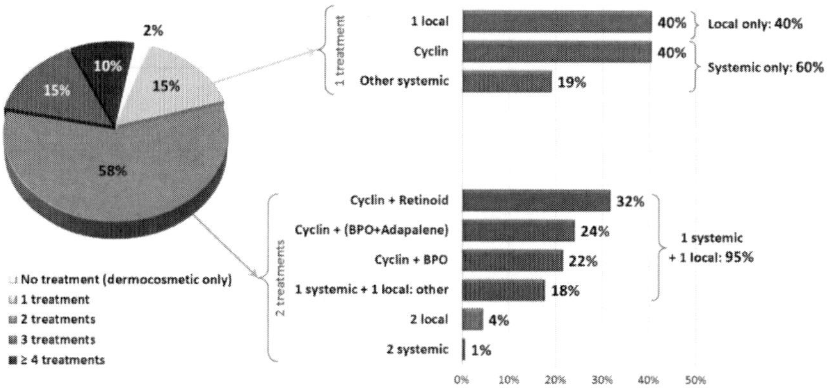

Figure 4. Regimen prescribed for Grade 4 patients (n=273).

Second Visit (58 ± 17 Days after)

All therapeutic regimens prescribed were efficacious as acne improved for 77% of patients at the second visit (reduction of one grade or more) ($p<0.0001$) (Table 4). We also noticed a decrease in the level of seborrhoea in 89% of cases ($p<0.0001$) (Table 3). For 94% of patients, dermatologists found it worthwhile to combine a drug treatment with a cosmetic product to improve patient comfort and tolerance while maintaining and/or enhancing its effectiveness. Moreover, 86% of patients were satisfied with the efficacy of the cosmetic product prescribed. Dermatologists noted the tolerance of treatments as "good" or "excellent" for 93% of patients and for 90% of patients by auto-evaluation.

Table 3. Clinical progress (GEA Grade) and seborrhoea score between baseline and Visit 2

No improvement (same grade)	22%
Improvement of 1 grade (reduction of 1 grade)	56%
Improvement of 2 grades	20%
Improvement of 3 grades	1%
Deterioration of 1 grade	1%

	Baseline Mean ± SD	2nd visit Mean ± SD
Seborrhea score (VAS 0-10)	4.6 ± 1.8	2.6 ± 1.5

Discussion and Conclusion

This survey evaluated the current management of 5809 European patients with acne by dermatologists in private practice. The results provide a better understanding of patient characteristics related to their acne severity and confirms the value, and ease of use of the

GEA scale ("Global Evaluation Acne Scale") [13]. For example, the presence of acne lesions on the trunk was more frequent for severer grades (66% versus 6%)(Table 1). For severer grades, males consulted more often than females and in contrary, for milder grades, females consulted more often than males (Table 1). This was perhaps either due to consultations for aesthetic reasons, or because the adult female population included some patients with premenstrual acne syndrome. This is supported by the fact that grades 2 and 3 acne are diagnosed for more than twice as many women, aged 30 years or more, than men.

This study indicated that European dermatologists do not usually prescribe medical treatments to treat grade 1 acne (in 44% of cases, they prescribe only application of the dermocosmetic product to patients with very mild acne); one drug treatment, usually a topical one to treat grade 2 acne (in 44% of cases, one treatment was prescribed to patients with mild acne) and two treatments (a combination of topical and systemic therapy) to those with grades 3 or 4 acne (in 48 and 58% of cases two treatments were prescribed to patients with moderate or severe acne respectively) (Figures 1-4). We also noticed that in 40% of cases, dermatologists prescribed several topical treatments (up to 3) associated with one or several systemic therapies (up to 2), as well as at least one cosmetic product (Table 2). The complexity of prescribing habits, particularly for young patients raises the question of adherence, which is a key factor for a successful treatment. Interestingly, data of the evolution of the clinical condition between the 2 visits (Table 4) seems to indicate that increasing the number of treatments in mild to moderate acne doesn't add any extra benefit.

Table 4. Clinical Progress for Grade 2 and 3 patients (n= 2441 / 2266)

Therapy / Grade 2	% of patients	GEA (Tf-Ti)*
No treatment	18%	-0.96 ± 0.64
1 treatment	44%	-0.85 ± 0.62
2 treatments	31%	-0.79± 0.64
3 treatments	6%	-0.84 ± 0.68

Therapy / Grade 3	% of patients	GEA (Tf-Ti)*
No treatment	6%	-1.36 ± 0.78
1 treatment	25%	-1.32 ± 0.71
2 treatments	48%	-1.23 ± 0.66
3 treatments	15%	-1.08 ± 0.68
4 treatments	5%	-1.07 ± 0.61

This study also demonstrated that the therapeutic regimens prescribed were efficacious (acne improved for 77% of patients (reduction of one grade or more at the second visit) (Table 3) and generally well tolerated, although these regimens are somewhat complex and differ from country to country (Table 2). Differences seen between eastern and western dermatologist's prescriptions were perhaps due to educational reasons, GDP level or problem of reimbursement.

These data highlight certain points that contradict the published recommendations [5, 6], indicating that dermatologists should not use antibiotics alone and that it is necessary to favour topical treatments with a single application a day to ensure patients use the treatment regularly. The development of bacteriological resistance and ensuing recommendations from health authorities limited the use of local and systematic antibiotics, favouring their use within the framework of combined therapy regimens [7, 11], Nevertheless, we noted in 12% of cases (687 prescriptions) only one local or systematic antibiotic was prescribed.

Finally, this study confirms that dermatologists prescribe dermocosmetic skincare as an integral part of acne management. A dermocosmetic product was prescribed alone for 44% of the patients with very mild acne, 18% of the patients with mild acne and 6% of patients with moderate acne. In 94% of cases, the dermatologists preferred to associate a dermocosmetic with their drug treatment to improve the tolerance of treatments, for patient comfort whilst maintaining and/or strengthening the overall efficacy of the regimen.

In conclusion, this study shows that European dermatologists frequently prescribe several treatments for acne, which is unfavourable for observance particularly for young patients with acne. Furthermore, in spite of published recommendations, local or systematic antibiotics are still often prescribed alone. Finally, a dermocosmetic product can be associated with prescription treatment, and may even provide good results in managing mild acne.

Acknowledgments

We would like to thank all the European dermatologists who participated in this survey, Martine Fortuné and Guénaëlle Le Dantec for their administrative support and Catherine Delva (SYLIA-STAT France) for the statistical analysis. We acknowledge editing assistance provided by Amy Whereat (Speak the Speech Consulting, Paris, France).

Conflict of interest: This observational study was sponsored by La Roche-Posay. Pr B. Dreno is consultant for La Roche-Posay and Sophie Seité employee of La Roche-Posay Pharmaceutical Laboratories.

Funding: This article was funded by La Roche-Posay Pharmaceutical Laboratories, France.

References

[1] Dréno B. Assessing quality of life in patients with acne vulgaris: implications for treatment. *Am J Clin Dermatol* 2006;7:99-106.

[2] Loney T, Standage M, Lewis S. Not just 'skin deep': psychosocial effects of dermatological-related social anxiety in a sample of acne patients. *J Health Psychol* 2008;13:47-54.

[3] Dréno B, Thiboutot D, Gollnick H, Finlay AY, Layton A, Leyden JJ, *et al*; Global Alliance to Improve Outcomes in Acne. Large-scale worldwide observational study of adherence with acne therapy. *Int J Dermatol* 2010;49:448-56.

[4] Dreno B, Daniel F, Allaert FA, Aube I. Acne: evolution of the clinical practice and therapeutic management of acne between 1996 and 2000. *Eur J Dermatol* 2003;13:166-70.

[5] Gollnick H, Cunliffe W, Berson D, Dreno B, Finlay A, Leyden JJ, *et al.* Global Alliance to Improve Outcomes in Acne. *J Am Acad Dermatol* 2003; 49: S1-S37.
[6] Thiboutot D, Gollnick H, Bettoli V, Dréno B, Kang S, Leyden JJ, et al. New insights into the management of acne: an update from the Global Alliance to Improve Outcomes in Acne group. *J Am Acad Dermatol* 2009; 60: S1-S50.
[7] Dreno B, Bettoli V, Ochsendorf F, Layton A, Mobacken H, Degreef H. European recommendations on the use of oral antibiotics for acne. *Eur J Dermatol* 2004;14:391-9.
[8] Auffret N, Revuz J, Poli F, Pawin H, Faure M, Chivot M, *et al.* Algorithm for treatment of juvenile facial acne. *Ann Dermatol Venereol* 2011;138:23-9.
[9] Dreno B, Daniel F, Allaert FA, Aube I. Acne: evolution of the clinical practice and therapeutic management of acne between 1996 and 2000. *Eur J Dermatol* 2003;13:166-70.
[10] Dréno B. Un algorithme thérapeutique dans l'acné : pourquoi ? *Ann Dermatol Venereol* 2010;137:S66-8.
[11] Dréno B, Bettoli V, Ochsendorf F, Perez-Lopez M, Mobacken H, Degreef H, *et al.* An expert view on the treatment of acne with systemic antibiotics and/or oral isotretinoin in the light of the new European recommendations. *Eur J Dermatol* 2006;16:565-71.
[12] Poli F. Acné : les soins d'hygiène. *Ann Dermatol Venereol* 2003; 130:148-50.
[13] Dréno B, Poli F, Pawin H, Beylot C, Faure M, Chivot M, et al. Development and evaluation of a Global Acne Severity Scale (GEA Scale) suitable for France and Europe. *J Eur Acad Dermatol Venereol* 2011;25:43-8.

In: Advances in Dermatology Research
Editor: James P. Vega

ISBN: 978-1-63482-226-8

Chapter 15

Ocular Rosacea: Recent Advances in Pathogenesis and Therapy

Alejandro Rodriguez-Garcia, MD*
Director of the Immunology & Uveitis Service
Senior Ophthalmic Research Coordinator
Instituto de Oftalmología y Ciencias Visuales
Escuela de Medicina y Ciencias de la Salud
TEC Salud. Tecnológico de Monterrey, México

Abstract

Ocular rosacea forms part of the clinical spectrum of rosacea. It is characterized by a chronic and recurrent inflammation of the eyelids, conjunctiva and cornea. Approximately 50% of rosacea patients present ocular manifestations, and the condition is most frequently diagnosed when cutaneous signs and symptoms are present. However in 20% of patients, ocular manifestations may precede the cutaneous disease. Most frequent ocular symptoms are: red eyes, burning, foreign body sensation, photophobia and blurred vision.

Chronic blepharitis with meibomian gland dysfunction is the most frequent ocular manifestation of the disease, and produces evaporative dry eye with consequent ocular surface damage. Corneal inflammation and scarring may be a cause of severe visual loss. In addition to therapeutic strategies for the cutaneous disease, ocular rosacea treatment involves, lid hygiene, topical macrolides and tetracyclines as eyelid gels or ointments, lubricant eye drops, and short-term topical steroids, depending on the severity of blepharitis, conjunctivitis and keratitis. Prognosis and visual outcome depend on the severity of the disease, early diagnosis and appropriate treatment.

* Correspondance: Instituto de Oftalmología y Ciencias Visuales. Centro Médico Zambrano Hellion (1er Piso Oriente). Av. Batallón de San Patricio No. 112. Col. Real de San Agustín. San Pedro Garza García, Nuevo León. C.P. 66278. MEXICO. Tel. 52(81) 8888-0551 y 0552. Fax 52(81) 8356-1799. E-mail: immuneye@gmail.com.

Definition

Ocular rosacea is defined as the clinical spectrum of ocular manifestations considered subtype-4 rosacea by the National Rosacea Society [1]. The syndrome is characterized by chronic inflammation involving the eyelids and to a variable extent, the conjunctiva and cornea [2, 3]. Its clinical course is one of exacerbations and remissions over a long period of time with poor correlation between the occurrence of ocular manifestations and the facial flushing. [4, 5]

History

The ocular manifestations of rosacea were recognized much later than the dermatologic ones. Rosacea was probably first evoked by the famous British writer Geoffrey Chaucer (1387) in his description of the Summoner's face in "The Canterbury Tales"[6] and painted one century later by the Florentine renaissance painter Domenico Ghirlandaio (1490), in "The Old Man and his Grandson"(Musée du Louvre, Paris), where he portraits a grandfather with a prominent rhinophyma. [7] The first person known to describe rosacea as a medical condition was a prominent medieval French surgeon, Dr. Guy de Chauliac (1300-1368) who called it "goutterose" which means, "pink droplet". [8] In the 18th century, the dermatologist J.J. Plenck (1738-1807) called it "gutta rosacea". [9, 10] Later on, both terms were replaced in the English literature by Batemann (1778-1821) who first called it "acne rosacea", [9, 10] a term that was later discarded due to the lack of evidence of a relationship between acne and rosacea. [11]

The first scientific description known of the ocular manifestations of rosacea came from Arlt (1864), who first noted conjunctivitis and keratitis in patients with facial disease. [12, 13] Sir W. Stewart Duke-Elder (1898-1978) first stated that "ocular rosacea is more common than reported, and is frequently undiagnosed," [14, 15] and affirmation that unfortunately is still valid today [16-18]. Only few case reports or literature reviews were written before 1980 in ophthalmology journals. [3, 13, 15, 19-21] But on the last two decades of the last century, the number of publications in both ophthalmologic and dermatologic journals started to raise, showing an increase scientific interest for the ocular manifestations of rosacea. [2, 5, 22-27]. Finally, from the last decade until present time, many reports reviewing particular aspects of ocular rosacea like, quality-of-life, pathophysiologic mechanisms and treatment modalities have increased the awareness, and improved our knowledge of the disease [28-37].

Epidemiology

Approximately 50% (range, 3 – 58%) of rosacea patients present ocular manifestations. [19, 38, 39] Ocular rosacea is most frequently diagnosed when cutaneous signs and symptoms of the condition are present. [40, 41] However, it may persist undiagnosed for a long period of time when cutaneous manifestations presented earlier in the course of the disease and are not prominent at the time of ophthalmic examination. [14, 18, 42] It is important to note that in 20% of patients, the ocular symptoms may be the initial manifestation of the disease, and in 27% of them, the cutaneous and ocular manifestations may occur simultaneously. [2, 19, 39]

Even though rosacea has been more commonly described in populations from the north and west of Europe, and in countries with a large European descent, particularly the United States, [11] there are no precise data on the prevalence variation among races. [5] It appears like rosacea may occur less frequently in other ethnic groups, particularly in dark-skin individuals. [25] Previous reports have found that approximately 4% of rosacea patients are of African, Latin, or Asian descent. [43]

In general, women without ocular involvement are more frequently affected than men, [13, 44] and although ocular rosacea appears to affect both sexes equally, the ocular manifestations tend to be more severe in man. [2, 35, 45] Ocular rosacea can appear at any age, including childhood. [31, 46, 47] Pediatric rosacea is a poorly defined condition, and it is probably underestimated as flushing and facial erythema are frequently confused with a "healthy glow" in children. [11] Ocular manifestations of rosacea in children are similar to adults, but sight-threatening complications are more frequently found at this age group. [47, 48] Children are likely to have a family history of rosacea, and the condition may persist through adulthood. [49, 50] In general, rosacea flushing usually initiates during the second decade of life, becomes troublesome at the third decade, and may continue to progress thereafter. [51] The peak incidence of the disease occurs later, between the fifth to seventh decades of life, when most cutaneous and ocular morbidity occurs. [52, 53] There appears to be a strong correlation between the degree of ocular involvement and the tendency to flush. [54]

Finally, ocular rosacea significantly affects the quality of life of affected patients [4].

Clinical Manifestations

Ocular manifestations are mainly present in the eyelids and the external ocular surface, comprising the conjunctiva and cornea, [2] and they can precede skin changes in a minority of patients; develop a the same time; develop later than skin manifestations; or occur independently from skin flushing. [55, 56] Most frequently, ocular manifestations occur after skin flushing, or coexist with an advanced cutaneous stage (subtype-3 or phymatous) of rosacea. [35] (Figure 1)

Problems range from minor irritation, dryness, and blurry vision to potentially severe ocular surface disruption and inflammatory keratitis. [35, 46, 57]

Ocular rosacea symptoms usually present bilaterally, but asymmetry or alternate inflammation is not uncommon. [58, 59] As would be expected, reports from ophthalmology clinics indicate a higher prevalence of ocular manifestations than dermatologic ones. [2, 5, 29, 45, 60] The most prominent symptoms of ocular rosacea are redness, tearing, foreign body sensation and irritation. [5, 35, 56]

Other symptoms equally important in these patients are: eyelid margin redness and pruritus, swollen eyelids, visibly dilated conjunctival vessels, mucus and/or watery discharge, grittiness, pain and burning, dryness, photophobia, blurred vision, recurrent hordeolum or chalazion, among others. [2, 5, 42, 56]

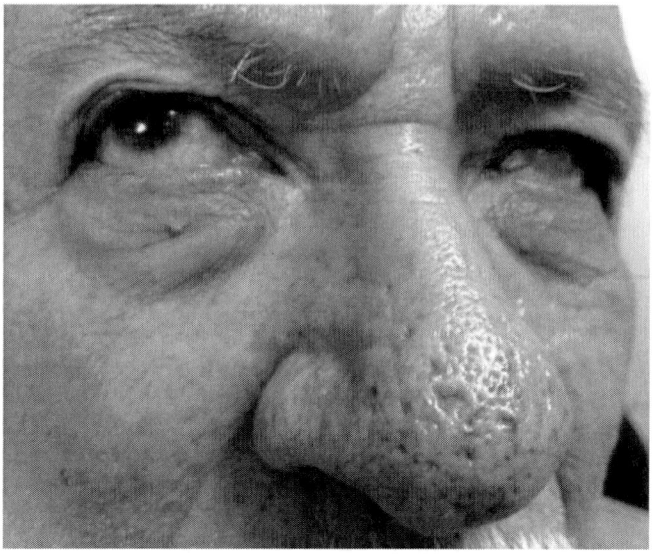

Figure 1. Patient with subtype-3 (Phymatous) rosacea showing a prominent rhinophyma, and severe ocular involvement OS>OD.

Symptoms most typically worsen early in the morning after awakening, but also by hostile environmental factors such as, air pollution, air conditioning and fans air flow, dry and hot climate, among others. [58, 59, 61, 62] These aggravates are related to meibomian gland inflammation and dysfunction (MGD), which typically worsen overnight to became more symptomatic early in the mornings, and to tear film instability causing evaporative dry eye. [53, 55, 60, 62-64].

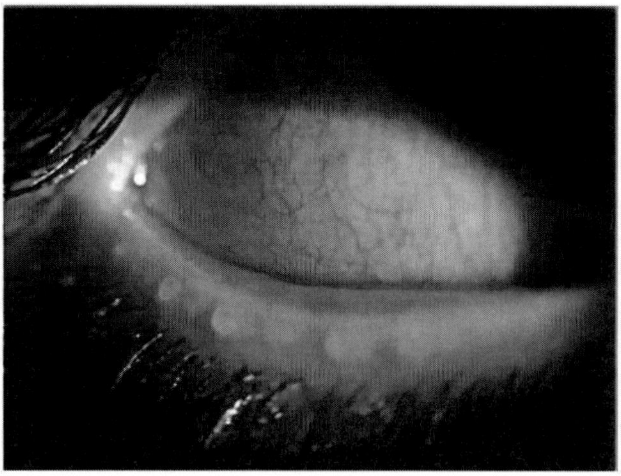

Figure 2. Inferior eyelid margin of a patient with ocular rosacea, showing grade-3 meibomian gland dysfunction with meiboum stagnation in most gland orifices.

Chronic blepharitis and conjunctivitis are most common signs of patients with ocular rosacea. [31, 57, 59] Signs may be divided according to the adnexa and ocular structure affected by the disease. (Table 1) Eyelid findings include, chronic anterior and posterior blepharitis, MGD, hordeolum and chalazion, eyelid margin erythema, crusting, scales, telangiectasias, meibomian duct obstruction with keratinization, squamous metaplasia, and lid border irregularity. [2, 5, 58] (Figure 2) Chronic blepharitis with associated MGD has been recognized as the most important feature of ocular rosacea. [28, 53, 65, 66] Meibomian gland dysfunction is seen in up to 78 to 83% of ocular rosacea patients, [5, 35] while approximately 60% of patients with chalazion have rosacea. [67]

The reported prevalence of most relevant signs of ocular rosacea is shown in Table 1.

Table 1. Ocular Rosacea Manifestations and Prevalence

Eyelids Manifestations	**Prevalence Range**	**References**
Blepharitis	47 – 93%	[5,13,35,42,55]
Meibomitis or meibomian gland dysfunction (MGD)	4 – 83.7%	[5,42,55]
Secretions (collarette, sleeves, crusts, scales)	56.3%	[35]
Telangiectasias	63 – 81%	[5,35,42]
Meibomian duct obstruction with keratinization	NA	---
Margin erythema	NA	---
Lid border irregularity	NA	---
Margin squamous metaplasia	NA	---
Hordeolum and chalazion	7.3 – 71.4%	[5,31,35,55]
Conjunctival Manifestations		
Hyperemia	45 – 86%	[5,13,35,42,55]
Papillary / follicular reaction	10.9%	[35]
Phyctenula	0.7%	[5]
Nodule	NA	---
Granuloma	0.7%	[5]
Bacterial conjunctivitis	16.3%	[35]
Cicatrizing conjunctivitis	9 – 20%	[5,57,69]
Corneal Manifestations		
Sicca or tear film instability	26 – 62.5%	[5,28,32,35,55]
Superficial punctate keratitis (SPK)	15 – 50.9%	[5,35,42,55]
Interstitial keratitis	28.5%	[31]
Pannus formation	20 – 65.2%	[31,35]
Vascularization and subepithelial infiltrates	6.5 – 67%	[5,13,35,42,55,63]
Vascularization and stromal thinning	7.2 – 10%	[35,42]
Recurrent epithelial erosion	5 – 12%	[5,42]
Ulceration	5 – 14.2%	[5,31,35]
Peripheral ulcerative keratitis (PUK)	9 – 19.4%	[35,42,63]
Scarring and leukoma formation	21 – 56.5%	[5,35,63]
Perforation	Case reports	[5,35]
Other Manifestations		
Episcleritis	8 – 8.1%	[5,63]
Scleritis	0.7%	[5]
Iritis	2 – 10%	[5,13,55]

NA = not available.

The conjunctiva frequently shows bulbar and tarsal hyperemia, a mixed follicular and papillary reaction, and to a lesser extent, phlyctenula, nodule and granuloma formation. [13,

35, 42, 68] Some patients may also experience from acute bacterial to chronic cicatrizing conjunctivitis. [57, 69]

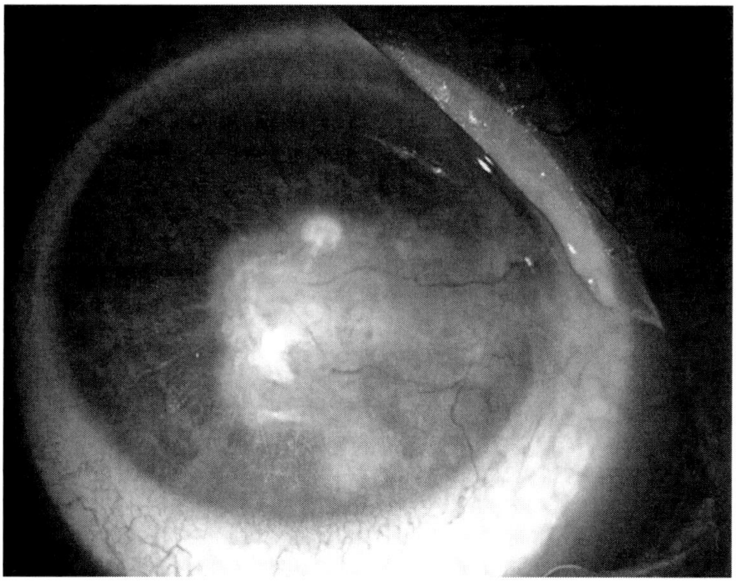

Figure 3. Large central corneal leukoma and stromal vascularization, obstructing the visual axis of a patient with chronic ocular rosacea.

Although site-threatening corneal findings are not common in patients with rosacea, the cornea has been involved in up to 50% of patients, and may vary from superficial punctate keratitis to severe corneal ulceration, scarring with dense leukoma formation, and even globe perforation. [5, 35] (Figure 3)

Other important corneal findings are: pannus formation, recurrent epithelial erosions, sub-epithelial infiltrates, interstitial keratitis, stromal thinning, vascularization, and peripheral ulcerative keratitis. [35, 53] (Figure 4)

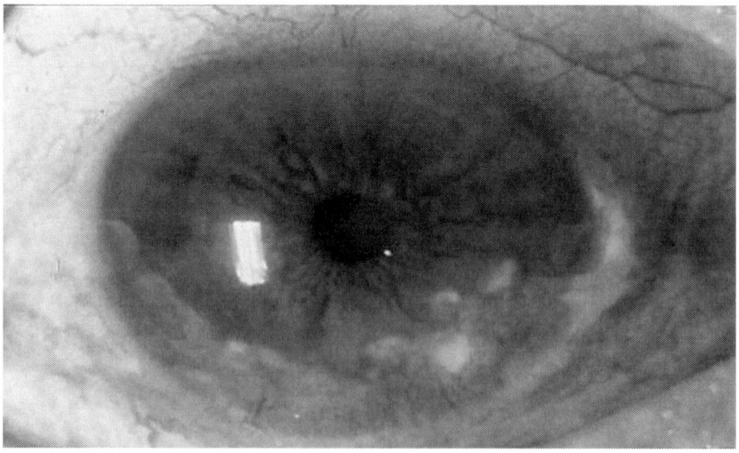

Figure 4. Inferior peripheral ulcerative keratitis with multiple corneal stromal infiltrates and vascularization in a patient with severe ocular rosacea.

As mentioned before, some of these corneal changes may produce serious visual impairment. Keratoconjunctivitis sicca associated with rosacea has been reported in as many as 40% to 56% of patients [55, 70]. This finding is due to a mixed form of lacrimal dysfunction (aqueo-mucinous deficiency and increased tear evaporation) [64, 70]. The evaporative part is directly related to chronic blepharitis and MGD seen commonly in these patients, and is responsible for symptoms exacerbations and aggravation of the ocular surface disease [5, 28, 35]. Other less frequent but not least important ocular manifestations of rosacea are episcleritis, scleritis and iritis [5, 40, 58].

Clinical Course, Stages and Grading

Ocular rosacea is considered subtype-4 of the disease by the National Rosacea Society Classification Committee, and the different subtypes do not necessarily follow one another in a consecutive manner [1]. Like the cutaneous disease, ocular rosacea is characterized by a chronic inflammation of the eyelids and ocular surface that waxes and weans throughout the clinical course of the disease [5, 45]. The role of known cutaneous triggers on ocular rosacea exacerbations is uncertain. In general, triggering factors are taken into account by ophthalmologists when following and managing the ocular inflammation [2, 5]. Ocular inflammation may last from weeks to months, and the longer the uncontrolled inflammation, the eye becomes more prone to sight-threatening complications due to corneal involvement [2, 58]. Skin manifestations may or may not be present at the time of ocular disease, and severity of skin flushing does not correlate with ocular manifestations [31, 59]. The National Rosacea Society has divided the clinical course of rosacea into one pre-rosacea stage, and 3 progressive stages of the disease. [71] Ocular changes are part of the second stage, along with cutaneous features like, persistent, spreading erythema; edema, papules, pustules; and enlarged pores. [71] (Table 2)

Table 2. Stages of Rosacea*

Stage	Symptoms and Signs
Pre-rosacea	Frequent flushing Irritation caused by topical preparations
Stage 1	Transient facial erythema that becomes more persistent Slight telangiectasias Increased skin sensitivity
Stage 2	Persistent, spreading erythema Edema, papules, pustules Enlarged pores Ocular changes
Stage 3	Large inflammatory nodules and furuncles Tissue hyperplasia, fibroplasias Rhinophyma

* Standard classification of rosacea: Report of the National Rosacea Society Expert Committee on the Classification and Staging of Rosacea. [1].

The severity of ocular manifestation of rosacea has also been analyzed by the National Rosacea Society Expert Committee on the Grading of Rosacea [71, 72] (Table 3). The purpose of grading the severity of the ocular manifestations is for specific recommendations on adequate therapeutic intervention.

Table 3. Grades of Ocular Rosacea*

Grade 1: Mild itch, dryness, or grittiness of eyes; fine scaling of lid margins; telangiectasia and erythema of lid margins; mild conjunctival injection (mild congestion of conjunctival vessels).
Grade 2: Burning or stinging of eyes; crusting or irregularity of lid margins, with erythema and edema; definite conjunctival hyperemia or injection; formation of chalazion or hordeolum.
Grade 3: Pain, photosensitivity, or blurred vision; se- vere lid changes, with loss of lashes; severe conjunctival inflammation; corneal changes, with potential loss of vision; episcleritis or scleritis; iritis.

* Standard grading system for rosacea: report of the National Rosacea Society Expert Committee on the classification and staging of rosacea. [71].

Pathophysiology

The pathophysiology of rosacea and its ocular manifestations is complex, and involves a closed interaction among innate immune defense mechanisms, innervation, adaptive immunity, and vascular biology. [73] Despite recent advances in our understanding of the complexities of neuro-immune communication, acute and chronic inflammation, immunity, and tissue repair mechanisms, the pathogenesis of rosacea remains inconclusive. [74-80]. Both, vascular dysregulation and altered immune system responses and consequent inflammatory changes have been majorly involved in the skin and the ocular surface. [81] Recent research has shown an upregulation of pro-inflammatory and vasoregulatory genes in rosacea patients [80, 82, 83]. The concept of an altered vascular function or a vascular hyperreactivity, is supported by the characteristic facial flushing, persistent erythema, and telangiectasias seen in these patients. [83] More recent studies point toward a vascular endothelial growth factor (VGEF)-mediated angiogenesis and lymphangiogenesis. [83, 84] Since IL-17 mediates the induction of VEGF in fibroblasts *in vitro*, there is a potential role of this cytokine in rosacea-associated angiogenesis [85, 86] Interestingly, increased vascular densities were correlated with the papulo-pustular and ocular rosacea subtypes [87]. Different chemokines have been shown to exert bimodal functions on the vasculature. Whereas interferon-inducible and CXCR3-binding chemokines such as CXCL9, CXCL10, and CXCL11 have been classified as angiostatic, CCL2, CCL11, CXCL1, CXCL8, CXCL12, and CXCL1 promote angiogenesis [88].

Nevertheless, the role of these chemokines in the vascular dysregulation, angiogenesis or lymphagiogenesis in rosacea remains to be elucidated.

On the other hand, alterations in the innate immune system responses include an overabundance of cathelicidin (an antimicrobial peptide), along with kallikrein-5 (KLK5), an enzyme involved in processing cathelicidin [78]. There is strong evidence for the role of proteases in rosacea, in particular, KLK5 which is able to activate signaling pathways, leading to the production of inflammatory mediators, cytokines, and LL-37 [78]. Kallikrein-5 also activates several matrix metallo-proteases, which cause shedding of several epithelial growth factor receptor (EGFR) ligands. These EGFR ligands may also induce more LL-37 production. However, the mechanism that enhances KLK5 in rosacea is not fully understood. [78]. In addition, it has been shown that toll-like receptor-2 (TLR2) activity of the innate immune system is upregulated in patients with rosacea [89, 90]. TLR2 activation leads to the expression of abnormally high levels of cathelicidin-LL37, which promotes leukocyte trafficking through the induction of CXCL8, and induce angiogenesis [77, 91]. In this respect, immunohistochemical staining for a variety of vascular markers and for toll-like receptor-4 (TLR4), performed to eyelid biopsies of ocular rosacea patients, and normal controls has shown a statistically significant staining for ICAM-1 and CD105 among arterioles but not venules on ocular rosacea patients compared to controls [34]. And the correlation between the number of TLR4 positive cells and each vascular marker was also statistically significant [34]. These findings suggest that ICAM-1 and CD105 mediate the vascular abnormalities seen in the eyelids of ocular rosacea patients, and that the innate immune system may govern the cutaneous effects of ocular rosacea. [34]

Ocular surface inflammation in patients with rosacea has also been related to increased levels of interleukin-1α (IL-1α), matrix metalloproteinase-8 (MMP-8), and gelatinase-B (pro-MMP-9) activity in the tears of these patients [24, 27, 92]. Gelatinase-B activity correlates with a delayed tear clearance and tear fluid concentration of interleukin-1α, a pro-inflammatory cytokine that has been reported to increase the production and activity of certain enzymes of the matrix metalloproteinase (MMP) family, including collagenases and gelatinases, like MMP-8 and MMP-9 [27]. These enzymes degrade extracellular matrix and may contribute to the development of eyelid and ocular surface irritation, recurrent corneal epithelial erosions, corneal vascularization and persistent epithelial defects, as well as corneal ulceration seen in some of these patients [27, 92, 93]. In addition, delayed tear clearance, a common feature of MGD present in almost all ocular rosacea patients, has shown a strong correlation with decreased corneal and conjunctival sensitivity scores [64, 94]. Although the cause of decreased ocular surface sensation has not been established, the inflammation of the ocular surface that develops in these patients is a possible cause [95]. Inflammatory factors, including IL-1 have been reported to alter sensory neural threshold [96]. The importance of a reduced ocular sensation is a decreased stimulation reflex to the lacrimal glands for tear production, which further decreases tear clearance rate, creating a vicious cycle [97, 98]. More recently, impression cytology combined with flow cytometry performed to samples from eyes with active ocular rosacea, showed a significant increase of HLA-DR and ICAM-1 expression by epithelial cells compared to normal eyes [28]. Both markers were well correlated with each other and inversely correlated with the tear break-up time (TBUT) and Schirmer test [28]. Also, the percentage of goblet cells in the conjunctiva was significantly decreased in rosacea patients compared with the normal group, with a significant negative correlation with both HLA-DR and ICAM-1 markers [28].The goblet cell deficiency has been further corroborated by significantly lower levels of the peptide core of the conjunctival mucins (M1/MUC5AC), as compared to normal controls [28].

A variety of rosacea triggers have been described including eyelid colonization with *Demodex* mites [99, 100] and *Staphyloccocus epidermidis* [101, 102]. A recent study looking at the concentration of cytokines and chemokines in tears of patients with *Demodex* blepharitis demonstrated increased levels of IL-2, IL-7, and IL-17 as compared with *Demodex*-free blepharitis, suggesting that specifically IL-17, may play a role in the inflammation of the lid margin and ocular surface [99]. *Helicobacter pylori* is well recognized as a causative factor for gastritis and duodenal ulcers, and rosacea has long been associated with gastritis [103]. The prominent English ophthalmologist Sir Stewart Duke-Elder stated, "digestive troubles have frequently been cited as a causal factor of rosacea" [14]. However, the proposed link of *H. pylori* to rosacea is intriguing but unproven so far [103, 104]. Few studies have been carried out to clarify this controversy. In an uncontrolled, non-comparative study of a short cohort of patients, eradication of *Helicobacter pylori* improved rosacea in some patients. Based on these results, it was then suggested that the organism may play a role in the pathogenesis of the disease [105]. On the contrary, a further well-controlled, comparative clinical assay was not able to establish a direct relationship between the organism and rosacea [106, 107]. Finally, the eradication of *Helycobacter pylori* from seven patients with ocular rosacea, whom at the same time had clinical and serological evidence of systemic infection with *H. pylori,* resulted in improvement of ocular symptoms far better than the cutaneous response, raising again the possibility of the pathogenic role of this microorganism in the disease [108].

The role of well-established clinical cutaneous flushing triggers such as, microbes, cold, heat, alcohol, coffee and caffeine-containing beverages, tobacco, spicy foods containing *Capsicum*, vasodilating medications and emotional stress, has not been well studied for ocular rosacea [79, 109]. However, it is generally assumed that they all can also contribute to the exacerbation of ocular signs and symptoms of rosacea.

The same is true for UV-light exposure, which directly decreases the competence of already dilated vasculature, increasing persistent erythema and telangiectasias. UV-irradiation also induces the expression of IL-1β, IL-6, IL-10, TNFα, and CXCL8 in a time and dose-dependent manner [110]. In particular, IL-1β and TNFα are known to induce the expression of a subset of pro-inflammatory chemokines (CXCL1, CXCL8, CCL20, CCL27) in keratinocytes [110]. CXCL8 may induce neutrophil recruitment [111]. However, the specific role of these cytokines and chemokines in the pathogenesis of rosacea and its ocular manifestations is unclear at the present time.

Diagnosis

Ocular rosacea is frequently undiagnosed because of its large diversity of non-specific clinical manifestations; the lack of specific diagnostic tests; and the difference in timing between the appearance of cutaneous and ocular signs and symptoms [16, 17, 32]. Indeed, ocular rosacea is most frequently diagnosed when cutaneous findings typical of rosacea are also present at the time of diagnosis [2, 45, 59].

Table 4. Differential Diagnosis of Ocular Rosacea

Ocular Disease	Similarities	Differences
Chronic blepharitis	Identical eyelid changes	Facial flushing and skin changes
Staphyloccocal blepharitis	Collarette secretion, eyelid erythema; conjunctival hyperemia.	Facial flushing and skin changes. Phlyctenula formation
Seborrheic blepharitis	Crusts and scaling, eyelid margin and conjunctival hyperemia, MGD, telangiectasias.	Foamy conjunctival discharge. Scaling, eczematous changes of paranasal, nasolabial, and extrafacial distribution.
Sebaceous gland carcinoma	Recurrent chalazia, MGD, eyelid margin erythema and irregularity, yellowish secretion.	Tendency to invade periocular region; pagetoid infiltration of the conjunctival epithelium or skin epidermis.
Meibomian gland dysfunction	Obstructed meibomian ducts, turbid or paste meiboum secretions; increased tear film break-up time, SPK.	Indistinguishable, apart from facial skin changes.
Recurrent chalazia	Identical hordeolum or chalazion characteristics.	Indistinguishable, apart from facial skin changes.
Allergic conjunctivitis	Conjunctival hyperemia, papillary reaction, watery discharge	Ocular pruritus, Horner-Trantas dots; tarsal giant papillae.
Bacterial conjunctivitis	Conjuntival hyperemia, mucopurulent discharge, sticky eyelids.	Indistinguishable, apart from facial skin changes.
Viral conjunctivitis	Conjunctival hyperemia, follicular reaction, watery discharge	Conjunctival pseudo-membrane or membrane formation
Chlamydia conjunctivitis	Chronic conjunctival hyperemia, mucopurulent discharge.	Follicular reaction, tarsal fibrosis, Herbert pits, trichiasis.
Ocular mucous membrane pemphigoid	Chronic red eye, foreign body sensation, graining and stinging.	Subepithelial fibrosis, fornix foreshortening, symblepharon formation, trichiasis/dystrichiasis.
Atopic keratoconjunctivitis	Chronic red eye, foreign body sensation, graining and stinging.	Pruritus, photophobia, tarsal papillae, subepithelial fibrosis, corneal conjunctivalization.
Keratoconjunctivitis sicca	Chronic red eye, foreign body sensation, graining and stinging.	Filamentary keratitis, low tear meniscus, reduced Schirmer test
Recurrent corneal erosion	Red eye, watery discharge, photophobia, foreign body sensation	Facial flushing and skin changes
Bacterial keratitis	Conjunctival injection, mucopurulent discharge, corneal stromal infiltrate, photophobia and blurred vision.	Facial flushing and skin changes
Peripheral ulcerative keratitis	Crescentric peripheral corneal ulceration, ciliary injection. Foreign body sensation, photophobia.	Indistinguishable, apart from facial skin changes
Episcleritis	Episcleral edema and vasodilation; ocular hypersensitivity.	Indistinguishable, apart from facial skin changes
Scleritis, autoimmune related	Scleral edema, vascular ingurgitation, ocular pain.	Indistinguishable, apart from facial skin changes
Acute iritis, idiopathic or autoimmue	Ciliary injection, photophobia, pain and blurred vision.	Indistinguishable, apart from facial skin changes

SPK = superficial punctate keratitis.

The problem arises when the patient experiences skin flushing much earlier in the course of the disease and by the time ocular manifestations occur, facial flushing may not be prominent or even absent. In such cases, a definitive diagnosis of ocular rosacea becomes a difficult task to the ophthalmologist due to the lack of specific ocular manifestations of the disease [16, 17]. Moreover, in many cases of ocular rosacea, the severity of ocular symptoms does not correlate to cutaneous findings, and skin manifestations are not a prerequisite for the ocular diagnosis [1, 3, 45, 56].

To complicate even more the diagnosis, many other ocular surface disorders may mimic ocular rosacea. (Table 4). According to the Report of the National Rosacea Society Expert Committee on the Classification and Staging of Rosacea, [1] the diagnosis of ocular rosacea should be considered whenever the following signs and symptoms are present in both eyes of any patient regardless of cutaneous manifestations: ocular redness, watery discharge, foreign body sensation, burning or stinging, dryness, itching at the palpebral margin; photophobia, blurred vision, swollen and erythematous eyelids with scaling; telangiectasias, eyelid margin irregularity, and chronic blepharitis with MGD; recurrent chalazion or hordeolum; keratitis, episcleritis, scleritis, and iritis [3, 11, 29, 72, 112].

In summary the diagnosis of ocular rosacea is established clinically and is often aided by dermatologic findings [58, 59]. There are no laboratory tests directly related to the diagnosis, but in some cases, eyelid margin scraping and culture for *Staphylococcus aureus* and coagulase-negative, *Demodex folliculorum*, and other potentially involved microorganisms can be performed [2, 3, 99].

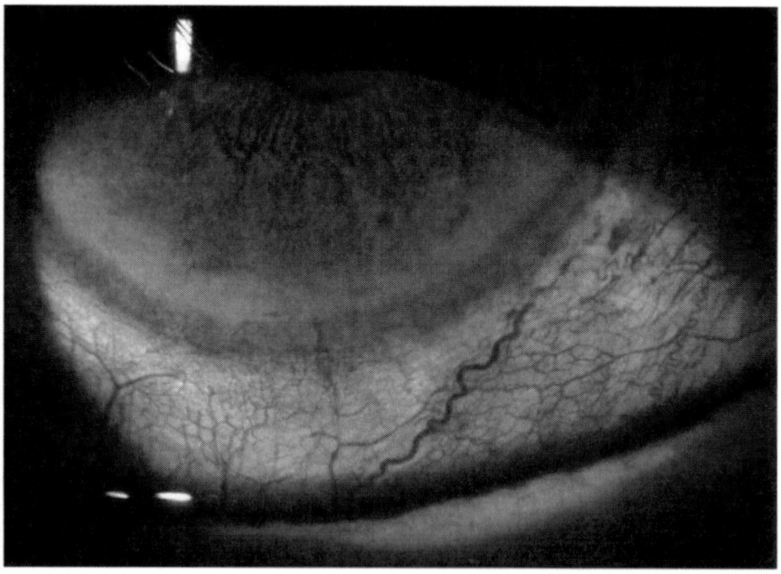

Figure 5. Positive inferior lisamine green staining pattern typical of chronic blepharitis with meibomian gland dysfunction associated to ocular rosacea.

From the ophthalmological perspective, the diagnosis of ocular rosacea can also be aided by careful examination of the eyelid margins looking for signs of chronic blepharitis, like secretions (collarette, sleeves, crusts and scales), telangiectasia formation, and posterior displacement, keratinization and/or inspissation of the meibomian gland excretory orifices

[66]. Also, manual expression of meibomian gland ducts need to be done, looking at the amount of functional glands, and the appearance of meiboum secretions for grading severity of MGD [66, 113, 114]. Meibography can also be performed with halogen trans-illumination, infrared light or confocal microscopy in order to measure meibomian gland atrophy and dropout [115-118].

Patients with ocular rosacea frequently experience an aqueous deficient type of dry eye [55, 70]. The Schirmer test, although unreliable because of its variability, [97, 119] and lack of repeatability, [120] has been used to demonstrate an aqueous tear deficiency in patients with ocular rosacea [55, 60]. Using fluorescein dye, the tear break-up time must be assessed, as well as corneal staining in order to measure tear film stability and corneal damage. [121] Other vital dyes, like lisamine green may be used to detect the amount of conjunctival cell damage due to dryness [122]. The typical staining pattern of the inferior interpalpebral quadrants seen in chronic blepharitis may also be considered for the diagnosis in patients with ocular rosacea [114] (Figure 5).

Histopathology

The first histopathologic analysis from the conjunctiva of patients with ocular rosacea was performed by Brown and Shahinian in 1978 [3]. They found that 6 out of 12 conjunctival biopsies stained positive for IgG, IgA, or IgM by direct or indirect immunofluorescence, and 5 out of 6 biopsies also stained positive for C3. At that time, they concluded that the significance of their findings was unclear postulating that possibly, local autoimmune mechanisms were responsible for at least part of the initial inflammatory signs or were the result of prolonged inflammation, and that these eyes might respond more violently to further episodes of the disease [3].

Although there are not specific immunohistopathologic features for ocular rosacea, the conjunctiva is frequently infiltrated by inflammatory cells. The conjunctival epithelium is attenuated and significantly infiltrated, mainly by lymphocytes-T (CD4+), phagocytic cells and antigen presenting cells (CD14, Mac-1) [23]. In the stroma, there is increased vascular dilation and large sub-epithelial infiltrates of chronic inflammatory cells with granulomatous changes, resembling a type IV hypersensitivity reaction. All cell types are present in larger proportions than normal controls, but especially T-helper (CD4+) lymphocytes. There is a 3.5-fold increase in the lymphocyte-CD4+ to CD8+ ratio in the conjunctiva of patients with rosacea [23].

Differential Diagnosis

The differential diagnosis of ocular rosacea is related to most common forms of chronic blepharitis, and/or ocular surface inflammatory diseases. (Table 4) Most frequently, ocular rosacea is misdiagnosed in patients with chronic staphylococcal and seborrheic blepharitis with meibomian gland dysfunction. Meibomitis-related keratoconjunctivitis (MRKC), characterized by sub-epithelial cellular infiltrates and superficial vascularization of the cornea associated to *Propionibacterium acnes* needs also be considered in the differential [123, 124].

Another very important diagnosis is sebaceous gland carcinoma, a disease frequently misdiagnosed as recurrent chalazia which needs to be biopsied for histopathology confirmation [58, 125, 126].

Other causes of infectious conjunctivitis with chronic or recurrent conjunctival hyperemia, as well as cicatrizing conjunctivitis may resemble ocular rosacea, like mucous membrane pemphigoid, pemphigus vulgaris, lichen planus, and atopic keratoconjunctivitis. [127-129]. On the other hand, many disorders resembling cutaneous rosacea may also exhibit ocular manifestations in a diverse clinical presentation. Diseases like acne vulgaris, seborrehic dermatitis, steroid rosacea, contact dermatitis, photodermatitis, systemic lupus erythematosus, dermatomyositis, mucous membrane pemphigoid, and pemphigus vulgaris. [11, 130]

Treatment

Ocular rosacea remains incurable and disease stabilization remains elusive despite its relatively common nature and its severe potential consequences [131]. Our limited understanding of the pahogenic mechanisms responsible for the onset and development of rosacea has resulted in an array of non-specific and less than optimal therapeutic strategies to minimize ocular damage [89, 131, 132]. Therefore, no precise treatment algorithm has become the standard of care, and ocular management remains empirical and limited to symptomatic control and resolution of complications only [132].

The treatment of ocular rosacea may be divided into three main categories: 1) avoidance of triggers to reduce exposure of the eyelids and ocular surface to the disease; 2) conservative measures to minimize the damage caused by rosacea and alleviate active symptoms; and 3) therapies to revert the damage that has already occurred [131]. Avoidance of known triggers of rosacea exacerbation such as, prolonged exposure to UV-sunlight; intake of alcohol and caffeine-containig beaverages; and physical or emotional stress among others, should be recommended to all patients with ocular rosacea [133]. Because most ocular rosacea patients suffer from chronic blepharitis and MGD, conservative measures intended to unclog the meibomian gland ducts, improve the outflow of meiboum, and stabilize the tear film through the application of warm compresses to the eyelids and lid hygenie (scrubs and massage) are mainstay therapy for these patients [66]. It is very important to instruct the patient to warm the eyelids with a hot-humid compress in order to liquefy the solidified meiboum in the gland ducts and to dilate the ducts. Then, the patient must massage the lids to mechanically force the meiboum and debris from the plugged or stagnant ducts, and to clean the eyelid margins [5]. Massage can be done by rubbing with the fingers or with special eyelid pads design for that purpose. [66, 134] Topical antibiotics such as bacitracin and erythromycin ointments, as well as fusidic acid viscous eyedrops, may be effective to control bacterial overgrowth and reduce staphylococci colonies from the eyelid margins [5, 135, 136]. Conventional management of chalazion and hordeolum with warm compresses, and incision with curettage when necessary should take place if these lesions occur [5, 67].

According to the National Rosacea Society Comittee, topical medication should be reserved for grade 1 (mild) disease; systemic medication for grade 2 (moderate) rosacea; and all patients with persistent grade 1 or 2 disease, or suspected to have grade 3 (severe) disease should be referred to the ophthalmologist [71]. From the ophthalmological standpoint, this therapeutic strategy is difficult to follow if we consider that the evaluation of the ocular manifestations of rosacea needs the expertise of an specialized physician, the use of a biomicrosocope for detailed assessment of the eyelid margins, the conjunctiva and the cornea, and the clinical tests like fluorescein and lisamine green staining, as well as the Schirmer test, among others [35, 72]. Since the ocurrence of ocular rosacea has been documented prior to cutaneous manifestations, and the severity of the ocular disease does not correlate well with the cutaneous findings, we recomend that all patients with rosacea who experience ocular signs or symptoms, regardless of the grade of disease progression, be referred to an ophthalmologist for a thorough evaluation and adequate management [35].

For patients with moderate to severe MGD and ocular surface disease characterized by lacrimal dysfunction with conjunctival and corneal epithelial irregularity or defects, appart from lid hygiene and topical management to the eyelids, patients also need artificial tears, gels, and lubricant ointments [28, 63, 70]. Since ocular rosacea patients suffer from decreased numbers of goblet cells, decreased tear production, and increased tear breakup time, which are all clinical features of chronic dry eye, lubricants are applied frequently and for prolonged periods of time therefore, preservative-free eyedrop formulations are preferred [70, 131]. Also, medications containing hyaluronic acid, chondroitin sulfate, aprotinine, and dexpanthenol, which are intended to reestablish and heal epithelial defects are frequently needed [137, 138]. Additionally, nutritional supplementation with fish oil and flax seeds containing omega-3 fatty acids has been reported to improve the symptoms of blepharitis, MGD, and dry eye [135, 139, 140-142].

If the ocular surface inflammation is significant, particularly in patients with rosacea keratitis, a short course of topical corticosteroids should be considered [133, 143]. Formulations like, preservative-free dexamethasone phosphate 0.1%, loteprednol etabonate 0.2% and 0.5%, and flurometholone phosphate 0.1%, are adequate for these patients when used for short periods of time and at the lowest possible concentration, under close monitoring of intraocular pressure [135]. It is important to note that patients with rosacea are prone to rapid corneal melting at high corticosteroid concentrations [135, 144] Topical corticosteroids are also useful in managing episcleritis and iritis associated to rosacea [2, 3, 131].

Other topical anti-inflammatory medications can also be used as adjunctive therapy for severe ocular rosacea. In a double-masked, randomized, comparative clinical trial, cyclosporine 0.05% showed a significant improvement in the ocular surface disease index (OSDI) scores, corneal staining patterns, tear break up time, and tear-production levels in patients with ocular rosacea and secondary chronic inflammation of the ocular surface and dry eye [145]. Moreover, a retrospective clinical study of chronic active ocular rosacea patients who failed to respond to various combinations of traditional therapies, showed a significant improvement in the ocular signs and symptoms in 31% of patients, and resolved the inflammation in 18% of them, after treatment with topical cyclosporine 0.05% and low-dose oral tetracycline for 6 months [146].

The indirect ocular effects of facially applied metronidazole, was prospectively studied in 20 patients with ocular rosacea. After 8 weeks of facial metronidazole 0.75% gel application, there was improvement in ocular signs and symptoms and the tear break-up time in ocular rosacea patients as compared to normal controls[147]. In another prospective study, metronidazole 0.75% gel was applied topically to one eyelid margin, while lid hygiene alone was perfomed to the fellow eye of 10 patients with ocular rosacea [26]. There was a significant improvement in the eyelid score, but not in the ocular surface inflammation of both the treated and control groups. When the pre-treatment and post-treatment eyelid and ocular surface scores were combined, there was a significant improvement in the treated eyes but not in the control eyes. No adverse effects on the metronidazole treatment group were encountered in this study [26].

Another alternative of topical therapy for ocular rosacea is azythromycin 1.5% eyedrops. In a propective and comparative study, a significant improvement in tear break up time, meibomian gland plugging, and Oxford score associated with symptom reduction was reported by all patients after one month of topical azythromycin therapy. [148] Except for mild burning after instilation, azythromycin 1.5% eyedrops were well tolerated by all patients [36]. In another retrospective trial, 16 children with ocular rosacea and phlyctenular blepharokeratoconjunctivitis were treated with lid hygiene plus azithromycin 1.5% eye drops: 3-day treatments (1 drop twice a day) every 10 days, reduced based on efficacy to one treatment every 15 days and then to one treatment per month [149]. Ocular inflammation was controlled by azithromycin alone in 15 patients; bulbar conjunctival hyperemia resolved completely within one month in all eyes, whereas phyctenules and keratitis took longer to improve, with complete resolution within 3 to 10 months post-therapy. Therapy was stopped after a median of 6 months (range, 4 to 10 months) without recurrence of inflammation [149].

Despite these promising results with different therapeutic modalities, a Cochrane Database Review of interventions in chronic blepharitis found no strong evidence for any of the treatments in terms of curing [150]. According to this analysis, commercial products are marketed to consumers and prescribed to patients without substantial evidence of effectiveness. The review suggests that further research is needed to evaluate the effectiveness of such treatments. Medical interventions and commercial products should be compared with conventional lid hygiene measures, such as warm compresses and eyelid margin washing, to determine effectiveness, as well as head-to-head to show comparative effectiveness between treatments [150].

More advanced and severe cases of ocular rosacea generally require oral antibiotics which remain the mainstay of therapy, even though the mechanisms of action of these medications are unclear and often non-specific [131]. Considerable controversy still exists of whether the improvement in ocular surface inflammation is due to the antimicrobial effect of these agents or their anti-inflammatory and anti-angiogenic properties [151, 152]. In either case, oral oxy-tetracycline, minocycline or doxycycline, initiated at full dose for several weeks, and then gradually decreased (titrated to clinical response); a combination of a 30mg dose of standard doxycycline and 10mg of sustained-release doxycycline, or a 40mg slow-release dose of doxycycline alone, have all shown to be effective in the treatment of ocular rosacea and chronic blepharitis with MGD [22, 37, 153-161]. Nonetheless, these medications require prolonged use and may be associated with side effects including, infections, allergy, multi-drug resistance, gastrointestinal distress, photosensitivity, among others [151, 155]. These inconveniences, rise the necessity for targeted therapeutic strategies with safer profiles, that can be well tolerated for prolonged periods of time. In this respect, a comparative study of the effects of tetracycline and doxycycline on ocular rosacea patients showed that tetracycline alleviated the symptoms faster, but doxycycline caused less gastrointestinal side effects and hence showed better compliance [162]. Another study showed relatively similar side effects of both tetracycline and doxycycline [5].

One small cohort clinical trial showed some clinical benefit of oral metronidazole (20-30mg/kg/day for 3 to 6 months), as adjunctive therapy in ocular rosacea children with MGD, keratitis, and corneal ulceration [163].

A recent Cochrane Database Review found that the majority of assessed rosacea treatment trials were at high or unclear risk of bias however, there was some evidence to support the effectiveness of topical metronidazole, azelaic acid, and oral doxycycline (100mg or 40 mg) in the treatment of moderate to severe rosacea, and cyclosporine 0.05% ophthalmic emulsion for ocular rosacea [164]. The review concluded that further well-designed, adequately-powered randomized controlled trials are required to elucidate the efficacy of different topical and systemic medications in the management of rosacea [164].

As we expand our knowledge on the pathogenic mechanisms that govern the ocular manifestations of rosacea, new and more specific therapeutic strategies with fewer side effects will emerge. Ideally, new therapies would focus on tackling the biochemical and immunological alterations that ultimately lead to chronic inflammation and damage to the eyelids and the ocular surface.

References

[1] Wilkin J, Dahl M, Detmar M, Drake L, Feinstein A, Odom R, et al. Standard classification of rosacea: Report of the National Rosacea Society Expert Committee on the Classification and Staging of Rosacea. *J. Am Acad Dermatol.* 2002; 46(4):584–7.

[2] Browning DJ, Proia AD. Ocular rosacea. *Surv Ophthalmol.* 1986; 31(3):145–58.

[3] Brown SI; Shahinian L Jr. Diagnosis and Treatment of Ocular Rosacea. *Ophthalmology.* 1978; 85(8):779–86.

[4] Awais M, Amwar MI, Iftikhar R, Iqbal Z, Shehzad N, Akbar B. Rosacea: The ophthalmic perspective. *Cutan. Ocul Toxicol.* 2014; 9:1-6.

[5] Akpek EK, Merchant A, Pinar V, Foster CS. Ocular Rosacea: Patients characteristics and follow-up. *Ophthalmology.* 1997; 104(11):1863–7.

[6] Chaucer G. The Summoner´s Tale. In: The Canterbury Tales. First edition. Caxton W, Editor. Westminster; c.1476-77, [G]8v. JRL 11567.

[7] Cadogan KJ. Domenico Ghirlandaio: Artist and Artisan. Yale University Press; April 10, 2001. ISBN-13**:** 978-0300087208.

[8] Chauliac, Guy De. Complete Dictionary of Scientific Biography; 2008. *Encyclopedia.com.* (January 4, 2015). http://www.encyclopedia.com/doc/1G2-2830900872.html

[9] Rolleston JD. A Note on the Early History of Rosacea. *Proc. Roy Soc. Med.* 1933; 26(4):327–9.

[10] Reyn A. Untersuchungen über Rosacea. Acta Derm Venereol. 1936; 17:366–75.

[11] Culp B, Scheinfeld N. *Rosacea: a review.* P T. 2009; 34(1):38–45.

[12] Artl F. Ueber acne rosacea und lupus. *Klin Monatsbl Augenheilkd.* 1846; 2329–30.

[13] Wise G. Ocular Rosacea. *Am. J. Ophthalmol.* 1943; 26(6):591–609.

[14] Duke-Elder WS. *System of Ophthalmology,* 2nd ed. vol. 8, pt 1. St. Louis: CV Mosby, 1965;536.

[15] Roper-Hall MJ. Ocular Aspects of Rosacea. *Trans Ophthalmol Soc UK.* 1966; 86:727–32.

[16] De Marchi SU, Cecchin E, De Marchi S. Ocular rosacea: an underdiagnosed cause of relapsing conjunctivitis-blepharitis in the elderly. *Br. Med. J. Case Rep.* 2014;2014.

[17] Vieira AC, Mannis MJ. Ocular rosacea: common and commonly missed. J *Am. Acad. Dermatol.* 2013; 69(6 Suppl 1):S36–S41.

[18] Blount BW, Pelletier AL. Rosacea: a common, yet commonly overlooked, condition. *Am. Fam. Physician.* 2002; 66(3):435–40.

[19] Goldsmith A. The ocular manifestations of rosacea. Br J Dermatol. 1953.

[20] Cowan MA. Rosacea and its treatment. *Trans Ophthalmol Soc UK.* 1966; 86:719-25.

[21] Herzog H. Zur Frage der Rosazeaerk-rankung, ins besondere der Rosazea keratitis. *Klin Monatsbl Augenheilkd.* 1974; 165:338–41.

[22] Frucht-Pery J, Sagi E, Hemo I. Efficacy of doxycycline and tetracycline in ocular rosacea. *Am. J Ophthalmol.* 1993 Jul 15;116(1):88-92.

[23] Hoang-Xuan T, Rodriguez A, Zaltas MM, Rice BA, Foster CS. Ocular rosacea. A histologic and immunopathologic study. *Ophthalmology.* 1990; 97(11):1468–75.

[24] Barton K, Monroy DC, Nava A, Pflugfelder SC. Inflammatory cytokines in the tears of patients with ocular rosacea. *Ophthalmology.* 1997; 104(11):1868–74.

[25] Browning DJ, Rosenwasser G, Lugo M. Ocular Rosacea in blacks. *Am. J. Ophthalmol.* 1986; 101(4):441–4.

[26] Barnhorst DA Jr MD, Foster JA, Chern KC, Meisler DM. Efficacy of topical metronidazole in the treatment of ocular rosacea. *Ophthalmology.* 1996 Nov 1;103(11):1880–3.

[27] Afonso AA, Sobrin L, Monroy DC, Selzer M, Lokeshwar B, Pflugfelder SC. Tear fluid gelatinase B activity correlates with IL-1alpha concentration and fluorescein clearance in ocular rosacea. Invest *Ophthalmol. Vis. Sci.* 1999 Oct 1;40(11):2506–12.

[28] Pisella PJP, Brignole FF, Debbasch CC, Lozato PAP, Creuzot-Garcher CC, Bara JJ, et al. Flow cytometric analysis of conjunctival epithelium in ocular rosacea and keratoconjunctivitis sicca. *Ophthalmology.* 2000 Oct 1;107(10):1841–9.

[29] Ghanem VC, Mehra N, Wong S, Mannis MJ. The prevalence of ocular signs in acne rosacea: comparing patients from ophthalmology and dermatology clinics. *Cornea.* 2003 Apr 1;22(3):230–3.

[30] Donaldson KE, Karp CL, Dunbar MT. Evaluation and treatment of children with ocular rosacea. *Cornea.* 2007 Jan;26(1):42-6.

[31] Chamaillard M, Mortemousque B, Boralevi F, da Costa CM, Aitali F, Taïeb A, et al. Cutaneous and ocular signs of childhood rosacea. *Arch Dermatol.* 2008 Feb 1;144(2):167–71.

[32] Lazaridou E, Fotiadou C, Ziakas NG, Giannopoulou C, Apalla Z, Ioannides D. Clinical and laboratory study of ocular rosacea in northern Greece. *J. Eur. Acad. Dermatol Venereol.* 2011 Mar 2;25(12):1428–31.

[33] Holzchuh FG, Hida RY, Moscovici BK, Albers MBV, Santo RM, Kara-José N, et al. Clinical treatment of ocular demodex folliculorum by systemic ivermectin. *Am. J. Ophthalmol.* 2011 Jun 1;151(6):1030–1.

[34] Wladis EJ, Carlson JA, Wang MS, Bhoiwala DP, Adam AP. Toll-like receptors and vascular markers in ocular rosacea. *Ophthal Plast Reconstr Surg.* 2013 Jul 1;29(4): 290–3.

[35] Patiño-Ramírez BE, Rodríguez-García A, Díaz JC, Perfecto Ávalos Y. Alterations of the ocular surface in patients with rosacea. *Rev. Mex Oftalmol.* 2012;86(2):86–96.
[36] Mantelli F, Di Zazzo A, Sacchetti M, Dianzani C, Lambiase A, Bonini S. Topical azithromycin as a novel treatment for ocular rosacea. *Ocul. Immunol Inflamm.* 2013 Oct;21(5):371–7.
[37] Sobolewska B, Doycheva D, Deuter C, Pfeffer I, Schaller M, Zierhut M. Treatment of ocular rosacea with once-daily low-dose doxycycline. *Cornea.* 2014 Mar;33(3):257–60.
[38] Starr PA, Macdonald A. Oculocutaneous aspects of rosacea. *Proc. Roy Soc Med.* 1969 Jan 1;62(1):9–11.
[39] Borrie P. Rosacea with special reference to its ocular manifestations. *Br. J. Dermatol.* 1953.
[40] Buechner SA. Rosacea: an update. *Dermatology (Basel).* 2005;210(2):100–8.
[41] Knox CMC, Smolin GG. Rosacea. *Int. Ophthalmol Clin.* 1997 Jan 1;37(2):29–40.
[42] Jenkins MS, Brown SI, Lempert SL, Weinberg RJ. Ocular rosacea. *Am. J. Ophthalmol.* 1979 Sep;88(3):618–22.
[43] Halder RM, Brooks HL, Callender VD. Acne in ethnic skin. *Dermatol Clin.* 2003 Oct;21(4):609–15–vii.
[44] Rulison RH. Rosacea: With a study of accompanying conditions. *Am. J. Med. Sci.* 1927.
[45] Webster G, Schaller M. Ocular rosacea: a dermatologic perspective. *J. Am. Acad. Dermatol.* 2013 Dec;69(6 Suppl 1):S42–3.
[46] Erzurum SA, Feder RS. Acne rosacea with keratitis in childhood. *Arch Ophthalmol.* 1993 Feb;111(2):228-30.
[47] Nazir SA, Murphy S, Siatkowski RM, Chodosh J, Siatkowski RL. Ocular rosacea in childhood. *Am. J. Ophthalmol.* 2004 Jan;137(1):138–44.
[48] Mavrakanas N, Schutz JS, Dosso AA. Pediatric ocular rosacea. *J. Ped Ophthalmol Strabismus.* 2010 Mar;47(2):117–20.
[49] Drolet B, Paller AS. Childhood rosacea. *Pediatr Dermatol.* 1992 Mar 1;9(1):22–6.
[50] Kroshinsky D, Glick SA. Pediatric rosacea. *Dermatol Ther.* 2006 Jul 1;19(4):196–201.
[51] Berg M, Lidén S. An epidemiological study of rosacea. *Acta Derm Venerol.* 1989 Jan 1;69(5):419–23.
[52] Marks R. Concepts in the pathogenesis of rosacea. *Br. J. Dermatol.* 1968 Mar 1;80(3):170–7.
[53] Quarterman MJ, Johnson DW, Abele DC, Lesher JL, Hull DS, Davis LS. Ocular rosacea. Signs, symptoms, and tear studies before and after treatment with doxycycline. *Arch. Dermatol.* 1997 Jan 1;133(1):49–54.
[54] Wilkin JK. Rosacea. *Int J. Dermatol.* 1985 Dec;24(10):670–1.
[55] Gudmundsen KJ, O'Donnell BF, Powell FC. Schirmer testing for dry eyes in patients with rosacea. *J. Am. Acad. Dermatol.* 1992 Feb 1;26(2 Pt 1):211–4.
[56] Barankin B, Guenther L. Rosacea and atopic dermatitis. Two common oculocutaneous disorders. *Can. Fam. Physician.* 2002 Apr;48:721–4.
[57] Tanzi EL, Weinberg JM. The ocular manifestations of rosacea. *Cutis.* 2001 Aug 1;68(2):112–4.
[58] Vieira ACC, Höfling-Lima AL, Mannis MJ. Ocular rosacea-a review. *Arq Bras Oftalmol.* 2012 Oct;75(5):363–9.

[59] Oltz M, Check J. Rosacea and its ocular manifestations. *Optometry.* 2011 Feb 1;82(2):92–103.
[60] Bakar O, Demircay Z, Toker E, Cakir S. Ocular signs, symptoms and tear function tests of papulopustular rosacea patients receiving azithromycin. *J. Eur. Acad Dermatol. Venereol.* 2009 May 1;23(5):544–9.
[61] Kligman AM. Ocular rosacea: current concepts and therapy. *Arch Dermatol.* 1997 Jan;133(1):89-90.
[62] Yáñez B, Morante V. Ocular rosacea and tear film stability. *ARVO Meeting Abstracts.* 2004 May 1;45(5):102.
[63] Yáñez B, Morante V. Rosácea ocular: clínica y alteraciones de la película lagrimal. *Folia Dermatol.* 2006;17(1):17–20.
[64] Nichols KK, Foulks GN, Bron AJ, Sullivan DA. Meibomian gland dysfunction. What is it, why does it occur and how may it be treated? TFOS. www.tearfilm.org. 2011 Mar 31;1–2.
[65] Hamada S, Khan I, Denniston AK, Rauz S. Childhood blepharokeratoconjunctivitis: characterising a severe phenotype in white adolescents. *Br. J. Ophthalmol.* 2012 Jun 19;96(7):949–55.
[66] Foulks GN, Nichols KK, Bron AJ, Holland EJ, McDonald MB, Nelson JD. Improving awareness, identification, and management of meibomian gland dysfunction. *Ophthalmology.* 2012 Oct 1;119(S):S1–S12.
[67] Lempert SL, Jenkins MS, Brown SI. Chalazia and rosacea. *Arch Ophthalmol.* 1979 Sep 1;97(9):1652–3.
[68] Blaustein BH, Gurwood AS. Recurrent phlyctenular keratoconjunctivitis: a forme fruste manifestation of rosacea. *Optometry.* 2001 Mar;72(3):179–84.
[69] Rahman MQ, Lim Y, Roberts F, Ramaesh K. Fibrosing blepharo-conjunctivitis following pyogenic granuloma in ocular acne rosacea. *Ocul. Immunol Inflamm.* 2010 Oct;18(5):346–8.
[70] Lemp MA, Mahmood MA, Weiler HH. Association of rosacea and keratoconjunctivitis sicca. *Arch. Ophthalmol.* 1984 Apr;102(4):556–7.
[71] Wilkin J, Dahl M, Detmar M, Drake L, Liang MH, Odom R, et al. Standard grading system for rosacea: report of the National Rosacea Society Expert Committee on the classification and staging of rosacea. *J. Am. Acad Dermatol. 2004* Jun;50(6):907–12.
[72] Powell FC. Clinical practice. Rosacea. *N. Engl. J. Med.* 2005 Feb 24;352(8):793–803.
[73] Steinhoff M, Bergstresser PR. Pathophysiology of rosacea: Introduction. *J. Invest Dermatol Symp Proceed.* 2011 Dec 1;15(1):1–1.
[74] Wilkin JK. Rosacea: pathophysiology and treatment. *Arch Dermatol.* 1994;130:359–62.
[75] Tisma VS, Basta-Juzbasic A, Jaganjac M, Brcic L, Dobric I, Lipozencić J, et al. Oxidative stress and ferritin expression in the skin of patients with rosacea. *J. Am. Acad Dermatol.* 2009 Feb;60(2):270–6.
[76] Steinhoff M, Buddenkotte JOR, Aubert J, Sulk M, Novak P, Schwab VD, et al. Clinical, cellular, and molecular aspects in the pathophysiology of rosacea. *J. Invest Dermatol Symp Proceed.* 2011 Dec 1;15(1):2–11.
[77] Yamasaki K, Gallo RL. Rosacea as a disease of cathelicidins and skin innate immunity. *J. Invest Dermatol Symp Proceed.* 2011 Dec 1;15(1):12–5.

[78] Meyer-Hoffert U, der J-MSO. Epidermal proteases in the pathogenesis of rosacea. *J. Invest Dermatol Symp Proceed.* 2011 Dec 1;15(1):16–23.

[79] Gerber PA, Buhren BA, Steinhoff M, Homey B. Rosacea: the cytokine and chemokine network. *J. Invest Dermatol Symp Proceed.* 2011 Dec 1;15(1):40–7.

[80] Aubdool AA, Brain SD. Neurovascular aspects of skin neurogenic inflammation. *J. Invest Dermatol Symp Proceed.* 2011 Dec 1;15(1):33–9.

[81] Sobottka A, Lehmann P. Rosacea 2009: new advances in pathophysiology, clinical staging and therapeutic strategies. Hautarzt. 2009 Dec 1;60(12):999–1009.

[82] Fimmel S, Abdel-Naser MB, Kutzner H. New aspects of the pathogenesis of rosacea. *Drug Discov Today*. 2008;5:103–11.

[83] Huggenberger R, Detmar M. The Cutaneous Vascular System in Chronic Skin Inflammation. *J. Invest Dermatol Symp Proceed.* 2011 Dec 1;15(1):24–32.

[84] Gomaa AHA, Yaar M, Eyada MMK, Bhawan J. Lymphangiogenesis and angiogenesis in non-phymatous rosacea. *J. Cutan Pathol.* 2007 Oct 1;34(10):748–53.

[85] Numasaki M, Fukushi J-I, Ono M, Narula SK, Zavodny PJ, Kudo T, et al. Interleukin-17 promotes angiogenesis and tumor growth. *Blood.* 2003 Apr 1;101(7):2620–7.

[86] Tartour E, Pere H, Maillere B, Terme M, Merillon N, Taieb J, et al. Angiogenesis and immunity: a bidirectional link potentially relevant for the monitoring of antiangiogenic therapy and the development of novel therapeutic combination with immunotherapy. *Cancer Metastasis Rev.* 2011 Mar 1;30(1):83–95.

[87] Aroni K, Tsagroni E, Kavantzas N, Patsouris E, Ioannidis E. A study of the pathogenesis of rosacea: how angiogenesis and mast cells may participate in a complex multifactorial process. *Arch. Dermatol Res.* 2008 Mar 1;300(3):125–31.

[88] Gerber PA, Hippe A, Buhren BA, Müller A, Homey B. Chemokines in tumor-associated angiogenesis. *Biol. Chem.* 2009 Dec 1;390(12):1213–23.

[89] Del Rosso JQ. Advances in understanding and managing rosacea: part 1: connecting the dots between pathophysiological mechanisms and common clinical features of rosacea with emphasis on vascular changes and facial erythema. *J. Clin. Aesthet Dermatol.* 2012;5(3):16.

[90] Yamasaki K, Kanada K, Macleod DT, Borkowski AW, Morizane S, Nakatsuji T, et al. TLR2 Expression is increased in rosacea and stimulates enhanced serine protease productionby keratinocytes. *J. Invest Dermatol.* 2010 Nov 25;131(3):688–97.

[91] Chen Q, Schmidt AP, Anderson GM, Wang JM, Wooters J, Oppenheim JJ, et al. LL-37, the neutrophil granule- and epithelial cell-derived cathelicidin, utilizes formyl peptide receptor-like 1 (FPRL1) as a receptor to chemoattract human peripheral blood neutrophils, monocytes, and T cells. *J. Exp. Med.* 2000 Oct 2;192(7):1069–74.

[92] Määttä M, Kari O, Tervahartiala T, Peltonen S. Tear fluid levels of MMP-8 are elevated in ocular rosacea—treatment effect of oral doxycycline. Graefes *Arch Clin Exp Ophthalmol.* 2006 Aug;244(8):957-62.

[93] Woessner JF. Matrix metalloproteinases and their inhibitors in connective tissue remodeling. *FASEB J.* 1991 May;5(8):2145–54.

[94] Afonso AA, Monroy D, Stern ME, Feuer WJ, Tseng SC, Pflugfelder SC. Correlation of tear fluorescein clearance and Schirmer test scores with ocular irritation symptoms. *Ophthalmology.* 1999 Apr;106(4):803–10.

[95] Stern ME, Beuerman RW, Fox RI, Gao J, Mircheff AK, Pflugfelder SC. The pathology of dry eye: the interaction between the ocular surface and lacrimal glands. *Cornea.* 1998 Nov;17(6):584–9.

[96] Schäfer M, Carter L, Stein C. Interleukin 1 beta and corticotropin-releasing factor inhibit pain by releasing opioids from immune cells in inflamed tissue. *Proc. Natl. Acad. Sci. USA.* 1994;91(10):4219–23.

[97] Jordan A, Baum J. Basic Tear Flow: Does It Exist? *Ophthalmology.* 1980 Sep 1;87(9):920–30.

[98] Heigle TJ, Pflugfelder SC. Aqueous tear production in patients with neurotrophic keratitis. *Cornea.* 1996 Mar 1;15(2):135–8.

[99] Kim JT, Lee SH, Chun YS, Kim JC. Tear cytokines and chemokines in patients with Demodex blepharitis. *Cytokine.* 2011 Jan 1;53(1):94–9.

[100] Randon M, Liang H, Hamdaoui El M, Tahiri R, Batellier L, Denoyer A, et al. In vivo confocal microscopy as a novel and reliable tool for the diagnosis of Demodex eyelid infestation. *Br. J. Ophthalmol.* 2014 Sep 24.

[101] Smolin G, Okumoto M. Staphylococcal blepharitis. *Arch. Ophthalmol.* 1977 May;95(5):812–6.

[102] Smith RE, Flowers CW. Chronic blepharitis: a review. *CLAO J.* 1995 Jul;21(3):200–7.

[103] Rebora A, Drago F. Helicobacter pylori and rosacea. *J. Am. Acad. Dermatol.* 2000 Nov 1;43(5 Pt 1):884–4.

[104] Mindel JS, Rosenberg EW. Is Helicobacter pylori of interest to ophthalmologists? *Ophthalmology.* 1997 Nov 1;104(11):1729–30.

[105] Utaş S, Ozbakir O, Turasan A, Utaş C. Helicobacter pylori eradication treatment reduces the severity of rosacea. *J Am Acad Dermatol.* 1999 Mar;40(3):433–5.

[106] Bamford JTJ, Tilden RLR, Blankush JLJ, Gangeness DED. Effect of treatment of Helicobacter pylori infection on rosacea. *Arch Dermatol.* 1999 Jun 1;135(6):659–63.

[107] Bamford JT, Tilden RL, Gangeness DE. Does Helicobacter pylori eradication treatment reduce the severity of rosacea? *J. Am. Acad Dermatol.* 2000 Mar 1;42(3):535–6.

[108] Daković Z, Vesić S, Vuković J, Milenković S, Janković-Terzić K, Dukić S, et al. Ocular rosacea and treatment of symptomatic Helicobacter pylori infection: a case series. *Acta Dermatovenerol Alp Pannonica Adriat.* 2007 Jun 1;16(2):83–6.

[109] Wilkin J, editor. Factors that may trigger rosacea flare-ups. National Rosacea Society; [cited 2015 Jan 11]. Available from: http://www.rosacea.org

[110] Brink N, Szamel M, Young AR, Wittern KP, Bergemann J. Comparative quantification of IL-1beta, IL-10, IL-10r, TNFalpha and IL-7 mRNA levels in UV-irradiated human skin in vivo. Inflamm Res. 2000 Jun;49(6):290–6.

[111] Meller S, Winterberg F, Gilliet M, Müller A, Lauceviciute I, Rieker J, et al. Ultraviolet radiation-induced injury, chemokines, and leukocyte recruitment: An amplification cycle triggering cutaneous lupus erythematosus. *Arthritis Rheum.* 2005 May;52(5):1504–16.

[112] Zug KA, Palay DA, Rock B. Dermatologic diagnosis and treatment of itchy red eyelids. *Surv Ophthalmol.* 1996 Jan;40(4):293–306.

[113] Driver PJ, Lemp MA. Meibomian gland dysfunction. *Surv Ophthalmol.* 1996;40(5):343–67.

[114] Tomlinson A, Bron AJ, Korb DR, Amano S, Paugh JR, Pearce EI, et al. The International Workshop on Meibomian Gland Dysfunction: Report of the Diagnosis Subcommittee. *Invest Ophthalmol Vis Sci*. 2011 Mar 30;52(4):2006–49.
[115] Arita R, Itoh K, Inoue K, Amano S. Noncontact infrared meibography to document age-related changes of the meibomian glands in a normal population. *Ophthalmology*. 2008 May;115(5):911–5.
[116] Yamaguchi M, Kutsuna M, Uno T, Zheng X, Kodama T, Ohashi Y. Marx line: Fluorescein staining line on the inner lid as indicator of meibomian gland function. *Am J Ophthalmol*. 2006 Apr;141(4):669–669.e8.
[117] Ibrahim OMA, Matsumoto Y, Dogru M, Adan ES, Wakamatsu TH, Shimazaki J, et al. In Vivo Confocal microscopy evaluation of meibomian gland dysfunction in atopic keratoconjunctivitis patients. *Ophthalmology*. 2012 Oct 1;119(10):1961–8.
[118] Ryan J Wise BS BA, MD RKS, Richard C Allen MD P. Meibography: A review of techniques and technologies. *Saudi J. Ophthalmol*. 2012 Dec 1;26(4):349–56.
[119] Nichols KK, Nichols JJ, Mitchell GL. The lack of association between signs and symptoms in patients with dry eye disease. *Cornea*. 2004 Nov 1;23(8):762–70.
[120] Feldman F, Wood MM. Evaluation of the Schirmer tear test. *Can. J. Ophthalmol.* 1979 Oct;14(4):257–9.
[121] Jones SM, Nischal KK. The non-invasive tear film break-up time in normal children. *Br. J. Ophthalmol*. 2013 Aug 9;97(9):1129–33.
[122] Uchino M, Yokoi N, Uchino Y, Dogru M, Kawashima M, Komuro A, et al. Prevalence of dry eye disease and its risk factors in visual display terminal users: the Osaka study. *Am. J. Ophthalmol*. 2013 Oct 1;156(4):759–66.
[123] Suzuki T, Sano Y, Yokoi N, Kinoshita S. Clinical entity similarities between meibomitis-related keratoconjunctivitis and ocular rosacea. *ARVO Meeting Abstracts*. 2011 Apr 22;52(6):1504.
[124] Suzuki T, Kinoshita S. Meibomitis-related keratoconjunctivitis in childhood and adolescence. *Am. J. Ophthalmol*. 2007 Jul 1;144(1):160–1.
[125] Zurcher M, Hintschich CR, Garner A, Bunce C, Collin JRO. Sebaceous carcinoma of the eyelid: a clinicopathological study. *Br. J. Ophthalmol*. 1998 Sep 1;82(9):1049–55.
[126] Wolfe JT, Yeatts RP, Wick MR. Sebaceous carcinoma of the eyelid: errors in clinical and pathologic diagnosis. *Am. J. Surg. Pathol*. 1984 Aug;8(8):597-606.
[127] Thorne JE, Jabs DA, Nikolskaia OV, Mimouni D, Anhalt GJ, Nousari HC. Lichen planus and cicatrizing conjunctivitis: characterization of five cases. *Am. J. Ophthalmol.* 2003 Aug;136(2):239–43.
[128] Akova YA, Rodriguez A, Foster CS. Atopic keratoconjunctivitis. *Ocul Immunol Inflamm*. 1994;2(3):125–44.
[129] Ata-Ali F, Ata-Ali J. Pemphigus vulgaris and mucous membrane pemphigoid: update on etiopathogenesis, oral manifestations and management. *J. Clin. Exp. Dent.* 2011;3(3):246-50.
[130] Olazagasti J, Lynch P, Fazel N. The great mimickers of rosacea. *Cutis*. 2014 Jul 1;94(1):39–45.
[131] Wladis EJ, Adam AP. Current and emerging therapies for ocular rosacea. *Touch Med Media*. 2013 Oct 23;:86–8.

[132] Del Rosso JQ. Advances in understanding and managing rosacea: part 2: the central role, evaluation, and medical management of diffuse and persistent facial erythema of rosacea. *J. Clin. Aesthet Dermatol.* 2012;5(3):26.

[133] Gupta AK, Chaudhry MM. Rosacea and its management: an overview. *J. Eur. Acad Dermatol Venereol.* 2005 May;19(3):273–85.

[134] Paranjpe DR, Foulks GN. Therapy for meibomian gland disease. *Ophthalmol Clin North Am.* 2003 Mar 1;16(1):37–42.

[135] Jackson WB. Blepharitis: current strategies for diagnosis and management. *Can. J. Ophthalmol.* 2008 Apr;43(2):170-9.

[136] Doughty MJ, Dutton GN. Fusidic acid viscous eyedrops-an evaluation of pharmacodynamics, pharmacokinetics and clinical use for UK optometrists. *Ophthalmic Physiol Opt.* 2006 Jul;26(4):343–61.

[137] Limberg MB, McCaa C, Kissling GE, Kaufman HE. Topical application of hyaluronic acid and chondroitin sulfate in the treatment of dry eyes. *Am. J. Ophthalmol.* 1987 Feb;103(2):194–7.

[138] Göbbels M, Gross D. Clinical study of the effectiveness of a dexpanthenol containing artificial tears solution (Siccaprotect) in treatment of dry eyes. *Klin. Monbl. Augenheilkd.* 1996 Aug 1;209(2-3):84–8.

[139] Rand AL, Asbell PA. Nutritional supplements for dry eye syndrome. *Curr. Opin. Ophthalmol.* 2011 Jul;22(4):279–82.

[140] Macsai MS. The role of omega-3 dietary supplementation in blepharitis and meibomian gland dysfunction (an AOS thesis). *Trans Am Ophthalmol Soc.* 2008 Jan 1;106:336–56.

[141] Barabino S, Rolando M, Camicione P, Ravera G, Zanardi S, Giuffrida S, et al. Systemic linoleic and gamma-linolenic acid therapy in dry eye syndrome with an inflammatory component. *Cornea.* 2003 Mar 1;22(2):97–101.

[142] Aragona P, Bucolo C, Spinella R, Giuffrida S, Ferreri G. Systemic omega-6 essential fatty acid treatment and PGE1 tear content in Sjogren's syndrome patients. *Invest Ophthalmol & Vis Sci.* 2005 Dec 1;46(12):4474–9.

[143] Stone DU, Chodosh J. Ocular rosacea: an update on pathogenesis and therapy. *Current Opinion in Ophthalmology.* 2004 Dec 1;15(6):499–502.

[144] Comstock TL, DeCory HH. Ophthalmic drug design based on the metabolic activity of the eye: soft drugs and chemical delivery systems. *AAPS J.* 2005;2012(4):E820–33.

[145] Schechter BA, Katz RS, Friedman LS. Efficacy of topical cyclosporine for the treatment of ocular rosacea. *Adv Therapy.* 2009 Jun;26(6):651–9.

[146] Perry HD, Wittpenn JR, D'Aversa G, Donnenfeld ED. Topical cyclosporine 0.05% for the treatment of chronic, active ocular rosacea. *ARVO Meeting Abstracts.* 2005 May 1;46(5):2660.

[147] Koçak-Altintas A, Koçak-Midillioglu I, Gul U, Bilezikci B, Isiksacan O, Duman S. Effects of topical metranidazole in ocular rosacea. *Ann Ophthalmol* (Skokie). 2005 Jun 1;37(2):77–84.

[148] Bron AJ, Evans VE, Smith JA. Grading of corneal and conjunctival staining in the context of other dry eye tests. *Cornea.* 2003 Oct;22(7):640–50.

[149] Doan S, Gabison E, Chiambaretta F, Touati M, Cochereau I. Efficacy of azithromycin 1.5% eye drops in childhood ocular rosacea with phlyctenular blepharokeratoconjunctivitis. *J. Ophthal Inflamm Infect.* 2013;3(1):38–8.

[150] Lindsley K, Matsumura S, Hatef E, Akpek EK. Interventions for chronic blepharitis. *Cochrane Database Syst Rev.* 2012 Jan 1;5:CD005556–6.
[151] Griffin MO, Fricovsky E, Ceballos G, Villarreal F. Tetracyclines: a pleitropic family of compounds with promising therapeutic properties. Review of the literature. *AJP: Cell Physiology.* 2010 Aug 26;299(3):C539–48.
[152] Agwuh KN. Pharmacokinetics and pharmacodynamics of the tetracyclines including glycylcyclines. *J. Antimicrob Chemother.* 2006 May 30;58(2):256–65.
[153] Bartholomew RS, Reid BJ, Cheesbrough MJ, Macdonald M, Galloway NR. Oxytetracycline in the treatment of ocular rosacea: a double-blind trial. *Br. J. Ophthalmol.* 1982 Jun 1;66(6):386–8.
[154] Stone DU, Chodosh J. Oral tetracyclines for ocular rosacea: an evidence-based review of the literature. *Cornea.* 2004 Jan 1;23(1):106–9.
[155] Marmion VJ. Tetracyclines in the treatment of ocular rosacea. *J. Royal Soc Med.* 1969 Jan 1;62(1):11–2.
[156] Frucht-Pery J, Chayet AS, Feldman ST, Lin S, Brown SI. The effect of doxycycline on ocular rosacea. *Am. J. Ophthalmol.* 1989 Apr;107(4):434–5.
[157] Quarterman MJ, Johnson DW, Abele DC, Lesher JL, Hull DS, Davis LS. Ocular rosacea: signs, symptoms, and tear studies before and after treatment with doxycycline. *Am. J. Ophthalmol.* 1997 Sep;124(3):426.
[158] Aronowicz JD, Shine WE, Oral D, Vargas JM, McCulley JP. Short term oral minocycline treatment of meibomianitis. Br J Ophthalmol. 2006 Jul 1;90(7):856–60.
[159] Lee H, Min K, Kim EK, Kim T-I. Minocycline controls clinical outcomes and inflammatory cytokines in moderate and severe meibomian gland dysfunction. *Am. J. Ophthalmol.* 2012 Dec;154(6):949–957.
[160] Souchier M, Joffre C, Gregoire S, Bretillon L, Muselier A, Acar N, et al. Changes in meibomian fatty acids and clinical signs in patients with meibomian gland dysfunction after minocycline treatment. *Br. J. Ophthalmol.* 2008 Jun 3;92(6):819–22.
[161] Ta CN, Shine WE, McCulley JP, Pandya A, Trattler W, Norbury JW. Effects of minocycline on the ocular flora of patients with acne rosacea or seborrheic blepharitis. *Cornea.* 2003 Aug 1;22(6):545.
[162] Frucht-Pery J, Sagi E, Hemo I, Ever-Hadani P. Efficacy of doxycycline and tetracycline in ocular rosacea. *Am. J. Ophthalmol.* 1993 Jul;116(1):88–92.
[163] Léoni S, Mesplié N, Aitali F, Chamaillard M, Boralevi F, Marques da Costa C, et al. Metronidazole: alternative treatment for ocular and cutaneous rosacea in the pediatric population. *J. Fr Ophtalmol.* 2011 Dec;34(10):703–10.
[164] van Zuuren EJ, Kramer S, Ben Carter, Graber MA, Fedorowicz Z. Interventions for rosacea. *Cochrane Database Syst Rev.* 2011 Jan 1;(3):CD003262–2.

Index

A

B

C

D

G

H

I

J

K

L

M

N

O

P

Q

R

S

W

Y

Z